MANAGED MENTAL HEALTH CARE

ADMINISTRATIVE AND CLINICAL ISSUES

MANAGED MENTAL HEALTH CARE

ADMINISTRATIVE AND CLINICAL ISSUES

Edited by

Judith L. Feldman, M.D.
Associate Chief,
  Central Psychiatric Programs
Harvard Community Health Plan,
  Boston, Massachusetts
Clinical Instructor in Psychiatry
Harvard Medical School
Boston, Massachusetts

Richard J. Fitzpatrick, Ph.D.
Chief, Mental Health Department
Peabody Center
Harvard Community Health Plan
Peabody, Massachusetts

Washington, DC
London, England

Note: The authors have worked to ensure that all information in this book concerning drug dosages, schedules, and routes of administration is accurate as of the time of publication and consistent with standards set by the U.S. Food and Drug Administration and the general medical community. As medical research and practice advance, however, therapeutic standards may change. For this reason and because human and mechanical errors sometimes occur, we recommend that readers follow the advice of a physician who is directly involved in their care or the care of a member of their family.

Books published by American Psychiatric Press, Inc., represent the views and opinions of the individual authors and do not necessarily represent the policies and opinions of the Press or the American Psychiatric Association.

Copyright © 1992 American Psychiatric Press, Inc.
ALL RIGHTS RESERVED
Manufactured in the United States of America on acid-free paper.
First Edition 95 94 93 92 4 3 2 1

Library of Congress Cataloging-in-Publication Data
Managed mental health care / edited by Richard Fitzpatrick and Judith L. Feldman — 1st ed.
    p. cm.
  Includes bibliographical references and index.
  ISBN 0-88048-355-5 (alk. paper)
  1. Mental health services—United States. 2. Managed care plans (Medical care)—United States. 3. Psychiatry—Practice—United States. I. Fitzpatrick, Richard, 1953–   . II. Feldman, Judith L., 1944–   .
  [DNLM: 1. Managed Care Programs—organization & administration—United States. 2. Mental Health Services—organization & administration—United States. WM 30 M2655]
  RA790.6.M28 1992
  362.2'0973—dc20
  DNLM/DLC
  For Library of Congress   91-47070
                                     CIP

British Library Cataloging in Publication Data
A CIP record is available from the British Library.

Table of Contents

Section I: Administrative Issues

Section II: Clinical Issues

Section III: Special Topics

Contributors

Bridie Aubel, R.N.
Staff Nurse, Behavioral Medicine Service, Department of
Psychiatry, Kaiser Permanente Medical Center, Hayward,
California

Haroutun M. Babigian, M.D.
Professor and Chairman, Department of Psychiatry, University
of Rochester School of Medicine, Rochester, New York

Peter Barglow, M.D.
Chief, Substance Abuse Services, Martinez Veterans
Administration Hospital, Martinez, California; Chief of
Educational Services in Substance Abuse, Department of
Psychiatry, University of California, Davis, School of Medicine;
Professor of Psychiatry, Northwestern University Medical
School, Chicago, Illinois

Jeffrey Becker, Esq.
Senior Partner in Health/Corporate Law, Epstein, Becker and
Green, P.C., New York, New York

Michael J. Bennett, M.D.
Massachusetts Medical Director, American Biodyne, San
Francisco, California; Assistant Clinical Professor of Psychiatry,
Harvard Medical School, Boston, Massachusetts

Maurice Bermon, M.D.
Chief of Mental Health Services, Rhode Island Group Health
Association, Providence, Rhode Island; Assistant Clinical
Professor, Psychiatry and Human Behavior, Brown University
School of Medicine, Providence, Rhode Island

Allan Bernstein, M.D.
Chief, Department of Neurology, Kaiser Permanente Medical
Center, Hayward, California

Thomas E. Bittker, M.D.
Medical Director, Truckee Meadows Mental Health System,
HCA Truckee Meadows Hospital, Reno, Nevada; Associate
Professor of Psychiatry, University of Nevada, Reno, Nevada;
formerly Medical Director, CIGNA Health Plan, Phoenix, Arizona

Theodor Bonstedt, M.D.
Staff Psychiatrist, Lee Mental Health Center, Ft. Myers,
Florida; Clinical Assistant Professor of Psychiatry, University of
Miami School of Medicine, Miami, Florida

Jonathan F. Borus, M.D.
Director of Psychiatry, Brigham and Women's Hospital, Boston,
Massachusetts; Associate Professor of Psychiatry, Harvard
Medical School, Boston, Massachusetts

Simon H. Budman, Ph.D.
Director of Mental Health Research, Harvard Community
Health Plan, Boston, Massachusetts; Assistant Professor of
Psychology, Department of Psychiatry, Harvard Medical School,
Boston, Massachusetts

Richard Caplan, M.S.W., L.I.C.S.W., M.P.H.
Manager, Substance Abuse Services, Harvard Community
Health Plan, Boston, Massachusetts

Doyle Carson, M.D.
Psychiatrist-in-Chief, Timberlawn Hospital, Dallas, Texas;
Associate Clinical Professor of Psychiatry, University of Texas
Southwestern Medical School, Dallas, Texas

Seeley Chandler, M.D.
Medical Director, Adolescent Inpatient Unit, Lutheran General
Hospital, Park Ridge, Illinois; Instructor, University of Chicago
Medical School, Chicago, Illinois

Robert A. Dorwart, M.D., M.P.H.
Chairman, Mental Health Policy Working Group, Malcolm
Weiner Center for Social Policy, John F. Kennedy School of
Government, Harvard University, Cambridge, Massachusetts;
Associate Professor, Harvard Medical School, Boston,
Massachusetts; Department of Psychiatry, The Cambridge
Hospital, Cambridge, Massachusetts

Sherrie S. Epstein, B.A., B.Sc.
Research Associate, Malcolm Weiner Center for Social Policy, John F. Kennedy School of Government, Harvard University, Cambridge, Massachusetts

Judith L. Feldman, M.D.
Associate Chief, Central Psychiatric Programs, Harvard Community Health Plan, Boston, Massachusetts; Clinical Instructor in Psychiatry, Harvard Medical School, Boston, Massachusetts

Richard J. Fitzpatrick, Ph.D.
Chief, Mental Health Department, Peabody Center, Harvard Community Health Plan, Peabody, Massachusetts

Gerald W. Frank, M.D.
Medical Director, Behavioral Medicine Service, Department of Psychiatry, Kaiser Permanente Medical Center, Hayward, California

Jay H. Glasser, Ph.D.
Professor of Biometry, School of Public Health, University of Texas Health Science Center, Houston, Texas

Roger L. Gould, M.D.
CEO, Interactive Health Systems, Princeton, New Jersey, and Santa Monica, California; Associate Clinical Professor of Psychiatry, UCLA School of Medicine, Los Angeles, California

Marie Lehn, R.N.
Staff Nurse, Behavioral Medicine Service, Department of Psychiatry, Kaiser Permanente Medical Center, Hayward, California

Bruce Lubotsky Levin, Dr.P.H., F.A.M.H.A.
Associate Professor of Epidemiology and Policy Analysis, The Florida Mental Health Institute, University of South Florida, Tampa, Florida; Adjunct Associate Professor, Department of Health Policy and Management, University of South Florida School of Public Health, Tampa, Florida; Adjunct Associate Professor, School of Public Health, University of Texas Health Science Center, Houston, Texas

Sharon Marshall, Esq.
Attorney-at-Law, New York, New York

Dale A. Masi, D.S.W., L.C.S.W.
President, MASI Research Consultants, Inc., Washington, DC;
Professor, University of Maryland School of Social Work,
Baltimore, Maryland

Nancy Molitor, Ph.D.
Director, Adolescent Intensive Treatment Program, Humana
Michael Reese HMO, Chicago, Illinois

Daniel Offer, M.D.
Director of Adolescent Research, Institute of Psychiatry,
Northwestern Memorial Hospital, Chicago, Illinois; Professor of
Psychiatry, Northwestern University Medical School, Chicago,
Illinois

Daniel Y. Patterson, M.D.
Private Practice, Wilmington Psychiatric Associates,
Wilmington, North Carolina; Associate Clinical Professor of
Psychiatry, Georgetown University Medical School, Washington,
DC; formerly Vice President for Medical Affairs and Corporate
Medical Director, American Psych Management, Inc.

Sylvia K. Reed, Ph.D.
Information Systems Director, Department of Psychiatry,
University of Rochester Medical Center, Rochester, New York

Alex R. Rodriquez, M.D.
Chief Medical Officer, Preferred Health Care, Ltd., Wilton,
Connecticut; Staff Psychiatrist, Naval Hospital, Groton,
Connecticut; Lecturer in Psychiatry, Yale University School of
Medicine, New Haven, Connecticut

James E. Sabin, M.D.
Associate Director, Teaching Center, Harvard Community
Health Plan, Boston, Massachusetts; Assistant Clinical
Professor of Psychiatry, Harvard Medical School, Boston,
Massachusetts

Susan C. Sargent, M.B.A., C.M.C.
President, GLS Associates, Philadelphia, Pennsylvania

S. Alan Savitz, M.D.
Medical Director for Mental Health, Aetna Health Plans, Salt Lake City, Utah

Kathleen Schneider-Braus, M.D.
Staff Psychiatrist, Jefferson County Human Services Department, Madison, Wisconsin; formerly Chief of Mental Health Services, Minneapolis Group Health Plan, Minneapolis, Minnesota

Steven S. Sharfstein, M.D.
Medical Director and Executive Vice President, The Sheppard and Enoch Pratt Hospital, Baltimore, Maryland; Clinical Professor of Psychiatry, University of Maryland Medical School, Baltimore, Maryland

Steve Stelovich, M.D.
Chief, Central Psychiatric Programs, Harvard Community Health Plan, Boston, Massachusetts; Instructor in Psychiatry, Harvard Medical School, Boston, Massachusetts

Linda Tiano, Esq.
Partner, Health/Corporate Law, Epstein, Becker and Green, P.C., New York, New York

Steven R. Tulkin, Ph.D.
Program Director, Behavioral Medicine Service, Department of Psychiatry, Kaiser Permanente Medical Center, Hayward, California

Robert A. Wise, M.D.
Medical Director of Mental Health and Substance Abuse, Blue Cross Blue Shield of Illinois, Chicago, Illinois

William R. Zwick, Ph.D.
Coordinator of Substance Abuse Services, Rhode Island Group Health Association, Providence, Rhode Island; Assistant Clinical Professor, Psychiatry and Human Behavior, Brown University School of Medicine, Providence, Rhode Island

Preface

We have been working in managed mental health care for a total of 23 years. Each of us came to this field with idealistic notions: a one-class system of care, national health insurance, treatment of mental illness in the private sector, and so on. We joined Harvard Community Health Plan, a "second generation" health maintenance organization (HMO). Now, as we watch the development of the fourth and fifth generations, we find ourselves part of big business. We have shifted right in the political and economic spectrum, poised between large health care corporations and even larger employers who purchase the care.

The literature on managed mental health care is growing. Surveys by professional groups now list "HMO" as a choice for "site of practice," so we don't have to check "other—please specify." We have our own professional organization, the Group Health Association of America. In November 1988, the American Psychiatric Association sponsored a 2-day conference on psychiatry and managed care. HMO mental health care now has a history reaching back at least 20 years. We even have our gurus, some of whom have graciously contributed to this book.

For many of us working in this area, the challenges of managed care have honed our thinking and stimulated our creativity. We hope this book will demonstrate the innovative and effective clinical and administrative techniques that have been developed and tested in managed systems. However, there are many serious concerns about mental health in managed care systems: Are these systems providing second-class care? treating long-term problems with short-term solutions? Are managed care clinicians caught in untenable conflict-of-interest situations? Are capitated or prepaid arrangements unethical? Are alternatives to hospital care unsafe? ineffective? Is utilization management intruding unduly into the practice of psychiatry?

Although we do not have definitive answers to these questions, we hope this volume will provide the reader with enough background knowledge and current understanding to approach these issues and to add data and experience to this exciting and growing field.

The book is roughly divided into three sections: administrative issues, clinical issues, and special topics. The authors of the chapters on administrative issues detail historical, economic, and managerial approaches to the understanding of managed care and mental health.

Those who contributed to the chapters on clinical issues either discuss a theoretical approach to treatment or describe a specific treatment program or approach that has been developed by the authors. This administrative/clinical division is far from complete. Chapters in the clinical section use managerial language (utilization, cost savings, systems), and those in the administrative section have clinical examples. This is no accident. Every managed care clinician is a clinical manager. Administrative and clinical concepts are inextricably intertwined. Since all mental health care is financed in *some* fashion, this confounding of economics and clinical care is universal, and not only attributable to managed systems. We hope that clinicians and administrators will be able to apply these concepts and ideas to other systems of care.

There is considerable variation in style and approach to the various topics covered in this volume. In part, this variability is because of differences in the writing styles of the authors. However, it is also related to the incompleteness of our knowledge and variability in the literature in managed care psychiatry. Many authors have done extensive studies themselves; others have done more informal surveys; and still others are just beginning to develop a theoretical framework with which to examine their topic. In addition, the field is changing rapidly as we write. Only a short time ago, HMOs were the dominant form of managed care. Now the picture includes employer-managed programs, self-insurance, utilization management companies, open-ended HMOs, and newer models yet to be named. Study and reflection lag behind innovation in this rapidly changing arena.

Although we were not able to cover every new area, we hope that the basic ideas, concepts, and studies in this volume will apply as well to the present and near future as they have to the recent past, and that others will continue the process of communicating as our field continues to develop.

We would like to thank our HMO teachers and mentors: Mike Bennett, Jim Sabin, Si Budman, Tom Pyle, John Ludden, Dan Patterson, Tom Bittker, and Don Berwick. We are also grateful to the officers and members of the American Psychiatric Association who supported our ideas and the development of this book. Many thanks also to our clinical colleagues and patients at Harvard Community Health Plan, and, of course, to our families.

Judith L. Feldman, M.D.   Richard J. Fitzpatrick, Ph.D.

Section I:

Administrative Issues

✦ 1 ✦

The Emergence of Prepaid Psychiatry

Thomas E. Bittker, M.D.

s with prepaid medicine, prepaid psychiatry has emerged from various traditions, each shaping practice according to its unique goals, values, and technologies. In the infancy of the health maintenance organization (HMO) movement, psychiatric service provision within HMOs was considered peripheral to the provision of basic, affordable medical services. The two sources of the HMO movement, prepayment and group practice, held in common the expectation that health care could be both affordable and of satisfactory quality (Bennett 1988). Prepayment, the provision of a set package of medical services by an identified provider for a predetermined fee, sprung from the challenge of delivering services to a geographically remote and often migratory population. The prepaid experiments of the early 1900s in the lumbering, mining, transportation, and construction industries were Spartan in dimension and scope, often resembling frontline military medicine much more than any form of civilian practice (Bennett 1988). There was neither the inclination nor the training to deal with psychiatric problems.

Group practice originated with the Mayos in the 1880s, who sought to improve both the quality of care for patients and the quality of the physician's ongoing training and experience by bringing together an array of specialties capable of approaching a patient's problem from a variety of perspectives and by coordinating a patient's care within one organizational setting. Later, the concepts of prepayment and group practice were married in behalf of farmers in rural cooperatives in Oklahoma, the employees of the Los Angeles County Water and Power Department, and the Boulder Dam employees (Mayer and Mayer

3

1985) as well as city government employees (Health Improvement Plan of Greater New York), and in behalf of a consortium of employers and consumers seeking an alternative to fee-for-service (FFS) medicine (Group Health Association of Washington, DC; Group Health Cooperative of Puget Sound). By the mid- to late 1950s, FFS providers practicing in the shadows of the rapidly growing HMOs conceived of a confederation of independent practitioners that would provide prepaid care in geographically separate offices, but under one organizational umbrella. The first of these systems, the San Joaquin Foundation for Medical Care, was born in 1954 and became the forerunner of other independent practice associations (IPAs; Nelson 1987). Although psychiatrists and other mental health professionals participated in these groups' staff and IPA practices, their prepaid services were confined largely to consultation, crisis intervention, and triage.

Psychiatric services were considered a luxury, too costly to incorporate into the benefit mainstream. Furthermore, indemnity coverage for mental health services was at that time sparse as well. The prepaid group was forced to rely on patient resources, the community mental health sector, or the public mental hospital, should the psychiatrically needy require more than a few visits for relatively circumscribed problems. For much of this early history of prepaid medicine—before 1960—clinical psychiatric interventions were perceived as requiring extensive time and labor to be effective. The few exceptions were found in military psychiatry and a nascent community mental health practice.

By the late 1960s, visionary insurers and state and federal government executives were becoming concerned by the then early evidence of a medical cost control problem developing in this country. Their concerns fostered several health care experiments that later matured to become staff and group model HMOs (e.g., the Harvard Community Health Plan, the Columbia Medical Plan, and the Arizona Health Plan). Each of these new plans sought to provide a basic mental health benefit package that would permit these plans to be competitive with the richer psychiatric benefits that were available in comparably priced indemnity plans. The problem for the new plans was to provide mental health coverage without inviting or encouraging patients with chronic mental illness to flood the system (see Chapter 5). Moreover, patients with alcohol and other drug abuse problems presented huge problems as well as possibilities in the form of care integrated among primary care internists, mental health and substance abuse specialists, and employers (see Chapters 18, 19, and 20).

The focus then became one of providing prompt access to time-limited services for problems deemed treatable within these time limits. Drug rehabilitation, court-ordered treatment, and the treatment of uncooperative patients were often specifically excluded by the benefit contracts in these pioneering efforts (Mayer and Mayer 1985). A psychiatric consultation to primary care remained the focus of intervention. Also, mental health benefits were included on the basis of riders that showed a decrease in medical utilization as a function of referral to mental health (Bittker 1985).

In 1969, Paul Ellwood, then of the American Rehabilitation Institute, seized on a perceived health care policy vacuum in the Nixon administration to advance a system of care that would provide incentives to promote health rather than to treat illness. The concept was embraced by President Nixon as an alternative to the Democratic proposals for national health insurance. Ultimately, the president signed the Health Maintenance Organization Act of 1973, a bill that promoted HMO development, but under conditions so restrictive that by 1977 only 183 plans were providing care to less than 7 million people (Mayer and Mayer 1985). This initial bill stipulated that plans seeking federal qualification were compelled to provide emergency and crisis intervention outpatient services of up to 20 visits per year. No inpatient care was required. However, most new plans included inpatient care of from 30 to 45 days or 60 to 90 days of partial care (see Chapters 2 and 3).

Cost-effective care disaggregated from the demonstrated maintenance of specific standards that guarantee minimum quality spawned serious legal and ethical questions (see Chapter 11). The American Psychiatric Association was initially concerned by the perceived discriminatory management of mental health care endorsed by the HMO Act of 1973. In 1983 an APA task force on Health Maintenance Organizations prepared a report on HMOs under the leadership of Daniel Patterson (see Chapter 21).

The report was largely descriptive of the state of HMO psychiatric practice extant and included recommendations intended to avoid the pitfalls of underutilization within the prepaid systems. Its tone was relatively positive regarding the promise of some of the innovations found and encouraged in prepaid systems. The report was never published. The expectation, however, that both general health care and mental health care could be provided at quality equivalent to that obtained in the indemnity world at costs substantially below that charged in the indemnity sector continued to attract the awareness of government, industry, and entrepreneurs.

By 1985 prepaid medical and behavioral health care had become a growth industry. For-profit providers aggressively pursued enrollees in an effort to capitalize on the inefficiencies and alleged cost-insensitivities of the FFS sector. As enrolled populations included people less interested in the idealism of community-based, prepaid practice and more concerned with receiving their full measure of care for premiums paid, the process of controlling costs became more challenging. Similarly, mental health providers recruited to the new systems were captured less by the ideals of an alternative system of care and more by the rewards of job security, predictable hours, pay, and benefits. The era of "productivity demands" had begun.

Thus, the growth of prepaid health and mental health care to the level that it now includes 31 million Americans in some managed care health system has been accompanied by substantial tensions for the participants. These have included an embarrassingly high number of recent health plan failures, high provider turnover, and an industry average membership turnover approaching 25% per year. Reflecting upon the past 20 years, however, permits an awareness of how the prepaid industry has shaped the focus and evolution of psychiatric practice. Whereas indemnity insurance limits reimbursement to specific interventions for specific medical diagnoses provided typically by doctoral-level health professionals in circumscribed settings, prepayment fosters opportunity for innovation in types of intervention problems treated and professionals and settings utilized (see Chapters 13, 16, and 20). In an effort to control cost exposure, the typical indemnity carrier will not, for example, reimburse for counseling provided by a social worker with a master's degree to the parents of an adolescent runaway who is living in a group home (see Chapter 17).

The prepaid carrier has the option of providing such an intervention as long as the intervention meets the prepaid plan's goal of cost-effective service delivery. Prepaid plans have rarely been so liberal in the interpretation of their mandate as to provide coverage for "social adjustment issues" or for living in nonmedical settings. However, current experience with capitation for patients with chronic illness has involved coverage of social and housing services as well as medical care (see Chapter 8). Many plans have extended the boundaries of treatment far beyond the hospital or outpatient clinic walls, using allied health professionals in the service of client problems that would rarely be reimbursed by an indemnity insurer. Prepaid health plans have developed psychoeducational groups focused on specific themes of personal development (e.g., divorce adjustment, widowhood, coping with terminal illness, or enhancing self-esteem; see Chapter 16). Others have experimented with technological enhancements of psychotherapy such as computer-facilitated group psychotherapy (see Chapter 22). The pressures of the prepaid setting continue to provide direct incentives for innovation in the development of specific treatment modalities (see Chapter 25) and in the application of these to specific patient populations. The mature integration of treatment choice to patient need is demonstrated in the advent of clinical algorithms.

Prepaid systems foster such innovation by bringing together a critical mass of members and professionals within one organization, by facilitating direct communication among providers and consumers, and by providing care based on the anticipated effectiveness of that care without the burden of the indemnity system's preoccupation with guild issues.

Inspired by the work of Benjamin Pasamanick, Donald Langsley, David Kaplan, and others, the pioneering efforts in prepaid psychiatry addressed the patient in crisis that had traditionally led to hospitalization (Pasamanick et al. 1967). The criteria for psychiatric hospitalization in prepaid settings fast became focused on whether the patient could function within his or her social support system between outpatient day treatment or home visits. If professional access could be provided on a 24-hour basis and if the prepaid plan were willing to provide crisis-residential care or a holding bed when needed, then hospital use could be reduced substantially. Incorporating these principles reduced inpatient hospitalization by an average of two-thirds when prepaid systems were compared with indemnity systems (Langsley and Kaplan 1968; Levin and Glasser 1984; also see Chapters 16 and 24).

The Industrialization of Psychiatric Services

Physician surpluses and escalating medical care costs have fostered an alliance among government, corporate America, and health insurers that has forged medicine's industrialization (see Chapter 4). These same forces have transformed psychiatry into an industry where pro-spective payment, automation, salaried employment for many, and central control of clinical activities stand poised to become the domi-nant mode of psychiatric practice (Bittker and Idzorek 1978). By dra-matically shifting the focus of care away from the hospital, reducing the duration of treatment, employing new technologies, relying on less expensive professionals, and providing group treatment experiences to supplant dyadic psychotherapy, pioneers in prepaid systems have constructed an almost insurmountable incentive for the indemnity industry to adjust its methods and further consolidate care (see Chap-ter 12).

The RAND Health Insurance Study provides a compelling argu-ment both to the economist and to the entrepreneur as to the cost im-pact of the prepaid approach. The study contrasted the utilization experiences of a Seattle population enrolled in FFS plans (with and without deductible payments) with those of people enrolled in a pre-paid plan (the Group Health Cooperative of Puget Sound; Craig and Patterson 1981). The findings have been abstracted below.

1. A 64% cost savings for mental health care, occurring when prepaid and FFS systems are compared.
2. An increased likelihood, by a factor of one-third, that a prepaid en-rollee will visit a mental health professional.
3. A more than threefold greater number of outpatient visits per 1,000 members of the FFS population.

Without countervailing research to demonstrate that the increased costs expended in the FFS system yield commensurate benefits, the private system of behavioral health care may be forced by cost consid-erations to adopt the methods and controls of the prepaid model.

Accompanying the changes in the economic nature of practice have come profound changes in the culture of practice itself. Professional values were nurtured in settings where the professional's primary al-liance was to the individual patient. The industrialization of psychiat-ric practice compels the professional to consider the well-being of the populations of persons at risk in the prepaid system and to conserve resources for the entire patient group. Under such conditions the pru-dent physician will be careful to deliver all *necessary* care, but expend not a penny in behalf of care that is merely *desired* by the patient (see Chapter 14). Economic rewards will be tied not only to professional skill and energies, but to the performance of the prepaid group at risk. Management of resources will rival clinical acumen as critical to group success. The ambitious professional may be seduced by the incentives to become a professional manager. The clinically oriented psychiatrist may need to become comfortable with collaborative and consulting roles, working as a part of a multidisciplinary team (see Chapter 9).

Although professionals affiliated with IPAs and preferred provider organizations (PPOs) may believe themselves shielded from the pressures operating on their colleagues practicing within group or staff model HMOs, this belief is likely to prove illusory. Economic incentives will direct patient flow to those systems of care that are most efficient (see Chapter 6).

To survive, the care of participants will be moved into centrally coordinated systems. Furthermore, the most successful systems will need to differentially reward the most cost-effective and quality proven professionals or professional groups either with a larger patient flow or with a larger percentage of the risk pool. The incentive systems that emerge may further challenge the traditional values of the professionals. Self-appraisal according to the principles of a highly internalized code of ethics may be supplanted by a group-centered and economically leveraged value system. How psychiatry copes with these pressures will be among the fundamental questions of its survival in the next century (see Chapter 21).

In summary, prepaid psychiatry has grown in the past quarter-century from its position as an appendage to a nascent prepaid medical industry to become the crucible in which the elements of revolution have been stirred. The revolution has emerged by adapting the innovations of community mental health practice to the private sector and by capitalizing on the factors contributing to psychiatry's industrialization. The forces that have sprung from the prepaid movement will be among the more important shaping the character of psychiatry in the next century.

References

Bennett M: The greening of the HMO: implications for prepaid psychiatry. Am J Psychiatry 145(12):1544–1549, 1988

Bittker TE: The industrialization of American psychiatry. Am J Psychiatry 142:149–154, 1985

Bittker TE, Idzorek S: The evolution of psychiatric services in a health maintenance organization. Am J Psychiatry 135:392–395, 1978

Craig TI, Patterson DY: A comparison of mental health costs and utilization under three insurance models. Med Care 19:184–192, 1981

Langsley D, Kaplan D: The Treatment of Families in Crisis. New York, Grune & Stratton, 1968

Levin BL, Glasser JH: A national survey of prepaid mental health services. Hosp Community Psychiatry 35(4):350–355, 1984

Mayer TR, Mayer GG: HMOs: origins and development. N Engl J Med 312:590–594, 1985

Nelson J: The history and spirit of the HMO movement. HMO Practice 1:75–85, 1987

Pasamanick B, Scarpitti F, Dinitz S: Schizophrenics in the Community. New York, Appleton-Century-Crofts, 1967

✦ 2 ✦

Economics and Managed Mental Health Care: The HMO as a Crucible for Cost-Effective Care

Robert A. Dorwart, M.D., M.P.H.
Sherrie S. Epstein, B.A., B.Sc.

This chapter provides a general background on the economics of mental health care as it pertains to the dilemmas of providing mental health services in managed care settings. There are several good general reviews of mental health economics (McGuire 1989; Schlesinger 1986). The evolution of the industry and its incorporation of psychiatric services also have been described, as have recent developments in reimbursement for services and their influence on mental health service delivery (Bennett 1988; Dorwart and Chartock 1988; Keeler et al. 1986; Scherl et al. 1988). In this chapter, we discuss briefly the concepts of supply and demand as used by economists in analyzing health care, with special reference to the dynamics of the health maintenance organization (HMO) model of service delivery. We then describe several major trends affecting health and mental health care, including the rising costs of care. Next, we outline the background of the major managed care models. After a brief discussion of HMO mental health benefit packages and their relationship to utilization and costs, we turn to a consideration of the economic advantages and disadvantages of HMOs. We conclude with some thoughts about the future of managed mental health care systems.

This work was supported in part by National Institute of Mental Health Grant No. K20 MH00848-01.

The HMO: Crucible of Health Care Pressures

The HMO may be viewed as a crucible—some would say pressure cooker—within which many forces converge to create a situation recently described by hospitals as a feeling of "contents under pressure" (American Hospital Association 1989). HMOs seek to strike a balance between demand for and supply of health care services, and they also are forced constantly to strike a balance between resources of primary medical care and those of subspecialty mental health care (Schlesinger 1989). HMOs are seen by many policymakers as a cost-containment device to ration care effectively and by others as a way to improve access to and comprehensiveness of care. At times these goals may conflict.

Demand for Mental Health Care

A number of studies have focused on the demand for mental health services, especially ambulatory mental health care (Horgan 1986; Manning et al. 1986). Despite some inevitable methodological flaws, these studies provide useful insights about the nature of demand for mental health services. One finding is that demand for mental health visits is responsive to price elasticity: the higher the price to the consumer, the lower the utilization. Price responsiveness decreases as income of patients increases and is more sensitive for mental health care than for general medical care. A concern among policymakers in interpreting these findings is that if price elasticity varies according to subgroups of patients or among insured populations, then restricting services results in trade-offs that may reduce needed care as well as "unnecessary" care. In the context of HMOs, this might be an especially difficult problem for patients who have major, chronic (costly) disorders, such as schizophrenia (Schlesinger 1986).

Other questions arise in relation to the demand for care. One involves the substitutability for inpatient care. Historically there has been a bias by insurers in favor of hospital care for the treatment of mental disorders, and observers disagree about the possible effects of trying to substitute ambulatory care coverage (McGuire 1981). HMOs are in a particularly good position to assess the effect of offering alternative benefit packages on demand for inpatient and outpatient care because of the flexibility of coverage benefits they may offer. For example, they can alter their mix of services provided and test whether providing day treatment service reduces the demand for inpatient care.

Another problem that concerns HMOs is that of latent demand. Epidemiologic studies suggest that there are many people in the population who have diagnosable psychiatric disorders but who receive no specialty mental health services (Shapiro et al. 1984). Theoretically, in an HMO there may be greater detection, referral, acceptance, and use of mental health services than in an insured general population because of the inherent screening of patients by primary care physicians. Will a prepaid health plan, by its very nature, attract patients with different psychological styles of health care utilization? If a particular HMO should attract patients because of the generosity of its benefit or the quality or style of care provided, it is said to experience adverse selection. Estimating the true demand for mental health services is difficult, though it is especially critical for HMOs because they operate on a fixed budget.

It has long been customary to distinguish between "need" and demand for services. The need for services usually refers to clinical manifestations of illness that meet established criteria and indications for medical treatment. Demand refers to the press of persons actually seeking care as measured, for example, by visits to the clinics and other requests for care. The studies of mental health care mentioned earlier underscore the discrepancy between need and demand. Demand may be reduced by the patient's inability to pay or lack of insurance. Actual utilization of services may be influenced by the provider's policy toward delivery of care.

An insured patient is said by economists to represent for the provider a "moral hazard"; that is, the insured person is more likely to seek care and the provider is more at risk to have to provide that care. From the insurer's or organization's viewpoint, then, the problem of managing or controlling demand may be viewed as one of structuring the insurance coverage or "benefits package" in order to reduce the moral hazard for providing mental health care, or else of controlling selection of enrollees in order to lower demand; the demand for care will be reduced if the generousness of insurance coverage is reduced. An insurer who offers better insurance coverage than a competitor may be vulnerable to increased demand because of adverse selection. An HMO functions both as insurer and as provider and thus is doubly "at risk." Other methods commonly used to alter the nature of demand include deductibles, copayments, delays in treatment, and, in mental health especially, limits on covered amounts of care, such as $1,000 per year for all outpatient care.

Supply of Care

Recently, attention of many policymakers has turned from altering demand to altering the supply of services. In its most drastic form, altering the supply of services in order to reduce costs of care or to modify patterns of utilization might involve denial or rationing of care. A service may be excluded entirely from the benefit package or it may be severely limited; for example, a hospital may close its emergency room or an HMO may provide little or no psychiatric hospital care (Levinson 1987). This latter tactic has been taken by HMOs in 10 to 20 states that do not have mandated minimum inpatient mental health benefits.

Another approach to restricting supply of care is utilization review, designed to assess the medical necessity for care, the appropriateness of specific services, and so forth. For indemnity insurers this function may be performed by a separate utilization review firm (Sederer and St. Clair 1989). For self-insured groups, this function may be done by the employer's personnel division. HMOs may do their own utilization management. In a majority of HMOs there is also a built-in screening mechanism that prevents the patient from receiving specialty mental health services until evaluation and referral by a primary care physician. Another approach, referred to as "large-case management" or "catastrophic medical management" because it focuses on the costliest cases, involves modifying authorized benefits in order to meet the needs of individual patients. Among the goals of such approaches commonly used by HMOs is to reduce costs by increasing efficiency, effectiveness, and flexibility of provision of services through control of utilization (American Psychiatric Association 1989).

Trends in Mental Health Care Policy

A number of major trends in mental health care extrinsic to managed care are creating pressures on mental health services. One trend has been deinstitutionalization and the concomitant increase in outpatient care provided by mental health centers, clinics, and private practitioners of all disciplines (Thompson et al. 1982). Following the scientific and medical advances of the 1950s that introduced psychotropic medications for the treatment of major psychiatric disorders, treatment practice increasingly emphasized outpatient care, crisis intervention, rapid detoxification, and reduced use of hospitalization. These developments in health and mental health care were consistent with the preferred approaches used by managed care systems.

A second trend has been privatization and the growth of private psychiatric hospitals, psychiatric units in general hospitals, and the spread of specialty treatment facilities and programs (Dorwart and Schlesinger 1988). The important features of this movement have been an emphasis on maximizing profits, increasing efficiency, ensuring customer satisfaction, and the use of marketing, advertising, and public relations techniques to increase visibility and name recognition to stimulate demand for services (Dorwart et al. 1988). Another aspect of this trend has been corporatization: the growth of companies providing mental health care. Some firms own both hospitals and HMOs and other forms of insurance intermediaries. These approaches, associated with contemporary business methods in the delivery of health care, are also compatible with many managed care practices.

The trend toward privatization of health and mental health care has many dimensions. One already noted is the growth of private psychiatric hospitals. Another is the spread of investor-owned companies, many of which operate HMOs or utilization management companies. Still another development is "franchising" or contracting by companies to provide specialized services, such as mental health and substance abuse services, to general hospitals. Another rapidly growing aspect involves the contracting by state and local governments with private providers to provide health and mental health care; we see, for example, a trend toward proposals that would either permit or in some cases require Medicaid recipients to receive care from managed care systems.

Another trend has been increasing competition, especially in the past decade, not only among HMOs but also between HMOs and other insurers and providers of care (Schlesinger 1989). Competition leads to pressures to reduce prices and costs, to increase efficiency and effectiveness of services, and to stimulate responsiveness and innovation of providers to the changing demands of patients. Together these major trends can be expected to influence significantly the delivery of mental health services.

HMO Psychiatry

The HMO Act of 1973 had encouraged profit-making corporations to enter the health maintenance field to increase competition among health care providers. Their entry was presumed likely to lower costs. The act had also welcomed a new entity that would become the Individual Practice Association (IPA; see next section). Despite this encouragement of for-profit corporations, when the federal government stopped funding HMOs in 1983, it claimed that federal requirements were forcing HMO costs up and that government subsidies discouraged private development of plans (Bennett 1988). To qualify for federal aid, HMOs were required to offer community rating (a premium rate based on the average cost for all subscribers in a geographic area rather than experience rating that would charge higher prices for poor risks), open enrollment (periods when anyone may join a community pool), and certain services. Employers approached by federally qualified HMOs were required to offer the plan as alternative health insurance to their employees. (This requirement was changed in the 1988 Amendments to the HMO Act; in 1995, employers will no longer have to offer the HMO option.)

A principal perceived barrier to the public joining prepaid plans had been their organizational form—a panel of physicians employed by the plan. Thus, the consumer usually had little or no choice of physician. A barrier to the physician was that he or she was not fully in charge and had to cope with a managerial overlay that might disagree with the amount or type of medical treatment the physician advised. In the 1980s, these conflicts gave rise to the renewal of the prepaid health plan served by doctors in practice—common in Europe and the United States early in the century (Abel-Smith 1988)—known as the Individual Practice Association, or IPA.

Organizational Model Types of HMO Plans

Staff model. The traditional method of organizing an HMO is one in which physicians are salaried employees who serve only those enrolled in the HMO, thus operating as a "closed panel." The staff plan has the best record in cost control. The evidence showing lower medical costs for people enrolled in HMOs than for those with conventional health insurance came from studies of these staff plans reported in

1978 (Luft 1978); a business analyst found staff/group plans more profitable than IPAs in 1987 (Vignola 1988). It usually offers both preventive and specialist care, although the latter may sometimes be contracted for elsewhere. The start-up capital is higher than for the IPA, and membership tends to grow slowly. The staff plan prospers if participants use few expensive services. A physician or nurse "gatekeeper" to control use and subspecialty or so-called out-of-plan referrals is common practice. This early model is no longer as popular as other models described in this section and now makes up a small proportion of the total number of HMOs (12% in 1986, according to InterStudy, the HMO research group based in Excelsior, Minnesota), although this still accounts for a large proportion of enrollees. Some staff model plans have grown very large, and their profitability has been attributed to their size (Brown 1983). CIGNA Healthplans of California, for example, had 415,000 members in 1987. They may use community hospitals or own or contract with selected facilities.

Group model. The group model HMO contracts for the services of physicians in a group practice. In a closed group, which often excludes psychiatrists, physicians usually are permitted to accept only HMO patients. Primary physicians may receive a capitation fee for each patient, usually accompanied by a bonus plan in which they are rewarded if costs are below those expected. Some group plans offer payment by fee for service, however, often in a profit-sharing plan, which encourages administering many rather than few services.

Group network. In this model, physicians may be drawn from a number of groups to contract with the HMO, but they are permitted to accept patients outside the HMO. Cost controls are difficult to administer unless the HMO patients dominate the physicians' practices. A core of primary medical practitioners refer patients as needed to specialist consultants for services like mental health care. These specialists may or may not be employed by or have specific contractual arrangements with the HMO.

Individual practice association (IPA). In the IPA model, a management organization markets the HMO benefits plan, collects payments, and pays bills. It contracts with independent physicians and surgeons who agree to a prepaid rate for services to the IPA's members. This model generally offers the prospective member a wider choice of physicians in a wider number of locations than in other types of managed care organizations, because the doctors continue to see patients in their own offices. Limited capital investment is needed, and start-up can be relatively quick. It bears a risk in that physicians may end their contracts and take patients with them. Risk is increased by practitioner variability. IPA professionals usually maintain more autonomy than doctors in traditional plans because they can retain their fee-for-service patients. They are generally paid by capitation. Management usually withholds a certain amount that is returned to the physicians at the end of the budget year if costs meet or are below the budget.

Preferred provider organization (PPO). Another plan model of recent origin is the preferred provider organization (PPO). This is not a separate legal entity but only an arrangement between a payer and a provider; the payer is usually an employer who contracts with providers for lower rates in return for a guaranteed volume of patients. In fact, HMO models have become less distinct as they try to respond to competition (Gabel et al. 1987).

The PPO form of managed care is growing rapidly, with several hundred established across the country. Many indemnity insurance companies offer the PPO as an alternative "product" to the traditional insurance and the HMO options, creating the so-called "triple-option" plans. PPOs offer the consumer the opportunity to choose his or her own provider, who in turn contracts with the PPO entity for reimbursement for services provided; the PPO thus approximates more a fee-for-service arrangement than does a closed panel HMO. Thus, the PPO is in some ways a "hybrid" or open-ended form of HMO.

Some observers believe that PPOs are evolving toward some new form of managed care. Many employers, seeing the rapid change taking place in the marketplace for health care services, choose to create their own versions of a PPO by selectively contracting with providers; they are in effect self-insuring their employees. Other employers or insurance companies have made arrangements with specialized utilization management companies to organize and monitor the care of their beneficiaries. Examples of such companies would be American Psych Management, a utilization review company, or Preferred Health Care, itself a subsidiary of a hospital management company. Another example is Private Healthcare, a firm that is owned by a consortium of insurance companies and that provides utilization review, case management, and PPO contracting services nationwide. There are more than 50 such companies currently operating in the United States in the mental health field, according to a survey of the American Psychiatric Association (Tischler 1990).

Ownership type. With the end of federal sponsorship of HMOs, a rapid increase in the number of for-profit HMOs came about. Private capital had been invested in HMOs earlier—InterStudy estimated that more private than government funds had been invested between 1974 and 1980 (Iglehart 1984)—and some nonprofit plans had converted to for-profit management. Major hospital management companies (Hospital Corporation of America, Humana, American Medical International, National Medical Enterprises) formed their own HMOs in an effort to preserve patient revenues rather than discount beds to other HMOs. Also, major indemnity plans, such as Blue Cross/Blue Shield, John Hancock, Metropolitan Life, and others have created managed care products. In a national survey of psychiatric hospitals in 1988, we found that 20% (mostly community general hospitals) reported that they "owned" a managed care organization (Dorwart et al. 1991). The advent of Diagnosis-Related Groups or DRGs (prospective pricing for Medicare patients by fixing prices paid for each diagnosis) reduced hospital occupancy after 1983 and made filling beds an urgent need for these companies. In 1984, some 60 new HMOs were started, and 50 formerly nonprofit plans became for-profit.

By 1986, the traditional staff and group model HMOs accounted for 26% of the 600 HMOs in the country and 43% of the 24 million members. IPAs made up 57% of the plans but only 36% of the membership.

Economics of HMO Profitability

Studies of HMOs conducted when most were largely nonprofit and selectively marketed to working populations who were receptive to preventive care had shown them to be less costly users of health care, principally because days of hospitalization were fewer than for populations receiving fee-for-service care. As plans have increased and both the types of plans and the participants have become more varied, their success in containing costs has come into question and their premiums have risen (Kinzer 1987; Stein 1989).

From the viewpoint of the HMO manager, the number of days of hospitalization per member per month is a critical number that management attempts to keep as low as possible by sometimes providing incentives to its physicians to treat patients out of hospital and by utilization review of those patients admitted for inpatient care. Also influencing profitability (critical for so-called nonprofit plans as well, which must maintain a balance between revenue and expenditure) are the number of enrolled members and the monthly premiums charged. Typically an HMO is not likely to show even a modest profit until it is at least 3 years old and has a membership of 50,000 or more (Group Health Association of America [GHAA] 1988). HMOs operate at thin margins, with profits and losses small overall. The trade association for group model HMOs, GHAA, conducts an annual survey, and in 1986 its data for some 180 plans showed profitable ones with a surplus of from 1% to 4% and most of those showing losses having revenues only about 4% below expenses.

The HMO's fixed budget encourages management to offer fewer expensive services than would be the case under an unmanaged indemnity plan. Paradoxically, the enrollees, however, have an incentive to demand more services since they are paying a fixed price and usually have small copayments and no deductibles. Thus controlling demand is a critical factor, leading managers to target membership to groups perceived to have low utilization rates. Firms with a predominantly white-collar work force may be approached rather than those with blue-collar workers on the assumption they will have less serious problems and fewer family members at risk for major psychiatric or addictive illnesses. Another way to target members is through the location of the HMO facility. If the location is in a growing suburb, it is likely to attract membership that is younger and healthier than might be found in an older city location. The prices charged and the services offered also help to select the target population. Better pricing for family coverage and services such as well-baby clinics may attract younger members.

Another method of favorably selecting members is used by HMOs even when they are federally qualified and thus obligated to offer community rating. HMOs can offer community rating by class; an employer can be given a rate based on its classes of employees—rates may vary by family size, age group, or types of employment (Luft 1986). Both the Health Care Financing Administration (HCFA) and Best's Review (Trauner 1987) reported that most HMOs were moving away from true community rating in the 1980s (D. Musgrave, HCFA, personal communication, December 1989).

The HMO's necessity to limit expensive services militates against the patient with psychiatric illness who may need a lengthy period of hospitalization. In 1986, the average length of stay for acute medical illness was 7 days, whereas the average length of stay in a private freestanding psychiatric hospital was 33 days.

Employers were not only obligated by the HMO Act to offer the HMO alternative where it was available, they welcomed the alternative because it was expected to exert competitive pressure on traditional health care providers. Although employers were not unconcerned about quality, they assumed quality would be determined by consumer satisfaction. Their main concern was cost; health insurance premiums were increasing at 20% per year from 1981 to 1983, eroding corporate profits. By 1983 more than 50,000 employers offered HMOs and thought they were saving money even when the numbers joining were small. However, by 1986 other insurers were becoming competitive with HMOs. Employees were attracted to HMOs because employers were increasingly shifting health care costs to them by increasing deductibles; HMOs had no deductibles and seemed to promise comprehensive coverage. The new models (IPA and network) also offered greater choice of physicians than in the past.

Quality of Care in HMOs

HMOs may still seek federal "qualification" that was originally required by the HMO Act before they could receive federal funding. Now, federal qualification for an HMO has come to represent a minimum standard; federal status as a proxy for quality assurance is often sought by HMOs as a marketing advantage to reassure prospective members they will receive an approved level of care. Companies negotiating health care for their employees have usually required federal qualification of an HMO they planned to offer; however, monitoring performance of HMOs once they have qualified for federal approval has never been a requirement.

The argument has been made that salaried physicians can provide as good quality of care as fee-for-service practitioners (Relman 1988). Primary and specialized care can be integrated and the administrative nuisances of fee-for-service practice avoided, allowing more time for patient care. Whether these benefits are realized, however, seems to depend on the organization's methods and objectives. HMO physicians have complained that the quality standards they would like to maintain are threatened by the HMO's need to contain costs (Hirschorn 1986; Scovern 1988). It has been argued that providing high-quality mental health care can be compromised in HMOs because many plans offer physicians financial incentives for keeping specialty referrals low, often putting unassertive or depressed patients at a disadvantage in securing the kind of health services they need (Buie 1987). A recent study faulted HMO primary care physicians for failing to recognize depression in many of their patients; the study found HMO doctors less likely than fee-for-service doctors to identify depressed patients (Wells et al. 1988). HMO subscribers may be told about the number of hospital days or outpatient visits allowed, but will not be told about pressures on physicians to discourage use of specialty services (Levinson 1987). That these abuses were common is evidenced by Congress's passage of a law in 1986 that would prevent hospitals and HMOs from using financial incentives to doctors to limit patient care—but only HMOs serving Medicare and Medicaid patients were included and the effective date for HMO inclusion in the law's requirements was postponed until April 1990.

The 20-year experience of Kaiser HMOs has shown their managers that providing mental health coverage for their 8 million subscribers has been cost-effective in preventing inappropriate overuse of general medical care (Cummings and Vandenbos 1981). In a capitated payment HMO such as Kaiser, overuse threatens economic viability. Identifying "overuse" and referring patients to appropriate care implies the existence of a sophisticated medical review evaluation system, however, which is not a feature of every HMO. Referral to appropriate psychiatric care is also problematic when specialty staffing is inadequate. In fact, a survey carried out by Kaiser in 1988 indicated that employers were hearing complaints about access to mental health care in HMOs (American Psychiatric Association 1988).

Rates of Utilization

A survey of some 8,000 members who had remained for 5 years in a prepaid group practice found the utilization of psychiatric services to be 3.7%—lower for children and adolescents (3%) and higher for adult men under 50 (4.3%) and for women (5.8%) (Kessler 1984). The age distribution in this HMO was much younger than that of the population as a whole, but findings were age-standardized (Kessler 1984).

A 1988 InterStudy report based on responses from 286 HMOs in

1985 found that 3.4% (680,000) of the 20 million members received some mental health treatment, and 7.4% of those treated were hospitalized—a small fraction (0.2%) of the overall membership (Shadle and Christianson 1988b). Costs for mental health treatment matched usage: 3.1% of costs overall were for mental health. The average inpatient episode for mental health cost $3,797—higher than average cost per case ($3,126) for all patients in community hospitals in 1985 (American Medical Association 1985). The average hospitalization for mental illness in the surveyed HMOs lasted 12.75 days.

Patterns of Psychiatric Care in HMOs

One advantage of HMO psychiatry is that it brings the delivery of psychiatric services closer to primary care medicine and this is especially so in staff model HMOs. In this way, medical etiologies and comorbidities associated with psychiatric disorder are more likely to be detected, resulting in an improved quality of services, than in settings where this approach is not taken. Another advantage is the tendency toward multidisciplinary practice and multimodal therapy associated with the group practice commonly used by HMOs. This means that multiple perspectives on a patient's problem are available through peer team evaluation and review, consultations are available, and the most appropriate treatments, whether they be medical, psychological, behavioral, or social, are likely to be more convenient than in a solo practitioner setting. This kind of staffing, together with the administrative support provided by the HMO organization, should result in better and possibly more cost-effective care. One way that care can be provided more cost-effectively is through the use of low-cost, nonphysician services or through the use of low-cost treatment approaches, such as group therapy. Both approaches were adopted by the Group Health Cooperative studied by RAND (Wells et al. 1986). Still another is through increased productivity of clinical staff, reported in the most recent study we have (Shadle and Christianson 1988a) to be 80% of staff time spent in direct care activity.

Along with the advantages of HMO psychiatry come several disadvantages. Because of the many types of plans and coverage programs, it is clear that both from an organization and a financing viewpoint there is little uniformity in services provided by HMOs. This makes it difficult for patients to evaluate knowledgeably the quality of benefits offered by HMOs even if the amount of benefits is specified. There appear to be more exclusions, a narrower range of service benefits, and less intensive short-term care by mental health providers in HMOs than in non-HMO insurance programs.

If reduced services deliver care more efficiently and appropriately, this could be viewed as a positive aspect of HMO psychiatry; however, if lower utilization per person reflects skimping on care—then it is a decided disadvantage. Currently, there are little available data on outcomes to judge the appropriateness of most HMO care. Data collected by the authors regarding hospital care provided by HMOs indicate that, although HMOs have been growing in market share in every region of the country and currently enroll some 30 million people, there appears to be surprisingly little use of psychiatric hospital services nationally by this group, compared to use by patients with other kinds of insurance (Dorwart et al. 1991).

We found that in 1988, roughly 3% of revenues of psychiatric hospitals were for patients from managed care organizations. Private nonprofit psychiatric hospitals reported 6% of revenues from these organizations and private for-profit psychiatric hospitals received 3% of revenues from this source. Public hospitals reported about 1% of their revenues derived from patients with this source of funding; however, in nearly half the states, state and county mental hospital facilities have no mechanisms for collecting such revenues. Similar small proportions were reported by general hospitals with psychiatric units (4%). Because nearly 15% of insured patients in the United States receive care through HMOs, there appears to be an underrepresentation of HMO patients in psychiatric hospitals. If this is true, one possible explanation would be the tendency for selection into HMOs of less seriously ill patients, a practice commonly referred to as skimming. Although the evidence is slim to support the claims of those who point to the possibility of reduced access for mental health care in HMOs, the issue is important and deserves further attention from mental health services researchers and health policymakers.

Conclusion

In this chapter we have reviewed several aspects of the economics of HMO psychiatry. Our review suggests that HMO psychiatry is growing and is rapidly becoming a major aspect of mental health services in the United States. At the same time, the important economic issues of selection and incentive structure surrounding the provision of mental health care in HMOs are different from traditional indemnity insurance arrangements, and there is some evidence that changing patterns of care are one result. There are not good data on the quality of services provided by mental health providers, whether in HMOs or elsewhere, but we believe evidence shows a reduced reliance of HMOs on hospital-based treatment for the mentally ill and a tendency toward briefer treatments in general. We have raised questions that deserve further study as managed care psychiatry evolves, concerning the trade-offs and the possible unintended consequences of pressures toward cost containment within the "pressure cooker" of HMO mental health departments. On the other hand, the pressures we ascribe to the HMO model of service delivery also could provide inducements for providers to find more creative and cost-effective ways to provide services without reducing quality of services—what we refer to as the "crucible" effect of HMOs on psychiatry. Whatever the long-term outcomes, there is a need for more and better studies of HMO psychiatry, including research using rigorous cost-benefit and cost-effectiveness designs and including measures of quality of care. Only in this way will we know whether HMO psychiatry is a healthy trend that will improve mental health services or an anemic one that will merely reduce utilization rates in order to lower costs of care.

References

Abel-Smith B.: The rise and decline of early HMOs. Milbank Q 66(4):694–719, 1988

American Hospital Association: Contents under pressure: management of psychiatric and substance abuse services. Annual Conference, Washington DC, June 7–9, 1989

American Medical Association: Economic Trends, Vol 1, No 2. Chicago, IL, Hospital Research and Educational Trust, 1985

American Psychiatric Association: HMO mental illness access criticized. Ecofacts. Washington, DC, American Psychiatric Association Office of Economic Affairs, December 1988, p 3

American Psychiatric Association: Interview with Mary Jane England. Ecofacts. Washington, DC, American Psychiatric Association Office of Economic Affairs, March 1989, p 4

Bennett MJ: The greening of the HMO: implications for prepaid psychiatry. Am J Psychiatry 145(12):1544–1549, 1988

Brown LD: Politics and Health Care Organization: HMOs as Federal Policy. Washington, DC, Brookings Institute, 1983

Buie J: Evidence of HMO flaws mounting. American Psychological Association Monitor 18(9):45, 1987

Cummings NA, Vandenbos GR: The 20-year Kaiser Permanente experience with psychiatric therapy and medical utilization. Health Policy Quarterly 1(2):159–175, 1981

Dorwart RA, Chartock LR: Psychiatry and the resource-based relative value scale. Am J Psychiatry 145(10):1237–1242, 1988

Dorwart RA, Schlesinger M: Privatization of psychiatric services. Am J Psychiatry 145(5):543–553, 1988

Dorwart RA, Epstein S, Davidson H: The shifting balance of public and private inpatient psychiatric services: implications for administrators. Administration and Policy in Mental Health 16(1):4–14, 1988

Dorwart RA, Schlesinger M, Davidson H, et al: A national survey of psychiatric hospitals. Am J Psychiatry 148(2):204–210, 1991

Gabel J, Jajich-Toch C, Williams K, et al: The commercial health insurance industry in transition. Health Aff (Millwood) 6(3):46–60, 1987

Group Health Association of America: HMO Industry Profile: Annual Survey, Vol. 3: Financial Performance. Washington, DC, Group Health Association of America, 1988

Hirschorn MW: Medical discord: some doctors assail quality treatment provided by HMOs. The Wall Street Journal, September 16, 1986, p 1

Horgan C: The demand for ambulatory mental health services from specialty providers. Health Serv Res 21(2):291–320, 1986

Iglehart JK: HMOs for profit and not-for-profit on the move. N Engl J Med 310(18):1203–1208, 1984

Keeler EB, Wells KB, Manning WG, et al: The Demand for Episodes of Mental Health Services. Santa Monica, CA, RAND Corporation, October 1986

Kessler LG: Treated incidence of mental disorders in a prepaid group practice setting. Am J Public Health 74(2):152–154, 1984

Kinzer DM: Is there a future for futurists? Massachusetts Medicine 2(1):24–31, 1987

Levinson DF: Toward full disclosure of referral restrictions and financial incentives by prepaid health plans. N Engl J Med 317(27):1729–1731, 1987

Luft HS: How do HMOs achieve their "savings"? N Engl J Med 298:1342, 1978

Luft HS: Compensating for biased selection in health insurance. Milbank Q 64(4):566–591, 1986

Manning WG, Wells KB, Benjamin B: Use of Outpatient Mental Health Care: Trial of a Prepaid Group Practice Versus Fee-For-Service. Santa Monica, CA, RAND Corporation, 1986

McGuire TG: Financing Psychotherapy: Costs, Effects and Public Policy. Cambridge, MA, Ballinger, 1981

McGuire TG: Financing and reimbursement for mental health services, in The Future of Mental Health Services Research (DHHS Publ No ADM-89-1600). Edited by Taube CA, Mechanic D, Hohmann A. Washington, DC, U.S. Government Printing Office, 1989

Relman AS: Salaried physicians and economic incentives. N Engl J Med 319(12):784, 1988

Scherl DJ, English JT, Sharfstein SS: Prospective Payment and Psychiatric Care. Washington, DC, American Psychiatric Association, 1988

Schlesinger M: On the limits of expanding health care reform: chronic care in prepaid settings. Milbank Q 64:189–215, 1986

Schlesinger M: Striking a balance: capitation, the mentally ill, and public policy, in Integrating Mental Health Services Through Capitation. Edited by Mechanic D, Aiken K. San Francisco, CA, Jossey-Bass, 1989

Scovern H: Hired help: a physician's experiences in a for-profit staff-model HMO. N Engl J Med 319(12):787–790, 1988

Sederer L, St. Clair R: Managed health care and the Massachusetts experience. Am J Psychiatry 146(9):1142–1148, 1989

Shadle M, Christianson JB: The organization of mental health care delivery in HMOs. Administration and Policy in Mental Health 15(4):201–225, 1988a

Shadle M, Christianson JB: The Organization and Delivery of Mental Health, Alcohol, and Other Drug Abuse Services Within Health Maintenance Organizations, Vol 1. Excelsior, MN, InterStudy, 1988b

Shapiro S, Skinner EA, Kessler LG, et al: Utilization of health and mental health services. Arch Gen Psychiatry 41:971–978, 1984

Stein C: HMOs feel the pinch, increase their rates. Boston Globe, March 9, 1989, p 33

Thompson JW, Bass RD, Witkin MJ: Fifty years of psychiatric services: 1940–1990. Hosp Community Psychiatry 33(9):711–717, 1982

Tischler GL: Utilization management of mental health services by private third parties. Am J Psychiatry 147(8):967–973, 1990

Trauner JB: The HMO identity crisis. Best's Review, 1987, pp 60–70

Vignola ML: HMOs. New York, Salomon Bros. Stock Research, May 1988

Wells KB, Manning WG Jr, Benjamin B: Use of outpatient mental health services in HMO and fee-for-service plans. Health Serv Res 21(3):453–474, 1986

Wells KB, Hays RD, Burnam MA, et al: Detection of depressive disorder for patients receiving prepaid or fee-for-service care. JAMA 262(23):3293–3302, 1988

✦ **3** ✦

Comparing Mental Health Benefits, Utilization Patterns, and Costs

Bruce Lubotsky Levin, Dr.P.H., F.A.M.H.A.
Jay H. Glasser, Ph.D.

Cost containment in health care has been a major preoccupation among policymakers, academicians, and health care professionals for a substantial portion of the post–World War II era. The search for a more comprehensive and coordinated approach for the organization, financing, and delivery of health services continues to evolve within the public and private sectors. Various strategies (including regulatory strategies, incentive reimbursement policies, and health care market reform) have been utilized in an attempt to deal with the escalating costs of providing health and mental health care.

Managed health care, an example of pro-competitive or health care market–based strategies, has utilized a number of mechanisms (including the utilization of alternative delivery settings, capitation payment, prospective payment, at-risk contracting, and utilization review mechanisms) to help redesign how medical care is delivered and reimbursed in America.

Alcohol, drug abuse, and mental disorders[*] comprise a multiplicity of conditions that continue to represent some of the most complex and least understood of all public health problems. Although nearly one out of five people annually suffers from a diagnosable mental disorder in the United States, only one out of five of these individuals actually

---

[*] The term "mental health" or "mental health services" throughout this chapter will refer to services for alcohol, drug, and mental disorders.

seeks treatment within the formal health care delivery system (Locke and Regier 1985; Robins et al. 1991). Furthermore, mental disorders result in staggering costs to society, which have been estimated to exceed $129 billion in annual direct and indirect costs in 1988 (Disease Prevention/Health Promotion: The Facts 1988; Rice et al. 1991).

The misuse of alcohol and other drugs represents a major hazard to the physical and mental health of Americans. At least 2.5 million people in the United States have serious drug problems, and an estimated 30 million Americans use illicit drugs. The annual economic (direct and indirect) costs to society have been estimated to exceed $85 billion for alcohol abuse and $58 billion for drug abuse in 1988 (Promoting Health/Preventing Disease: Year 2000 Objectives for the Nation 1989; Rice et al. 1991; U.S. General Accounting Office 1988).

Total mental health spending represents approximately 14% of the estimated $542 billion in national health expenditures for 1989. However, firms have been spending as much as 20 cents of every health care dollar on mental health services, by far the fastest growing health care cost in the United States (Wallace 1987). Concerns over insurance costs for mental health services have contributed to reductions in mental health benefits under private health insurance.

In this chapter, we will present the most recent findings from a national study that examined the organizational structure, benefits coverage, costs, and utilization of mental health services within one particular model of managed health care: health maintenance organizations (HMOs; Levin and Glasser 1988; Levin et al. 1988). We will also assess recent changes in HMO mental health services in comparison to earlier national HMO mental health surveys (Levin and Glasser 1979, 1984; Levin et al. 1984).

Background

Although insurance coverage for physical disorders has been traditionally based on the medical necessity for treatment, insurance coverage and reimbursement for mental disorders has been treated substantially differently, based on the duration of treatment (Seltzer 1988). Consequently, insurance coverage for mental health services has remained limited, expensive, and not equivalent to coverage for other medical disorders (American Psychiatric Association 1986; Sharfstein et al. 1984). Although coverage for mental health disorders has become more prevalent in employee health benefit plans, the actual benefit provisions have remained highly variable. For example, although the number of employees with mental health benefits increased from 1979 to 1984, there also was a rise in out-of-pocket costs (through copayments and deductibles) associated with mental health service coverage (Brady et al. 1986).

In an attempt to increase the availability of insurance coverage for mental disorders, state legislatures in 40 states have chosen to mandate the provision of benefits covering mental health treatment. By the end of 1987, 27 states regulated mental health benefits, whereas 38 states regulated alcohol and drug abuse benefits. Whether these laws were passed as mandatory benefit packages or required options, the benefits generally differed by state, included multiple levels of coverage limitations, and continued to emphasize inpatient mental health benefits structures rather than outpatient mental health benefits (Levin 1988a).

Mental health services within HMOs emerged in the 1970s through a number of pioneering projects conducted within individual health plans in the 1960s and through the passage of federal HMO legislation in the early 1970s (Avnet 1962; Glasser 1965; Shapiro and Fink 1963).

A number of informative case studies were reported in the literature during the 1960s, 1970s, and 1980s that described mental health service coverage and utilization within individual health plans as well as comparative studies on the cost and utilization of mental health services in an HMO and fee-for-service plan (e.g., Bittker and Idzorek 1978; Budman et al. 1979; Craig and Patterson 1981; Diehr et al. 1984; Fink et al. 1969; Follette and Cummings 1967; Goldberg et al. 1970; Goldensohn 1972; Goldensohn et al. 1969; Green 1969; Harrington 1975; Locke et al. 1966; Patterson 1976; Sachs 1972; Williams et al. 1979).

Comparative studies have examined the use of mental health services for members in an HMO compared to a fee-for-service plan. One study randomly assigned members of a general population to an HMO or several fee-for-service insurance plans (Wells et al. 1986). HMO enrollees were found equally likely to visit a mental health provider during the year, but were found to incur significantly less total ambulatory mental health costs compared to fee-for-service enrollees. These case studies, however, remain limited in their generalizability to a specific HMO setting.

Reed and associates (1972) provided the first examination of mental health coverage, costs, and service utilization within more than one HMO. Their landmark text was later updated by Reed (1975) and by Sharfstein and associates (1984). It was not until 1978 that a study was undertaken that examined the organizational characteristics, benefit coverage, and the utilization of mental health services within HMOs throughout the United States (Levin and Glasser 1979). This study revealed that nearly 90% of the 123 responding HMOs provided a minimum of 30 days (per member per year) for inpatient mental health care and a minimum of 20 visits (per member per year) for ambulatory mental health care through basic or supplemental benefit packages. HMOs reported lower physical and mental hospitalization but higher ambulatory utilization compared to more traditional fee-for-service health insurance plans. The mean staffing ratios (full-time equivalent per 10,000 members) in the plans studied were 1.06 psychiatrists, 0.58 psychologists, and 0.80 psychiatric social workers within group practice model HMOs.

An expansion of this national HMO study provided information on alcohol and drug abuse as well as mental health coverage, service utilization and costs, and organizational characteristics of the mental health components within 205 HMOs throughout the United States (Levin and Glasser 1984; Levin et al. 1984). The 1982 national study revealed that 94% of the HMOs offered mental health coverage as part of their basic health plan benefits, whereas more than 50% of the HMOs offered coverage for alcohol and drug abuse services. However, the mental health benefits offered were more limited than HMO medical care benefits, and the coverage for alcohol and drug abuse was limited even further.

In 1985 a national HMO study was conducted by Shadle and Christianson (1988), methodologically based on previous national studies (Levin and Glasser 1979, 1984; Levin et al. 1984). Although results reflected similar trends in mental health benefits coverage and service utilization, differences in the data were attributed, in part, to the different years of data collection, differing response rates for specific variables, and the use of different measures and terms (e.g., outpatient visits compared to ambulatory encounters).

Our focus in this chapter will be on presenting the highlights from the most recent national HMO mental health study, which sought to identify the level of participation by HMOs in providing mental health benefits, to examine the kinds of organizational models used by HMOs that provide mental health services, and to identify the factors associated with the level of coverage, costs, and utilization of mental health services. Factors hypothesized to influence HMO mental health benefits, costs, and service utilization included external or environmental variables, general HMO characteristics, HMO organizational characteristics, and HMO mental health organizational characteristics. We will also discuss changes in HMO mental health service coverage over the past decade.

Methods

The most recent national study of HMO mental health services utilized a survey research approach (Levin and Glasser 1988; Levin et al. 1988). The survey instrument utilized was a self-administered mail questionnaire, developed with the assistance of 24 administrators, medical directors, and mental health directors from American HMOs. The survey instrument was then pretested on a random sample of HMOs, stratified by HMO enrollment size and by federal qualification status.

Following a review of the pretest results, the final instrument was constructed, which contained 36 questions (utilizing subcategories where appropriate) designed to ascertain basic organizational characteristics, benefit structures, and utilization and cost of mental health services within all operational HMOs in America. Health plan benefit brochures and annual reports were also collected to increase data verification and promote standardized definitions of terms.

Careful attention was given to the reliability of the data collected throughout the study. This was accomplished through the use of pretest and follow-up techniques. Although the data were collected through mail questionnaires without on-site interviews, a combination of open-ended and closed-ended questions was used in the pretest instrument to allow maximum collection of information from the HMOs. This preliminary design of the pretest instrument permitted the identification of ambiguities, shortcomings, and areas of bias within the instrument.

Follow-up letters were mailed 4 weeks after the initial mailing, and telephone contact was initiated 3 weeks later. Subsequent contact was dependent upon the specific circumstances of each HMO.

In calculating the mean utilization rates for mental health ser-

vices, each individual HMO rate was weighted by that plan's enrollment size, producing a weighted average that reflected the utilization
experience of a typical HMO enrollee. In order to be considered for
analysis, HMO respondents had to provide data for all three mental
health hospital variables (annual hospital days per 1,000 enrollees,
annual hospital admissions per 1,000 enrollees, and average length of
stay per enrollee). This procedure was included so that the interrelated measures would all be calculated on a common set of respondent
HMOs.

Results

Questionnaires were initially sent to a total of 610 HMOs. Of these, 15
health plans had folded or were no longer operating as HMOs, and 171
organizations were either preoperational or operational for less than 1
full year. The remaining 424 HMOs met the study criteria of having
been operational for 1 year or more and having an enrollment in excess of 500 people. The 424 HMOs, in 1986, served approximately 23
million enrollees. A total of 304 of the 424 HMOs completed and returned the self-administered questionnaire, a 72% response rate. The
responding HMOs represented approximately 86% of the total number
of people enrolled in operational HMOs in 1986. They form the basis
for the analyses that follow.

General HMO Organizational Characteristics

Almost one-half (46%) of the 304 responding health plans had enrollments of fewer than 25,000 members, with the median enrollment
being approximately 28,000 members. More than half (52%) of the
HMOs had been operational for less than 6 years. Sixty-eight percent
of the health plans were federally qualified HMOs. More than two-
fifths (43%) of the health plans were individual practitioner association (IPA) model HMOs, whereas 53% of the health plans were
for-profit organizations. These and other selected general HMO characteristics have been summarized in Table 3–1.
   Nearly one-third (30%) of the HMOs were located in Public Health
Region V, which includes Wisconsin, Illinois, Michigan, Indiana, Ohio,
and Minnesota (see Figure 3–1). The largest HMO enrollment (nearly
7 million members) was located in Public Health Region IX, which in-

Table 3–1. Distribution of selected HMO organizational characteristics

HMO organizational characteristics	Frequency	%
Enrollment size		
< 9,999	62	20.39
10,000–24,999	78	25.66
25,000–49,999	72	23.68
50,000–74,999	38	12.50
75,000–99,999	14	4.61
> 100,000	40	13.16
Total	304	100.00
(Mean 65,369)		
(SD 174,055)		
(Median 27,603)		
HMO model		
Group	68	22.37
Staff	53	17.43
IPA	131	43.09
Network	52	17.11
Total	304	100.00
Health plan age (years)		
1–5	159	52.30
6–10	77	25.33
11–15	46	15.13
16–20	10	3.29
> 21	12	3.95
Total	304	100.00
(Mean 7.55)		
(SD 7.95)		
(Median 5.00)		
Federal qualification status		
Qualified	207	68.10
Not qualified	97	31.90
Total	304	100.00
Profit status		
Nonprofit	143	47.04
For-profit	161	52.96
Total	304	100.00
Competing HMOs in service area		
0–5	143	47.99
6–10	96	32.21
11–15	35	11.75
16–20	10	4.36
> 21	11	3.69
Total	298	100.00
HMO service area population		
50,000	6	1.97
50,001–100,000	14	4.61
100,001–250,000	34	11.19
250,001–500,000	44	14.47
> 500,001	206	67.76
Total	304	100.00

Source. Excerpted from Levin 1988b.

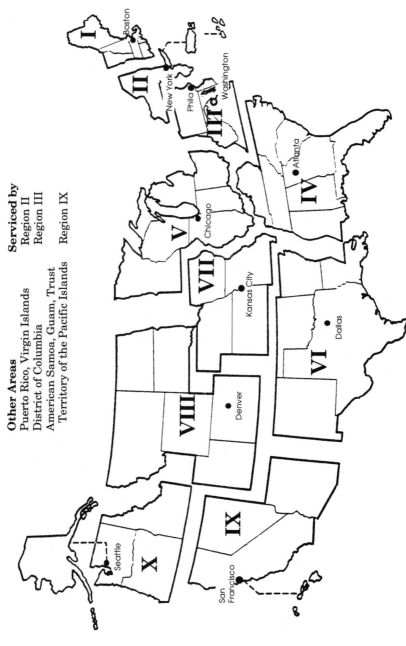

Other Areas
Puerto Rico, Virgin Islands
District of Columbia
American Samoa, Guam, Trust
Territory of the Pacific Islands

Serviced by
Region II
Region III

Region IX

Figure 3-1 United States Public Health Service Regions. Reprinted with permission from *U.S. Department of Health and Human Services Directory, 1990.*

cludes Hawaii, California, Arizona, Nevada, and Guam. California and Florida were the states with the most operational HMOs.

Mental Health Service Coverage and Benefits

The HMO Act of 1973 and subsequent amendments provided the legal and financial foundation for the establishment of HMOs throughout the United States (Introduction to Alternative Delivery Mechanisms 1986). These laws required federally qualified HMOs to provide for short-term outpatient evaluative or crisis intervention mental health services and to provide for the medical treatment and referral services for alcohol and drug abuse or addiction (United States Congress 1973, 1976, 1978, 1981).

Although federal HMO legislation does not specifically address inpatient mental health service coverage within federally qualified HMOs, nearly all responding HMOs (97%) offered mental health hospital coverage as a part of their basic health plan benefit. Nearly three-fifths (58%) of the HMOs offered 30 days (per member per year) of hospital mental health coverage, whereas nearly four-fifths (79%) of the HMOs offered 20 visits (per member per year) of ambulatory health coverage.

Federal HMO legislation also does not specify the minimum coverage levels for alcohol and drug abuse services within federally qualified HMOs. Nevertheless, two-thirds (66%) of the responding HMOs offered alcohol and drug abuse (hospital) benefits. Almost one-third (31%) of the health plans offered only detoxification and emergency drug abuse intervention services, and 3% of the HMOs did not offer any basic or supplemental alcohol and drug abuse benefits. HMOs that were more likely to offer alcohol and drug abuse benefits had enrollments of under 50,000, had been operational for less than 16 years, were federally qualified, and were IPA-model HMOs. Forty-five percent of the health plans had alcohol and drug abuse benefits separate from their mental health benefits. The annual median benefits for HMO alcohol and drug abuse coverage were 30 hospital days (per member) and 20 ambulatory visits (per member). Nearly one-half (48%) of the HMOs offered supplemental or multiple mental health benefits.

Despite the apparent provision of mental health service coverage, HMOs have used various methods to limit the use of these benefits: specified coverage exclusions (see Figure 3–2); restrictions on the

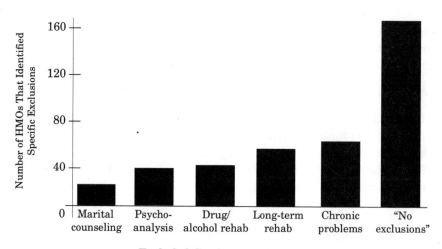

Figure 3–2. Specified HMO mental health service exclusions ($N = 304$). *Note:* Some HMOs indicated more than one service exclusion.

number of hospital days and ambulatory visits; the use of copayments, deductibles, and fees; supplemental or rider options with higher premiums; annual and lifetime benefit and cost limitations; mandatory "waiting" periods between hospital admissions; limitation of facility and human resources; restricted access to services; and a combination of these methods. Most HMOs (85% for mental health services and 95% for alcohol and drug abuse services) provided for hospital coverage *without* deductible or copayment requirements. Ambulatory coverage involved a mean copayment of $15.00 per visit for mental health treatment and $13.00 per visit for alcohol and drug abuse treatment.

Table 3–2 presents the annual mean hospital and ambulatory mental health benefit coverage (per member) by five general HMO characteristics: health plan enrollment size, federal qualification status, HMO model type, health plan age, and health plan profit status. Both hospital and ambulatory mental health benefits increased with HMO enrollment size. For-profit HMOs reported offering significantly lower hospital mental health benefits compared to nonprofit HMOs.

Mental Health Organizational Structure

HMO mental health services were provided through a variety of organizational structures, including internal provisions (e.g., a department), external provision (e.g., referral agreements and contractual arrangements with private practitioners and community facilities), and a combination of internal and external provision mechanisms. Approximately 15% of the HMOs provided mental health services primarily through an internal component. About 32% of the HMOs provided mental health services primarily through a combination of an internal component and referral to external providers. More than half (53%) of the HMOs contracted externally for mental health services, and private practitioners were the most frequently chosen providers of these services.

Table 3–2. Annual mean mental health coverage benefits by selected HMO organizational characteristics

HMO organizational characteristics	Annual mean hospital and ambulatory mental health coverage	
	Hospital benefits (days per member)	Ambulatory benefits (visits per member)
Enrollment size		
< 9,999	32.02*	19.68*
10,000–24,999	32.66	25.58
25,000–49,999	48.82	26.24
50,000–74,999	47.65	23.65
75,000–99,999	64.67	73.15
> 100,000	43.70	30.13
Federal qualification status		
Qualified	39.64	27.83
Not qualified	45.38	25.44
HMO model		
Group	43.05	30.66
Staff	49.66	21.90
IPA	39.82	23.79
Network	34.42	35.54
Health plan age (years)		
1–5	38.41	25.22*
6–10	38.97	21.78
11–15	45.16	21.74
16–20	65.60	89.50
> 21	60.42	49.58
Profit status		
Nonprofit	46.83*	26.84
For-profit	36.82	27.39
Entire population	41.41	27.13
N	292	287

* Tests of significance of differences within groups, $P < .05$.

One-fourth of the HMOs (25%) organized their mental health services within a formal departmental unit, whereas 16% of the HMOs reported that mental health services were organized through liaison or team approaches that involved professionals from several different departments within the health plan organization (see Figure 3–3). Larger HMOs (enrollments in excess of 50,000 members) were more likely to have mental health departments, whereas smaller HMOs (enrollments of fewer than 50,000 members) were more likely to use liaison or team approaches. Unlike the other HMO models, the IPA-model HMOs generally did not use either departmental or team approaches to organize their HMO mental health component. Rather, they utilized independent practitioners through their individual private offices.

Nearly half (47%) of the HMOs reported having no director or designated coordinator of either their mental health department or of their mental health services and benefits. Under these circumstances, the medical director was responsible for the mental health services. The majority (61%) of health plans without mental health directors were IPA-model HMOs. Of the remaining HMOs that had mental health directors, 63% were psychiatrists, 25% were psychologists, and 12% were either nurses or social workers. Mental health directors were most often found in HMOs with enrollments in excess of 50,000 members and in for-profit group model HMOs and nonprofit staff model HMOs (see Figure 3–4).

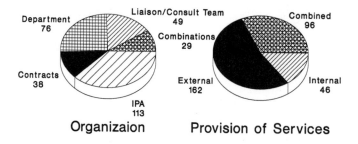

Figure 3–3. Organization and provision of HMO mental health services (*N* = 34).

The survey instrument also sought information regarding HMO psychiatrist affiliation, psychiatrist reimbursement, and type of psychiatric practice of HMO mental health providers. Of the psychiatrists employed by the HMOs responding to the national survey, 85% held contractual arrangements with the health plans (through a variety of reimbursement mechanisms), whereas 15% were HMO employees. Additionally, 60% of the HMO psychiatrists were affiliated with a single or multiple group practice, whereas 40% were solo practitioners.

HMO psychiatrists were reimbursed for their services through a variety of methods, including fee-for-service (44%), capitation (20%), salary (18%), and contract (18%).

Nearly two-fifths (38%) of the HMOs indicated that they permitted self-referral to mental health services, whereas nearly three-fifths (57%) of the HMOs reported that they referred all of their health plan members to mental health services only through the authorization of a primary care provider. Five percent of the HMOs permitted referral to mental health services through employers, friends, or clergy.

Costs and Utilization of Services

Responding HMOs reported total expenditures for mental health services, hospital costs, and ambulatory costs. The annual median expenditure for mental health services (as a percentage of total HMO costs) was 5%. The annual mean hospital and ambulatory costs for HMO

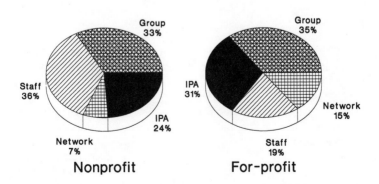

Figure 3–4. Distribution of model types by status in HMOs with mental health directors.

mental health services appear in Table 3–3. The annual mean hospital and ambulatory costs for HMO alcohol and drug abuse services appear in Table 3–4 for those health plans that were able to separate their alcohol and drug abuse service costs from their mental health service costs. Hospital costs for alcohol and drug abuse services were generally highest for HMOs with enrollments of fewer than 10,000 members.

HMOs also reported annual mean utilization for hospital and ambulatory mental health services (see Table 3–5) and for hospital and ambulatory alcohol and drug abuse services (see Table 3–6). The utilization of hospital mental health services was highest for HMOs with enrollments of fewer than 10,000 members. Additionally, HMOs that were not federally qualified reported significantly higher hospital mental health service utilization compared to the utilization rates reported by federally qualified HMOs. Finally, IPA-model HMOs reported higher hospital mental health use rates compared to all other

Table 3–3. Annual mean HMO mental health service costs for 1982 and 1986

Annual mean costs for mental health services	National survey year	
	1982 (n)	1986 (n)
Hospital costs		
Per member (month)	$ 0.46 (189)*	$ 0.97 (245)
Per episode	$2,802 (189)*	$3,319 (246)
Per day	$ 262 (189)*	$ 301 (249)
Ambulatory costs		
Per member (month)	$ 0.60 (189)*	$ 0.93 (249)
Per visit	$56.06 (189)*	$58.10 (254)

* 1986 dollars.

Table 3–4. Annual mean HMO alcohol/substance abuse service costs, 1986

Annual mean costs for alcohol/substance abuse	National survey year
	1986 (n)
Hospital costs	
Per member (month)	$ 0.59 (95)
Per episode	$2,684 (93)
Per day	$ 249 (93)
Ambulatory costs	
Per member (month)	$ 0.52 (87)
Per visit	$45.10 (87)

Table 3–5. Annual mean HMO mental health service utilization for 1978, 1982, and 1986

Annual mean utilization for mental health services	National survey year		
Hospital utilization	1978 (n)	1982 (n)	1986 (n)
Days (per 1,000)	65 (49)	32.13 (195)	36.90 (264)
Admissions (per 1,000)	6 (49)	3.00 (195)	3.27 (264)
Length of stay (per admission)	10.41 (49)	10.20 (195)	11.61 (264)
Ambulatory utilization			
Physician encounters (per member)		0.29 (199)	0.22 (269)
Total encounters (per member)		0.30 (199)	0.28 (270)

Table 3–6. Annual mean HMO alcohol/substance abuse service utilization, 1986

Annual mean utilization for alcohol/substance abuse	National survey year
Hospital utilization	1986 (n)
Days (per 1,000)	22.6 (103)
Admissions (per 1,000)	2.05 (103)
Length of stay (per admission)	11.32 (103)
Ambulatory utilization	
Physician encounters (per member)	0.14 (86)
Total encounters (per member)	0.15 (86)

HMO models (see Table 3–7). The utilization of alcohol and drug abuse services was generally highest for HMOs with enrollments of fewer than 10,000 members.

HMO mental health hospital and ambulatory service utilization rates were found to differ significantly by (geographic) region (see Figures 3–5 and 3–6).

Significant differences were found in the utilization of hospital mental health services for selected environmental variables (mandated mental health benefits), general HMO characteristics (federal qualification status and HMO model type), HMO organizational characteristics (physician affiliation, type of physician practice, and physician reimbursement), and HMO mental health organizational characteristics (existence and discipline of a mental health director, number of affiliated mental hospital facilities, location of mental health services, affiliation of the psychiatrist, internal/external provi-

Table 3–7. Annual mean hospital and ambulatory mental health utilization rates by selected HMO organization characteristics

HMO organizational characteristics	Annual mean hospital mental health utilization rates**			Annual mean mental health ambulatory utilization rates	
	Days per 1,000 members	Admissions per 1,000 members	Length of stay per admission	Total ambulatory physician encounters per member	Total ambulatory encounters per member
Enrollment size					
<9,999	41.22	3.56	12.03	0.22	0.27
10,000–24,999	39.58	3.40	11.70	0.24	0.28
25,000–49,999	34.98	3.17	11.69	0.21	0.28
50,000–74,999	31.21	2.92	11.06	0.18	0.26
75,000–99,999	36.26	2.88	12.64	0.24	0.30
>100,000	37.32	3.40	11.08	0.23	0.29
Federal qualification status					
Qualified	34.15*	3.23	10.87*	0.21	0.28
Not qualified	43.56	3.36	13.38	0.24	0.28
HMO model					
Group	34.29*	3.18*	11.21	0.23	0.31
Staff	29.80	2.63	11.68	0.20	0.30
IPA	42.20	3.61	11.80	0.22	0.26
Network	35.70	3.28	11.60	0.23	0.27
Health plan age (years)					
1–5	38.01	3.36	11.66	0.21	0.25*
6–10	37.34	3.30	11.44	0.25	0.33
11–15	33.97	2.91	11.87	0.21	0.28
16–20	36.78	3.38	11.76	0.18	0.26
>21	32.39	3.22	10.94	0.23	0.31
Profit status					
Nonprofit	37.20	3.12	12.20*	0.22	0.29
For-profit	36.62	3.40	11.06	0.22	0.27
Entire population	36.90	3.27	11.61	0.22	0.28
N	264	264	264	269	270

* Tests of significance of differences within groups, $P = .05$.
** To be included in this table, respondents had to provide data for all three hospital utilization variables.
Source. Excerpted from Levin 1988b.

sion of mental health services, organization of the mental health services component as a department, and hospital and ambulatory benefits offered by the HMO). Current research efforts are addressing the influence of these four types of variables upon predicting the rate of mental hospitalization and the costs associated with mental health services.

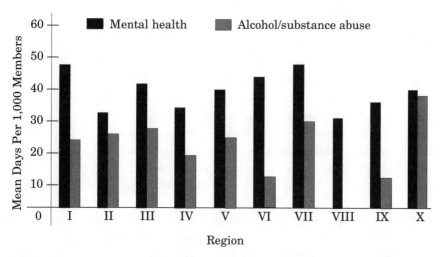

Figure 3–5. HMO mental health, alcohol, and substance abuse hospital utilization rates by region. *Note:* No responses were reported for alcohol and substance abuse utilization in Region VIII.

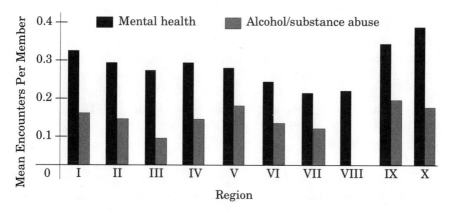

Figure 3–6. HMO mental health, alcohol, and substance abuse ambulatory utilization rates by region. *Note:* No responses were reported for alcohol and substance abuse utilization in Region VIII.

Discussion

The organization, financing, and delivery of health and mental health care in the United States remain in an era of major transition. In attempting to deal with the rapidly changing systems of health care financing in America, there has been a trend in indemnity insurance plans toward more limited insurance coverage for mental health care (Brady et al. 1986).

Since their development in the early 1900s as prepaid medical care plans, HMOs continue to evolve. The experience reported here, together with the earlier national studies (Levin and Glasser 1979; Levin et al. 1984), clearly demonstrate the dynamics of HMO development over the last two decades. The emergence of multiple coverage options and specified health benefit "carveouts" provide an added exigency to examine the consistency of trends as a basis for forecasting benefits, costs, and utilization in mental health services delivery.

The early 1970s marked the national emergence of alternative health care delivery systems, with the significant proliferation of HMOs. In 1978, there were 181 HMOs (operational for at least 1 year) with a total enrollment of 7.5 million members. The results of the 1978 national HMO study revealed that a majority of the health plans were group model HMOs that had been in operation for 5 years or less, were not federally qualified, and had enrollments of fewer than 15,000 members (Levin and Glasser 1979).

The second generation of HMOs emerged in the early 1980s with the steady growth of IPA-model HMOs as well as the growing affiliation of HMOs with national HMO systems. In 1982, there were 237 HMOs (operational for at least 1 year) with a total enrollment of 10.4 million members. The 1982 national HMO study revealed that nearly one-third of the HMOs were IPAs, nearly one-half were operational for 6 to 20 years with enrollments of under 50,000, and most were nonprofit health plans (Levin and Glasser 1984; Levin et al. 1984).

The mid-1980s marked the evolution of a third generation of HMOs, particularly for-profit health plans. This national study surveyed 304 HMOs (operational for at least 1 year) with a total enrollment of 23 million members in 1986. Results indicated that nearly one-half of the health plans were IPAs with enrollments under 25,000 that had been operational for less than 5 years and were structured as for-profit organizations. Nearly three-quarters of these health plans were federally qualified HMOs.

The current shift in HMO organizational structure is toward a mix of organizational models or hybrids (Levin and Levin 1986). The older HMOs continue to be a dominant factor in total enrollment. These HMOs are predominantly organized as group practice, nonprofit health plans. Similar to the general medical care delivery system, HMOs are affected by the current trend of affiliation with national health care firms. The number of HMOs has doubled nearly every 4 years since the late 1970s. However, HMO consolidation will increase as large insurers will acquire underfinanced HMOs, particularly IPA-model HMOs.

There appear to be several possible factors that influence mental health benefit design, including perceived competition, federal regulations, and state-mandated benefit laws. There has been a noted convergence toward a median mental health benefits coverage of 30 inpatient days (per member per year) and 20 ambulatory visits (per member per year). However, individual HMO benefit packages demonstrate considerable heterogeneity. Furthermore, the actual benefits offered by HMOs may or may not resemble the actual services available to enrollees within any given health plan. For example, although a health plan might provide up to a maximum of 60 days of hospital mental health coverage per enrollee per year, the use of 15 to 20 days of mental health hospital care may activate utilization review controls within the organization. This mechanism, in turn, may lead to the provision of alternative (nonhospital) mental health care either within or outside of the health plan, so that the absolute 60-day mental health hospital benefit is never fully utilized.

Nevertheless, recent emphasis specifically on alcohol and drug abuse treatment is reflected in a trend toward both increased inclusion of a substance abuse program within HMOs nationally and the separation of mental health and alcohol/drug abuse benefits within HMOs (Levin, in press, a, b).

Utilization of ambulatory mental health services has remained fairly stable, but there has been an 11% rise in inpatient days over the 4-year period (1982–1986). The increasing admission rate, length of stay, and thus increasing hospital days (from 1982 to 1986) are reflected in an increase of more than $500 in each inpatient episode of mental health care (Levin et al. 1988). Most importantly, the increased inpatient mental health utilization is occurring in the face of a 16% decrease in general medical inpatient days.

Although many utilization mechanisms have been implemented to control the use of physical and mental health services (including case management, utilization review boards, restructuring benefits, external provider and management contracting, and utilization of less costly treatment settings as well as less costly treatment providers), there has been no consensus on model systems for HMO mental health services.

Data from this study indicate a great majority of HMOs throughout the United States provide a minimum level of coverage for mental health treatment, but that the coverage varies more than the coverage provided for physical health services. HMO coverage for alcohol and drug abuse treatment is more restrictive than for mental health treatment. Although federal and selected state HMO legislation require certain minimum coverage for mental health services, minimum benefits, in practice, often become maximum benefit levels. Additionally, HMO federal legislation fails to specify guidelines for hospital mental health benefits as well as for hospital and ambulatory alcohol and drug abuse benefits.

A fourth generation of HMOs is evolving in the 1990s. HMOs are adopting open-ended or point-of-service options in an attempt to provide increased access to providers of care while maintaining the ability to control costs. Concurrently, health plans as well as insurers have developed multiple-option initiatives that can serve employers as a total replacement product. These exclusionary offerings often reduce or eliminate the availability of other competitive health plans to employee groups.

Many employers are also selecting to self-insure and introduce more experimentation with managed health care hybrids. For example, employers are increasingly "carving out" or separating mental health benefits from all other health benefits, in part to isolate the costs of mental health care. One strategy currently being utilized to control mental health care expenditures is utilization management, including preadmission certification, concurrent review, and high-cost case management (Tischler 1990).

Thus, these fiscal, organizational, and service delivery arrangements for providing mental health services are reflected in the current diversity of benefits, referral mechanisms, costs, and service utilization among existing HMOs.

As competition within the mental health sector increases and intensifies, there will be an increased need to develop more extensive and reliable information systems that contain demographic, organizational, utilization, and cost data as well as quality-of-care data. However, current data collection mechanisms within many health plans appear to be rather limited and incomplete (Levin, in press, a, b). The federal government currently has no reporting requirements with regard to mental health services within HMOs. The long-term impact of a lack of a standardized data base, from a national perspective, poses serious problems for all concerned with effective decision making regarding mental health service delivery. These limitations in data underscore the need to extend the parameters on which information regarding mental health services is collected.

One attempt to provide accountability in managed care organizations nationally was initiated several years ago under the auspices of the Joint Commission on Accreditation of Healthcare Organizations (JCAHO). The program sought to establish certification standards for HMOs. However, the JCAHO recently discontinued the program, apparently generating little national interest in the program initiative (Kirshner 1990).

In light of epidemiologic surveys indicating the potential demand for mental health services in the general population, the conflicting trends of norms and standards of care confront the issues of cost containment and benefits management. Timely data sources are necessary to monitor the anticipated pressures of organization, utilization, and costs of HMO mental health services.

References

American Psychiatric Association: The Coverage Catalog. Washington, DC, American Psychiatric Press, 1986, pp 1–21

Avnet HH: Psychiatric Insurance: Financing Short-Term Ambulatory Treatment. New York, Group Health Insurance and the American Psychiatric Association, 1962

Bittker TE, Idzorek S: The evolution of psychiatric services in a health maintenance organization. Am J Psychiatry 135:339–342, 1978

Brady J, Sharfstein SS, Muszynski IL: Trends in private insurance coverage for mental illness. Am J Psychiatry 143:1276–1279, 1986

Budman SH, Feldman JL, Bennett MJ: Adult mental health services in a health maintenance organization. Am J Psychiatry 136:392–395, 1979

Craig TJ, Patterson DY: A comparison of mental health costs and utilization under three insurance models. Med Care 19:184–192, 1981

Diehr P, Williams SJ, Martin DP, et al: Ambulatory mental health services utilization in three provider plans. Med Care 22:1–13, 1984

Disease Prevention/Health Promotion: The Facts. United States Office of Disease Prevention and Health Promotion. Palo Alto, CA, Bull Publishing Company, 1988, pp 12–19, 308–321

Fink R, Shapiro S, Goldensohn SS, et al: The "filter down" process to psychotherapy in a group practice medical care program. Am J Public Health 59:245–260, 1969

Follette W, Cummings NA: Psychiatric services and medical utilization in a prepaid health plan setting. Med Care 5:25–35, 1967

Glasser MA: Prepayment for psychiatric illness. Am J Psychiatry 121:736–741, 1965

Goldberg ID, Krantz G, Locke BZ: Effect of a short-term outpatient psychiatric therapy benefit on the utilization of medical services in a prepaid group practice medical program. Med Care 8:419–428, 1970

Goldensohn SS: A prepaid group practice mental health service as part of a health maintenance organization. Am J Orthopsychiatry 42:154–158, 1972

Goldensohn SS, Fink R, Shapiro S: Referral, utilization, and staffing patterns of a mental health service in a prepaid group practice program in New York. Am J Psychiatry 126:689–697, 1969

Green EL: Psychiatric services in a California group health plan. Am J Psychiatry 126:681–688, 1969

Harrington RL: Systems approach to mental health care in a HMO model (unpublished 2-year report for the National Institute of Mental Health Project MH-24109). Santa Clara, CA, Kaiser Permanente Medical Care Program, 1975

Introduction to Alternative Delivery Mechanisms: HMOs, PPOs, and CMPs. Washington, DC, National Health Lawyers Association, 1986

Kirshner E: Three vie for vacant HMO accreditation mantle. Healthweek 4:8, 1990

Levin BL: State mandates for mental health, alcohol, and substance abuse benefits: implications for HMOs. GHAA Journal 9:48–69, 1988a

Levin BL: Continued changing patterns in coverage and utilization of mental health, alcohol, and substance abuse within HMOs. GHAA Journal 8(2):17–29, 1988b

Levin BL: Mental health services within a national HMO alliance. HMO Practice (in press, a)

Levin BL: Utilization and costs of substance abuse services within a national network of group practice health plans. HMO Practice (in press, b)

Levin BL, Glasser JH: A survey of mental health service coverage within health maintenance organizations. Am J Public Health 69:1120–1125, 1979

Levin BL, Glasser JH: A national survey of prepaid mental health services. Hosp Community Psychiatry 35:350–355, 1984

Levin BL, Glasser JH: Mental health services in managed care: a national perspective of HMOs. Paper presented at the American Psychiatric Association meeting on Psychiatry and Managed Care Systems: A Resource Symposium, Washington, DC, November 18–20, 1988

Levin BL, Levin JD: Differential HMO organizational structures. GHAA Journal 7:43–49, 1986

Levin BL, Glasser JH, Roberts RE: Changing patterns in mental health service coverage within health maintenance organizations. Am J Public Health 74:453–458, 1984

Levin BL, Glasser JH, Jaffee CL Jr: National trends in coverage and utilization of mental health, alcohol, and substance abuse services within managed health care systems. Am J Public Health 78:1222–1223, 1988

Locke BZ, Regier DA: Prevalence of selected mental disorders, in Mental Health, United States, 1985 (DHHS Publ No ADM-85-1378). Edited by Taube CA, Barrett SA. Rockville, MD, National Institute of Mental Health, 1985, pp 1–6

Locke BZ, Krantz G, Kramer M: Psychiatric need and demand in a prepaid group practice program. Am J Public Health 56:895–904, 1966

Patterson DY: Psychiatric practice in an HMO. Psychiatric Opinion 13:27–31, 1976

Promoting Health/Preventing Disease: Year 2000 Objectives for the Nation. Washington, DC, Office of Disease Prevention and Health Promotion, 1989, pp 4-1–4-21

Reed LS: Coverage and Utilization of Care for Mental Considerations Under Health Insurance: Various Studies, 1973–1974. Washington, DC, American Psychiatric Association, 1975

Reed LS, Myers ES, Scheidmandel PL: Health Insurance and Psychiatric Care: Utilization and Cost. Washington, DC, American Psychiatric Association, 1972

Rice DP, Kelman S, Miller LS: Estimates of economic costs of alcohol and drug abuse and mental illness, 1985 and 1988. Public Health Rep 106:280–292, 1991

Robins LN, Locke BZ, Regier DA: An overview of psychiatric disorders in America, in Psychiatric Disorders in America: The Epidemiologic Catchment Area Study. Edited by Robins LN, Regier DA. New York, Free Press, 1991, pp 328–342

Sachs BC: An experience in providing mental health care in a comprehensive prepaid group practice plan. J Am Med Wom Assoc 27:186–196, 1972

Seltzer DA: Limitations on HMO services and the emerging redefinition of chronic mental illness. Hosp Community Psychiatry 39:137–139, 1988

Shadle M, Christianson JB: The organization of mental health care delivery in HMOs. Administration and Policy in Mental Health 15:201–225, 1988

Shapiro S, Fink R: Methodological considerations in studying patterns of medical care related to mental illness. Milbank Q 41:371–399, 1963

Sharfstein SS, Muszynski IL, Myers E: Health Insurance and Psychiatric Care: Update and Appraisal. Washington, DC, American Psychiatric Press, 1984

Tischler GL: Utilization management of mental health services by private third parties. Am J Psychiatry 147:967–973, 1990

United States Congress: Health Maintenance Organization Act of 1973. Public Law 93-222. 87 STAT. 914, 1973

United States Congress: Health Maintenance Organization Amendments of 1976. Public Law 94-460. 90 STAT. 1945, 1976

United States Congress: Health Maintenance Organization Amendments of 1978. Public Law 95-559. 92 STAT. 2131, 1978

United States Congress: Health Maintenance Organization Amendments of 1981. Public Law 97-35. 95 STAT. 572, 1981

United States General Accounting Office: Controlling Drug Abuse: A Status Report. Special Report from the Comptroller General of the United States. Washington, DC, Superintendent of Documents, 1988

Wallace C: Employers turning to managed care to control their psychiatric care costs. Modern Healthcare 17:82–84, 1987

Wells KB, Manning WG Jr, Benjamin B: Use of outpatient mental health services in HMO and FFS plans: results from a randomized controlled trial. Health Serv Res 21:453–474, 1986

Williams SJ, Diehr P, Drucker WL, et al: Mental health services: utilization by low income enrollees in a prepaid group practice plan and in an independent practice plan. Med Care 17:139–151, 1979

✦ 4 ✦

Contracting and Managed Care Payment Options

Susan C. Sargent, M.B.A., C.M.C.

As managed care systems become increasingly popular, more and more providers are entering into contracts for "managed care payments," not realizing that this term became an oxymoron for providers in the 1980s. Similar to "jumbo shrimp," "managed care payment" has not been a logical or actualized set of concepts. Hospitals, physicians, and other mental health and chemical dependency providers, faced with increasing competition for insured patients, have looked to health maintenance organizations (HMOs), preferred provider organizations (PPOs), insurers, and employers as potentially large sources of referrals through managed care arrangements. However, too many providers have been unable to "manage" within these various arrangements on two accounts: to provide the necessary care or, having provided it, to be paid reasonably for their services.

Providers in the 1990s must focus on their ability to *design* the payment options that will work for them and their patients, rather than react to managed care offers that mysteriously arrive in the mail requiring signature within 48 hours. The design of the best managed care contracts will, in turn, rest on a template for approaching and evaluating managed care opportunities. In this chapter, one such template is presented: the Six Steps for Managed Care Contracting. These steps include 1) the preparation, 2) the proposal, 3) the negotiation, 4) the contract, 5) the implementation, and 6) the evaluation/renegotiation. However, before I discuss the approach in detail, its operating definitions and tenets must first be presented.

Operating Definitions and Tenets

Recognizing that the terms within managed care contracting have been defined in as many ways as there are contracts, I have incorporated the following definitions into this chapter:

✦ *Utilization management:* Interventions designed to limit payments for services covered under benefit plans to those that are deemed medically necessary and appropriate (e.g., preadmission certification, concurrent review).

✦ *Case management:* Interventions targeted at high-expense episodes of care (e.g., hospitalization), where clinical direction of the cases is provided, to arrange and provide coverage for alternative, less expensive treatments and/or settings.

✦ *Managed care:* Comprehensive oversight of care for each episode, encompassing utilization management, case management, provider selection, and cost-containment measures.

Although each managed care contract will be unique, there are five underlying operating tenets that should ensure that the provider's needs are ultimately addressed:

1. The best contract will be a function of each provider's goals for securing managed care arrangements (e.g., a hospital that hopes to secure patients for a variety of inpatient, partial hospitalization, and outpatient services will need to secure a contract with a purchaser whose insurance coverage extends to this breadth of services and affords the discretion to actually move patients among the services).

2. The best contract may be different for each set of services (e.g., utilization management [as a service offered by the provider], employee assistance, inpatient and outpatient care, residential care, and patient assessment/diagnosis).

3. The best contract will be priced to allow for expansion or retrenchment over time. This may be accomplished through the negotiation of short-term contracts or through the negotiation of long-term contracts with provisions for service and/or pricing alterations over time.

4. The best contract will be market-sensitive. It will avoid placing the provider at greater risk than the market is demanding (e.g., a hos-

pital should not offer to enter into high-risk, capitated contracts when the market is content to contract for discounted per diem charges).

5. The best contract approach will entail a range of pricing options and prices within which the provider can comfortably negotiate (i.e., a hospital or group of physicians should clearly know the upper and lower end of the price range within which they can secure the contract and either maximally profit or break even before negotiating with a managed care system).

In sum, the provider should be adopting a proactive rather than a reactive approach to contracting for managed care, keeping in mind the desire to *design* the best arrangements. The purpose of the following approach is to assist the provider with the design; the approach will not answer all of the questions but will instead raise them in a logical format for consideration with each individual opportunity.

Six Steps for Managed Care Contracting

The Preparation

Objectives

Managed care contracting is a means to an end for a provider. The real key is defining that "end" (i.e., the organization's or clinician's objectives). These objectives might include but not be limited to:

✦ Securing a specific geographic or demographic market share in a particularly competitive marketplace. For example, managed care is one means for increasing adult admissions, should a hospital have a larger proportion of elderly patients than is desired.

✦ Securing a larger share of patients in a managed care–saturated marketplace.

✦ Diversifying revenues within a payment mix that is heavily reliant on a few payment sources. For example, a hospital in a community primarily insured by Blue Cross/Blue Shield may wish to seek managed care relationships with commercially insured employers or PPOs for purposes of securing higher levels of reimbursement and relying less on a single payment source.

✦ Generating revenues in other than fee-for-service arrangements.

These might include payments for evaluation, diagnosis, and refer- ral services on the basis of a fee per covered person per month, re- gardless of whether or not the clinician's services are sought and used. This has benefits for all parties: the purchaser has a fixed, budgeted amount for these services, the clinician has a fixed reve- nue from the purchaser, and the patient has ready access to a known provider.

Information Base

Having defined the objectives, the second most critical activity is es- tablishing a solid information base upon which to design a contracting strategy. The information will be both quantitative and qualitative, and will be derived from both internal operations and external market sources. Compiling and maintaining this information will be an ongo- ing activity and should encompass at least four major categories: utili- zation data, charge and cost data, target market information, and competitor analysis.

Utilization data. Facilities should collect data on the average lengths of stay (ALOS) by type of service (e.g., adolescent unit, adult residential services); average numbers of services per episode and the average elapsed time (e.g., 18 day hospital sessions over a period of 6 weeks); seasonal variations in utilization; utilization patterns by payor; utilization patterns among privately insured populations (e.g., admissions per thousand covered lives); and other utilization data rel- evant to the services that may be encompassed in managed care ar- rangements. Individual outpatient providers should document their own treatment patterns relative to average numbers of visits by type of patient (e.g., adolescents, adults with depression) as well as the types of visits (e.g., half-hour psychotherapy visits, group therapy). This will form the foundation for evaluating managed care opportuni- ties relative to the provider's established practice patterns. For exam- ple, a managed care system may have an ALOS of 12 days versus a hospital's existing ALOS of 21 days; this will entail either a reevalua- tion of the unit, a designation of short-term beds, or a determination that the potential managed care arrangement should be rejected.

Charge and cost data. A review and inventory of the costs and charges associated with each of the services offered by a facility or provider should be developed, with variations by payor or by contract noted. For example, some payors will reimburse hospitals on a global per diem basis (i.e., a fee that encompasses the hospital's per diem amounts plus the ancillary costs and the fees of the physicians). Others will pay for each unit of service separately. Both types of payment policies and costs need to be noted to ensure a thorough understanding of the provider's pricing options when negotiating with managed care providers. For individual practitioners, the variable charges by type of visit as well as the basis for the charges need to be understood prior to evaluating a managed care proposition. Accepting discounted fees for patients who are already in treatment may only result in the practitioner having to work harder for the same income. This then needs to be weighed against the likelihood of losing these patients to another preferred practitioner. In addition, the provider should understand the impact that increased patient volume may have on the costs per unit of service, as well as the historical increases in costs and charges over the last 5 years.

Target market information. An inventory of large employers, insurers, HMOs, PPOs, utilization managers, and employee assistance programs (EAPs) should be developed and updated quarterly, as the owners and players among all of these purchasing entities are changing continually. In addition, the provider should collect as much information as possible about each purchaser's employee/subscriber demographics; existing and proposed health benefit plan provisions; historical utilization and costs; EAP roles and responsibilities; utilization management provisions by health plan; labor/management issues and time frames; existing managed care arrangements for other services; and any conflicting incentives relevant to the proposed services (e.g., the absence or presence of provisions for a primary care physician gatekeeper). This information will assist the facility and individual practitioner in understanding the key variables within any given contract, as well as the competing opportunities in the marketplace.

Competitor analysis. Hospitals should develop and update an inventory of their primary competitors by type of service, location, and target market; typical charges and utilization patterns by service; and the perceived strengths and weaknesses of competitors in the marketplace (e.g., the basis upon which referral sources differentially decide where patients will be referred). For individual practitioners, the competitive evaluation may more appropriately focus on specialty services or credentials that will be important in the managed care contracting process (e.g., child and adolescent services, intensive outpatient chemical dependency services).

The accumulation and analysis of this information will be a lengthy and time-consuming process, but need not be expensive. Information may be readily available in health care cost reports, facility brochures, business coalition reports, state licensure/certification records, and state health planning documents. In addition, valuable, more qualitative information can be garnered from attendance at peer professional functions (e.g., psychiatric society meetings), as well as from media releases and local business publications. Regardless of the source, the information enables a provider to clearly identify the uniqueness of its services, charges, and resources in the managed care marketplace, while additionally highlighting which services should be included or excluded from the contracts. Should decisions ultimately be made to not enter the managed care market, the data are equally valuable for marketing individual practices or facilities, as well as pricing and promoting the services.

Services and Providers

Spectrum of services. Having defined the objectives and assessed the internal and external data relevant to a managed care system, the range of services to be provided and the provider settings must be determined. "Services" in this regard may include but not be limited to:

✦ Intake, evaluation, and referral services.
✦ Patient care services, cutting across mental health and chemical dependency services and ranging from outpatient care to partial/day hospitalization, residential care, or psychiatric intensive care.
✦ Employee assistance services.
✦ Utilization management, case management, and quality assurance services.

Service delivery settings, depending on the distribution of the target market populations and the managed care objectives of the provider, may need to be geographically dispersed, multidisciplinary, and distributed among modalities.

Provider settings. Assuming that a provider has determined the scope of services to be offered in the managed care marketplace, the next set of decisions will need to resolve how best to provide for or arrange for the provision of these services. A solid and candid evaluation of the services offered by the provider and the provider's competitors will produce a listing of those services, times, and locations that are already available and germane to the managed care product. At the same time, however, there may be some services currently offered by the provider that, upon reflection, should be excluded. Reasons for this exclusion might include inflexibility of charges, lengths of stay, patient mix, or inappropriateness for managed care programs (e.g., long-term residential care for schizophrenic patients.)

Furthermore, there may be additional services that will be desirable for the provider to develop. The risks associated with starting a new service based solely on assumptions regarding managed care contracting will be high; however, there may be other market factors that, in combination with a managed care population, will contribute to the support of developing such services as day hospital programs for children and adolescents, intensive outpatient chemical dependency programs, or additional sites for existing outpatient capabilities. Alternately, the plans for these programs may be developed and held until threshold numbers of managed care lives have been contracted.

The decision making for these potential programs will rest on a delicate balance of 1) the volumes of patients needed to ensure the financial viability of a service, 2) the percentage of all patients in the community using these services that the provider will need to attract, and 3) the need to have a specific new service to successfully compete for the contracts *and* survive once secured.

Finally, the risks associated with establishing new services and/or locations may be diminished by the opportunity to contract with other existing providers as part of the managed care network of services. This moderates the financial risk, but may pose additional risk as potential competitors are brought into the contracting process. Further, control over the quality of care, approach to service delivery, and accessibility of services becomes increasingly complicated, thereby endangering the overall success of the contract and achievement of the objectives set forth by the provider. However, as a short-term strategy for ensuring access to the full spectrum of services until new services can be developed or network partners acquired, subcontracting for services can serve to provide the necessary competitive advantage.

Patient Flow and Payment Options

The two most critical elements of any managed care contract are 1) the design of patient flow systems and 2) the formulation of payment strategies. The successful orchestration of these elements will, in turn, rest squarely on the availability of clinical leadership and managerial talent.

Patient flow. Merely having the full spectrum of services distributed by discipline, modality, and location will not ensure success in any managed care contract. Rather, the criteria for admission, discharge, and transfer among services become the necessary "clinical glue." This provides for the smooth flow of patients into the services, through the most cost-effective and appropriate levels of care, and, to complete the cycle, return to the original referral sources.

Patient flow into a managed behavioral system is a key component of contracting that is frequently overlooked by providers and contractors. Recognizing that mental health and chemical dependency services are very different from most medical services, providers must educate a managed care contractor early in their discussions by "walking" hypothetical patients through all of the potential entry points. For example, with chemical dependency treatment, referrals may be made by EAPs, law enforcement officials, general practitioners, school counselors, families, and self-referral. Depending on the managed care system, the various access points may dictate different utilization management and treatment decisions that need to be made explicit.

Further, integration of behavioral health services into the flow of patients through the *medical* system will need to be clearly delineated so as to avoid surprises on the parts of the patients, their families, the providers, the payors, and the purchasers. For example:

An open-panel HMO asked for competitive bids from multiple providers for a capitated mental health and chemical dependency benefit. Services were incorporated into a system placing heavy reliance on primary care physicians as gatekeepers. Two providers were awarded contracts. They, in turn, were told that they would need to compete for designation as the mental health/chemical dependency provider with each primary care physician. Upon designation, each provider's capitation basis would be derived from the primary care physicians' enrolled population. Given the HMO's strength in one of the provider's geographic markets as opposed to the other, both the resultant patient

flow and payment flow differed greatly from what had been anticipated. Further, both providers were listed as participating providers in
the HMO's brochures; thus, purchasers and enrollees were not aware
of the limited choice of providers until services were needed.

Once patients have gained access to services, the provider or facility must design criteria and support systems (e.g., medical records). In
this way, both the global, systemic issues as well as the day-to-day
operational concerns can be addressed and resolved prior to meeting
with potential managed care contractors. This, in turn, contributes to
1) the design of the proposal, 2) the clinical confidence and presentation of clinical issues with potential managed care contractors, and 3)
the smooth transition to operations once the contract is awarded. It
should be noted, however, that each managed care plan may require
the provider to custom-fit the patient flow mechanisms to ensure the
greatest satisfaction for all parties.

Payment options.   Historically, payors, insurers, and patients have
borne the risk for paying for health care services. That is, they have
agreed within a predetermined benefit plan to pay for the covered services that are necessary for good medical care, as determined by the
provider. However, within the managed care arena, efforts are frequently made to share the risk with utilization managers and providers, primarily through capitated payment options—agreeing to deliver
or monitor the delivery of a predetermined scope of services to an enrolled population for a negotiated price per person. To the degree that
fewer services are used than anticipated, the provider or the utilization manager generates revenues in excess of costs; to the degree that
more services are used, the provider or utilization manager loses. Although there are many managed care contracts that rely on capitated
mental health/chemical dependency benefit structures, there are
many more that work well within a range of payment options, the
most risky and last choice for providers undergoing capitation.

Keeping in mind that the payment options will need to be customized to each specific contract and set of services, options for structuring payment mechanisms within managed care arrangements include
but are not limited to the following:

◆ Agreeing to comply with existing utilization management provisions of the managed care purchaser as a preferred or exclusive pro-

vider at full fees. This option assumes that the provider is in a good competitive utilization and charge position; that the health plan benefits afford enough latitude to generate and document savings; that there are incentives for employees/subscribers to use the provider's services; and that the provider has a strong reputation in the community.

◆ Agreeing to comply with existing utilization management provisions as a preferred or exclusive provider at discounted fees.

◆ Agreeing to comply with existing utilization management provisions as a preferred or exclusive provider within a sliding scale of fees.

◆ Cooperating with existing utilization management provisions with a fixed fee-per-admission, whether on a full fee, discounted fee, or Diagnosis-Related Group (DRG) basis.

◆ Contracting to perform triage, referral, and case management services on a capitated basis in concert with one of the service payment options above, whether on a full fee, discounted fee, or fee-per-admission basis.

◆ Contracting on a capitated basis to provide all of the services described above, including the internalization of all utilization management provisions.

By starting with the least risky arrangements, providers and purchasers alike have the opportunity to become acquainted with the needs and requirements of each other's systems while generating modest savings. Purchasers and insurers hope to avoid the disgrace and embarrassment of selecting providers who are financially unable to provide the contracted services within the capitated amounts, almost as much as the providers want to avoid financial ruin. However, providers have repeatedly entered into capitated contracts without considering the following basic arithmetic:

A capitated contract for 600,000 lives at a rate of $2.00 per person per month can generate substantial annual revenue for a provider: $14.4 million. However, for every nickel per month error in the provider's capitation rate, there is an annualized difference of $360,000. From a utilization perspective, a hypothetical inpatient utilization rate of 41.2 days per thousand as opposed to the 40 days upon which the capitation rate is based will generate a similar loss, depending on the provider's costs per day.

Hence the risk associated with capitation cannot be overlooked; providers must weigh all of the options and consider alternate pricing and payment strategies. Regardless of the payment and pricing system selected, the provider will need to ascertain the parameters within which a managed care contract will be struck. That is, the provider must *know* the price at which to depart from the contracting process, as well as the price that will ensure the greatest latitude for performance. Equally critical will be the time frame associated with the pricing mechanism. The best contracts will have periodic opportunities for evaluating the utilization and cost experience and adjusting the pricing, whether as a short-term contract or a condition within a longer term contract.

Systems Requirements

The support systems required to implement the proposed managed care arrangements should be anticipated prior to submitting a proposal, and incorporated into the pricing considerations. Although each contract will necessitate different combinations of systems, almost all will require the installation of systems to ensure quality assurance, patient tracking, payment tracking, communications (especially for utilization and case management services), and performance tracking. The latter data system for tracking performance should enable the provider to monitor the utilization and cost of services provided within each contract and compare the performance with the provisions of the contract. For example, several providers around the country have contracted with employers and/or utilization management firms for a targeted hospitalization rate (e.g., 40 days per thousand). The providers must be able to track this utilization and differentiate inpatient days from partial hospitalization sessions, so as to produce a pure hospitalization rate at periodic performance reviews. This is based on the assumption that many insurer data systems have not focused on the intricacies of behavioral health services and have only recently started to cover and pay for partial or day hospitalization benefits. Incorporation of partial utilization with inpatient data will result in dissatisfaction on the part of the contractor, unless carefully tracked and documented by the provider.

Similarly, quality assurance systems linked to the clinical criteria and patient tracking systems will be important for documenting performance in existing contracts and/or competitively differentiating providers in subsequent negotiations. As most health benefit plans are unclear as to the quality of care within the behavioral health arena, credible quality assurance initiatives on the part of the provider will be regarded highly by potential contractors, as well as by the clinical staff, in the treatment of managed care patients. Quality assurance initiatives and documentation might include the assignment of case managers to every patient entering the system, the tracking of patterns of care throughout the continuum of services in comparison to more traditional treatment approaches, cost savings and readmission rates associated with the use of partial hospitalization services, and the effective design and utilization of clinical criteria in the assignment of patients to both modalities and clinical team members.

As is evident from the length of the previous discussions, preparation is everything in managed care contracting. Providers who commit 75% of their effort to preparation will find the balance of the six steps for managed care contracting consuming only 25% of their effort.

The Proposal

The submission of a proposal for a managed care contract may encompass a single, comprehensive document or several documents, as is more often the case. Although truly competitive situations may set the format, content, and criteria for the proposals, managed care contractors frequently request sequential documents over the course of several months, in concert with site visits and extensive clinical and administrative interviews. This pacing should be anticipated by the provider and regarded as a series of hurdles—the more a contractor comes back and wants to know about a provider, the farther along is the proposal process. In addition, the provider has the opportunity to learn more about the contractor, its priorities, and its criteria for judging the overall success of the effort.

Regardless of the pace or style of the proposal process, most proposals eventually encompass the following key components:

✦ Statements of the provider's and purchaser's objectives for the managed care contract.
✦ Delineation of the services and modalities to be included and specifically excluded, both in terms of service delivery and health plan coverage.
✦ Specification of the actual providers.

✦ A brief discussion of the provider's philosophical and technical approach to providing the specified services, including a superficial delineation of how patients will move through the systems.
✦ A statement of the approach to payment that is being proposed (e.g., discounts, excluding any discussion of specific prices).
✦ An explanation of the provider's and purchaser's provisions for utilization management and quality assurance.
✦ Statements of the reporting requirements on both sides of the transaction (e.g., utilization reports for the contractor, enrollment updates for the provider).
✦ Actual pricing approaches, upper parameter amounts, and underlying assumptions.

The proposal should be descriptive, selectively specific, and intentionally loose in such areas as patient flow, quality assurance provisions, and payment arrangements. In so doing, the provider and contractor can arrive at agreement on the concepts and general approaches to the delivery of services within the proposal process, while leaving the specifics open for the negotiation and contracting process.

Negotiation and the Contract

Having successfully maneuvered through the preparation and proposal process, a provider should enter the negotiation and contracting process with serious consideration given to the retention of outside legal counsel. Although many providers are both skilled and experienced in managed care contracting, the changes in the state and federal laws regarding the liabilities and risks inherent to this contracting process warrant both the expense and effort of securing counsel knowledgeable of health care contracting, managed care systems, insurance law, and corporate and tax law.

The decision to have counsel perform the actual negotiations will be an individual one, made on a case-by-case basis by providers utilizing different management styles. However, the goal of the negotiation is to secure the managed care contract that best addresses the objectives of the provider.

Equally important will be the list of "deal-breakers," or those contractual concerns upon which the provider will not consider negotiating or budging past a certain point. One such concern might revolve around utilization management (e.g., the provider may stipulate participation, only if the purchaser agrees to have all preadmission certifications and concurrent reviews performed by physicians).

Assuming the satisfactory resolutions of both the provider's and purchaser's concerns, attention must be paid to the mutual designation of the schedule and basis for evaluating and renegotiating the contract. Managed care contracts frequently have been for 2 years, with specific periodic reviews and targets for both utilization and cost. However, providers may also wish to incorporate process-oriented targets, given the reliance on patient and payment flow considerations in the overall success of the effort. For example, a hospital may warrant offering a discount to a PPO only if the charges are reimbursed within 30 days; payment after 30 days will be stipulated at the hospital's full fees. Or a physician may agree to participate only if patient eligibility within the insurance plan can be confirmed at the time of treatment with follow-up documentation received within 1 week.

Implementation and Evaluation/Renegotiation

Once the contract is secured, it must be implemented. Again, the greater the effort spent in preparing for the proposal and contract process, the easier will be the implementation. Specific concerns for the implementation phase, however, will include the following:

◆ Clinical and administrative personnel from both parties should assemble to explicitly come to agreement on the systems requirements, objectives and expectations for the contract, and criteria for evaluating it, on the parts of both the provider and purchaser.

◆ Specific statements of objectives, expectations, systems requirements, evaluation milestones, necessary actions for implementing the contract, dates, and responsibilities should be prepared and distributed, with specific dates for reviewing these items.

◆ At least every 6 months, the contractor and provider should meet to review the progress to date, problems, resolutions, and milestones for the subsequent 6-month period. This does not entail a renegotiation of the contract but rather a "maintenance check" on the expectations and issues inherent to both sides.

◆ At least annually, the goals for the managed care contracting process should be reexamined, restated as necessary, and distributed to key clinical, administrative, and board members, for purposes of clarity in the overall direction of the provider.

✦ Finally, the contract should be specifically reviewed by both parties and their counsel and modified to reflect changes in state/national law, pricing provisions, service/provider definitions, and other key concerns. Having met periodically over the course of the contract, the parties should be able to minimize the conflict—not necessarily to avoid it, but to enter and exit the renegotiations with relatively few surprises.

In conclusion, the fine points of each managed care contract will be legion, as the experience shared on both sides of the contract over time will be broad. The best approach for a provider is to have an approach—one that covers most of the issues most of the time and leaves much time and room for covering those unexpected issues. In so doing, the provider will be transposing the term "managed care" from that of an oxymoron to one that truly meets the needs of patients and their families.

✦ 5 ✦

Managing Psychiatric Exclusions

Theodor Bonstedt, M.D.

When Freud wrote "a poor man has just as much right to help for his mind" (Freud 1919/1953), he may not have realized that if psychiatric treatment is to be offered to large numbers of people, there also may have to be some limitations. Even before the advent of managed care in mental health, the public psychiatric clinics of the 1950s and 1960s searched desperately for ways of cutting their waiting lists (Bonstedt 1965). It was well known that in some of these public clinics, everyone had to fit into a group therapy schedule, whereas in other clinics, patients who were not judged to be good candidates for psychotherapy because of their character disorder would be assigned to a medication clinic with 15-minute appointments and psychiatrists assigned on a rotating basis (MacLeod and Middelman 1962).

In recognizing that the subject of limited versus unlimited mental health coverage inevitably starts an intense and emotionally charged debate, one also recognizes that as a matter of fact, within managed care, psychiatric exclusions are present and are here to stay. They came into usage in Kaiser health maintenance organizations (HMOs) in the 1950s, as many small employers did not want broad benefits. A decision was made to deal with this problem by benefit design *and* through exclusions applicable to the then-emerging mental health coverage (D. Y. Patterson, personal communication, November 1989). With the spread of HMOs in the 1970s, this practice came to the attention of the professional associations (notably, the American Psychiatric Association) and—not surprisingly—led to criticism.

But it is not only in HMOs that psychiatric exclusions exist within managed care (although that is where their impact is felt the most—within private practice). In many community mental health centers, since their inception in the 1960s, internal policies have been excluding some aspects of clinical area (e.g., a psychiatrist treating a patient may prescribe medication, but any psychotherapy beyond medication-related issues has to be secured from another, often quite independently functioning mental health professional at the center). Similarly, whenever a patient's move from one program within the center to another becomes necessary, a change in treating professionals may be mandated by internal policy. Significantly, though, internal policies are not as visible and assailable as legal contracts governing HMOs, preferred provider organizations (PPOs), and so on, and generally different segments of the population are affected.

It is essential to study the various types of exclusions as they affect various parts of our health system, reflecting different degrees of rational and ethical planning. The exclusions discussed in this chapter are usually based on contract language (as in an HMO health benefits summary). The relevant phrase typically reads "psychiatric conditions that are chronic or not likely to respond to short-term treatment are not a covered benefit."

Summary of Governmental Insurance Mandates

In my correspondence with all 50 states in the United States, it became apparent that currently a great majority of the states have no statutory rules against exclusions based on need for chronic psychiatric care. The main attention of the current state laws is focused on parity for mental health, and a minimum "package" of mental health benefits to be offered by each health insurance system, including all HMOs (i.e., a specified number of covered hospital days and outpatient visits per calendar year, possibly with a yearly dollar "cap"). The exclusions discussed in this chapter set in motion a different limitation that usually summarily terminates psychiatric benefits after their expiration. To our knowledge, only Virginia and Massachusetts specifically forbid "chronic" exclusions, whereas a few other states (Kansas, Wisconsin) specify that exclusions in mental health may apply "only to the same extent as it applies in any other condition." If the present trend continues, there might be an attempt in the near future, in an increasing number of states, to curtail the "chronic" exclusions in psychiatry, although any prediction in this regard does not seem possible. Because state laws are constantly changing, any reader wanting detailed information on a particular state should contact that state's Insurance Department directly.

Interpretation of Exclusions

Following is a list of exclusions currently in existence in HMOs in the United States (Bonstedt and McSweeney 1985). In administrative practice, the exclusionary language of a particular contract has to be explained (interpreted) as local policy. The following is a discussion of such interpretations.

Diagnosis. An example from an Ohio HMO is "diagnosis by psychiatrist, psychologist or qualified mental health professional of DSM III-R 301.00 through 301.90" (a personality disorder).

   This sounds objective, until one considers that even with DSM III-R and the new behavioral criteria, the issue of primary versus secondary diagnosis in psychiatry, and the choice of diagnosis per se, remains strongly subject to the bias of the individual diagnostician, his or her training and environment, and his or her countertransference. Such a criterion promotes lack of objectivity to an unacceptable degree. This can be seen in forensic psychiatry, where, for example, court battles erupt between qualified psychiatrists, psychologists, or other practitioners declaring the defendant to have a personality disorder, and to therefore be responsible—or to have a psychosis and therefore not be responsible—for his or her actions. Another measure of difficulty is determining what is the primary diagnosis. An example would be when a person primarily with a passive-aggressive personality disorder suffers anxiety attacks subsequent to being left by a spouse. Faced with such a patient, the provider might be tempted to single-handedly terminate his or her psychiatric benefits by declaring the patient to have primarily a passive-aggressive personality disorder.

Duration of illness. One HMO was recently refusing coverage to any person with "a psychotic illness over 6 months duration." The problem with this interpretation is how to define "illness" in operational terms—at best it brings us back to the concept of "diagnosis" and its own dubious status. As an example, this criterion would exclude a person who manifested auditory hallucinations following an acute stress and was restored to good reality testing with antipsychotic medication over several outpatient visits, and who then decided to stop taking antipsychotic medication. With life circumstances still stressful and with psychotic symptoms returning after a few months, this patient would lose all psychiatric benefits 6 months after the onset of symptoms. These efforts to stipulate diagnosis and duration are similar to recent attempts to define chronicity in the political arena (Menninger and Hannah 1987) where four dimensions have become part of various formulas: diagnosis or severity of illness, duration, disability, and number of hospitalizations. As the heterogeneity of the chronic mentally ill population becomes apparent, attempts to define such a population (here, for provision of service on the national level) face a similarly difficult process of operationalization.

Number/duration of hospitalizations. An arbitrary number of psychiatric hospitalizations over a particular time period is fixed (e.g., 4 psychiatric hospitalizations in the 4 years preceding the time of the administrative decision to terminate benefits). The aggregate length of these hospitalizations may or may not be stated.

The recent utilization of psychiatric benefits in the plan. In one HMO, an exclusion criterion consists of "full utilization of one year's mental health benefits," or "history of treatment in the year prior to admission to the plan, which would indicate the probability of utilization of above." This type of exclusion borders on the unethical, because a Catch-22 exists—if you use your benefits in a certain year, you get none the next—meaning you (the plan member) were never really entitled to them!

Degree of disability. In practice, this exclusion may have two meanings: one is that the particular person has been receiving disability benefits for mental illness from a socially appropriate agency—social security, the civil service system, an insurance company administering disability benefits, and so on. However, I also met up with another meaning in a particular HMO where all that was necessary was that it would be "the opinion of the HMO treatment team" that a patient meets the criteria for disability benefits due to his or her mental condition, excluding mental retardation, "as this would indicate a chronic condition (evidence of disorder for longer than two years)." An agency with the social mandate to determine disabilities would appear to offer a more impartial judgment than a provider team that could be accused of conflict of interest.

Lack of cooperation. Under review here is cooperation offered by the patient who may refuse treatment, ignore reminder letters, miss appointments, or skip medication. The courts have often determined that a person capable of informed consent may refuse to take medication except in emergencies; and the "right to refuse treatment" has become a celebrated cause in American psychiatry in recent years. Along the same lines, the Social Security Administration will not consider even trying to force a person to undergo psychiatric treatment in a situation where, without the treatment, psychiatric disabilities are bound to continue. Yet an HMO contract may represent a new territory, a situation where not only the providers but also the subscribers are contractually bound. In the absence of any legal decision to the contrary, it is presumably quite appropriate to declare "lack of cooperation in treatment" as a criterion of chronicity—as long as 1) such lack of cooperation is of a reasonably significant degree and is documented, and 2) such lack of cooperative behavior is not directly and solely determined by the very disorder or illness that is to be treated. (In some cases, a causation of this type may be very difficult to determine and may therefore require more time for review.)

Opinion of provider, team, department, and so on. The rules of one HMO state:

> If it is the opinion of the treatment team that the patient's condition is not subject to improvement through short-term acute treatment, the patient would not be eligible for the treatment of that specific disorder. Other unrelated disorders may be eligible for treatment.

In addition to the problem of diagnosis mentioned previously, there is also the issue of what is "related" or "unrelated" in diagnostic terms, and which conditions are or are not subject to such improvement. These are issues with low levels of agreement between different providers. This exclusion is further complicated if "treatment team" is not defined.

Second opinion. In my own HMO in Cincinnati, Ohio (Health Maintenance Plan), we had used an outside psychiatrist of prominent standing in the community to certify "chronicity" long before we got around to compiling our own interpretations of psychiatric exclusions. We have retained this clause ("outside consultant") because it seems impossible for a few concise criteria to reflect the complexity of these problems. By using outside consultants, we avoid any appearance of conflict of interest, excessive subjectivity, or bias. In our experience, the choice of such an objective consultant was never questioned, even though he or she was picked and paid by the medical group serving the HMO.

Outpatient versus inpatient versus total exclusions. Over the years, our HMO has found that a "total" exclusion produces the fewest clinical and administrative complications, and so we tend to use it except in special situations. Inpatient benefits may be eliminated with heavy utilizers while leaving outpatient benefits still available for these patients. This works initially, but over the years it creates a backlog of heavy outpatient utilizers whose care becomes discontinuous every time they have to be hospitalized outside of the HMO system. Similar discontinuity occurs when a patient is referred to an outside agency for a long-term outpatient therapy (we do this when therapy is expected to last for more than 20 visits within a year) while inpatient benefits are left intact. Often a therapist outside the HMO will recommend hospitalization one-sidedly and quickly whenever a serious problem arises, and the HMO provider has then no recourse but to hospitalize. Thus, coordination of care is the key problem.

Child exclusions. Exclusions used with adult subscribers are generally not suitable for mentally ill children—partly because of different clinical reality, but primarily because of the dependent nature of the child's relationship, which necessitates intensive participation by parents in any successful psychiatric treatment. Consequently, at our HMO we have established a separate set of psychiatric exclusions for children. The threshold number of psychiatric hospitalizations is smaller, more cooperation is required, and certain diagnostic groups are indeed excluded as such (i.e., pervasive developmental disorders).

Substance abuse. The area of chemical dependency also needs to be singled out as it may require a modified approach in exclusionary

policy. Because in this case the "offset effect" is relatively best documented and the field has its own identity, the provider needs to be
more flexible in applying exclusionary policy. Specifically, a heavier
reliance is justified upon the judgment and the recommendations of
the substance abuse counselor, who may be more inclined to consider
the changing motivation and compliance of a particular patient, the
existing family support, and field-specific phenomena such as "hitting
the bottom," "breakthrough," and so on. Finally, it is my impression
that substance abusing patients are less likely to relapse once they are
told that noncompliance may affect their coverage.

Analysis of Exclusions:
Toward a Rational and Ethical Set

A review of ideological premises is necessary when exclusions are
listed or compared. For a long time there has been evidence that a
small percentage of psychiatric patients may use up a disproportionately large share of the budget of an HMO. A medical group
may want to provide a quality psychiatric service in the most cost-
effective manner. Spreading resources too thin lowers quality, and
organizations need a consistent rationale for setting priorities. The
relatively few individuals who cost the most become, in effect, a low
priority in a program using exclusion. (Paradoxically, not only many
"sicker" patients end up in this group, but also some of the "healthier"
ones, e.g., intellectual people with family or occupational problems
who desire long-term, insight-oriented psychotherapy). The quality of
service is essential to obtain not only for the human satisfaction of
patients and providers, but also to secure the offset effect upon medical utilization (Borus et al. 1985).

Reliability.　In order to be effective, the "criteria of chronicity" (a
term that has been used interchangeably with "psychiatric exclusions") should be easy to apply by different observers, providers, and
administrators, with a high degree of agreement as to what is the
meaning of a particular criterion or exclusion.
　　It is for this reason that psychiatric diagnosis is of very limited usefulness, as I mentioned previously. Duration of illness is also unreliable in these terms.

Objectivity/verifiability/legal usefulness. As much as possible, exclusions should not be subject to the bias of the local provider or the person reviewing the case. The phenomenon of countertransference is well known in psychiatry, often leading to a change in diagnosis or other expert opinion regarding a difficult patient a practitioner has had in treatment for a long time. The training or "school of thought" of the particular psychiatric provider (and even the prevailing orientation in a particular psychiatric community) also contributes to such bias—as well as the pressures for productivity in a stressed and understaffed mental health department.

On the other hand, objectivity is enhanced when the various interpretations or criteria used to make judgments about patients are of specific behavior that can be easily verified or consensually validated (e.g., count of hospitalizations, count of calendar years, reference to the opinion of an outside expert on the subject in question). Some people like to call this approach "operational"—the field of the definable, the testable, and the repeatable, an orientation dependent on both the scientific method and clinical experience (Weiss 1970). Insisting upon operational criteria not only makes them more objective and verifiable, but it also makes it much easier to defend the administrative decision to exclude a patient when this decision is litigated by an attorney who argues that the person in question should continue to be treated by HMO psychiatric providers in spite of limitations in the contract.

Range of Efficient (Operational) Exclusions

Number/duration of hospitalizations. A time-proven criterion in our HMO has been "4 or more psychiatric hospitalizations in the previous 4 years (or 90 days of hospitalization in 2 successive years within the previous 5 years)." Here an attempt is made to pinpoint either an evident frequency of hospitalization as such or an existing tendency toward one or more prolonged hospitalizations in recent times as an established determinant of future hospitalizations (Solomon et al. 1984).

Years ago one might have been concerned about inappropriate hospitalizations taking place and being counted, but this is becoming rapidly less relevant as peer review and utilization management is becoming more effective and changed state mental health laws make inappropriate hospitalization much less likely. Necessary documentation requires medical history as provided by the patient or the previous attending psychiatrist. If this information is received verbally from a source other than the patient, it should be discussed with the patient (to allow for correction of any information considered inaccurate). Yet if doubt exists about the accuracy of information given by the patient, special effort should be made to obtain information from family, former providers, and other available sources. A note about the obtained history is then placed in the appropriate clinical file and an effort made to reconcile the existing factual information about the number of hospitalizations, and so on. Generally, it should not be necessary for a provider to wait for written information from hospitals and other sources that may take a long time to arrive.

Degree of disability. If a patient has been declared eligible to receive disability benefits because of his or her mental condition (exclusive of mental retardation), this would indicate to our HMO a chronic condition, and thus an exclusion from psychiatric services. Under this clause, the disability has to be certified by a duly established social agency (Social Security Administration, Veterans Administration, etc.). This requirement recognizes that in our society the issue of medical disability has its own due process between and among employers, workers, their physicians, and insurance agencies, who in turn use their own neutral physicians (often with an appeal process and special examination designed for that purpose). In my opinion, it would be a mistake to use only managed care providers for this review, who would be less qualified to determine disability in general (and also more biased). If disability information is received verbally, the providers should put a note about this information in the appropriate clinical file.

Lack of cooperation. With increasing pressure for lessened expense and more cost-effectiveness in health care, we are becoming ever more inclined to apply the clause of lack of cooperation to patients. On this, the chapter from an agency manual states,

> If a subscriber has signed him/herself out of an inpatient facility without the authorization of the agency psychiatrist or has not cooperated with recommended outpatient treatment directed at preventing future hospitalization, the subscriber would not be eligible for psychiatric services under the (agency) Certificate, provided that such failure to coop-

erate is not due to the mental condition for which the patient is being treated.

The patient's files should clearly show that after the initial evaluation the patient was informed of the goals and objectives of the treatment, the amount of the treatment, the expected duration of treatment, and so on; that the patient was warned that failure to cooperate may result in termination of benefits; and that the patient was competent to understand the information and the consequences of failing to cooperate. There should also be documentation of the failure of the patient to cooperate, such as missing appointments or refusal to take prescribed medication. I realize that this is the one criterion or interpretation that could be abused by stretching or pursuing the instances of noncooperation into smaller or less significant encounters. It is for this reason that our HMO would not apply this clause lightly, and never due to an isolated instance of this type.

Second opinion.   The provider or group selects an outside psychiatric consultant with a reputation in the community for fairness and impartiality who is asked to see the patient in question and to render an opinion as to whether or not he or she has a chronic psychiatric illness. We have had a chance to use several psychiatrists in that capacity. Although they vary a great deal in what they use as criteria for evaluating patients, they seem to stress the global concept of repeated and extensive psychiatric treatment, combined with unemployment that somehow results from psychiatric illness. In this connection, when our final set of interpretations of psychiatric exclusions was worked out, we used two such outside psychiatric consultants, seeking a consensus that was eventually reached.

Special cases.   As I mentioned previously, a provider may elect partial exclusion when the inpatient benefits remain unaffected but the patient is referred outside of the HMO for long-term therapy. This is done in the presence of a profound character or neurotic disorder for which very few professionals would advocate brief therapy.

Our HMO does recommend a separate set of "criteria of chronicity" for children under age 18. In view of this, I would also make it a point to review the case of each child upon his or her reaching adulthood at 18, to determine if adult criteria of chronicity would then apply. For the latter determination, any relevant information is used that may have accumulated in the files of the agency since the child was declared "chronic."

Documentation

The administrative expression of determination of "chronicity" is a letter signed by the medical director stating that a determination has been made that a particular person has fulfilled the contractual criteria of "chronic psychiatric problems or conditions which . . . are not subject to significant improvement through short-term treatment" (quotation from contract; Bonstedt and McSweeney 1985). A termination date is then listed, following which the agency will no longer pay for psychiatric care. This date is worked out jointly between the provider and the director of the department of psychiatry, with the agreement of the medical director. The medical director has to be involved in setting the tone or approach for this area of determination of exclusions. In any agency, such policies will have to reflect the overall orientation of the organization; if the procedures are questioned, it is the medical director who carries the final responsibility.

Impact of Exclusions

The existence of psychiatric exclusions in a managed care program complicates the functioning of the mental health providers. Many providers perceive such exclusions as inherently inhumane or detrimental to quality care, and these concerns have to be addressed when a staff member is hired and subsequently oriented to a particular job. For optimum performance, it is essential that the staff member not see this issue as a "black or white" one, because that may cause morale problems. These issues need to be discussed at various organizational levels, such as staff meetings of the psychiatry department, periodic meetings of key mental health personnel with the governing board, and so on. The purposes of exclusions should be well known to all providers, the latter having a major input into the decision to limit the service to a particular patient. By this time, a mental health professional may be sufficiently involved in treatment of that particular patient to have developed a relationship, and these issues must be considered as well.

A clinically difficult case may by the same token offer an opportunity to apply an exclusion and terminate the service at an earlier time. Here the training of the professional, and his or her supervisor, will be important. Similarly, a very positive relationship between patient and therapist may make it difficult for the mental health provider to sanction a termination based on official exclusion, even though it clearly applies on administrative grounds. Consequently, cases of "bootlegged patients" may be discovered during the regular departmental peer review. It will also make a difference if the provider is salaried, fee-for-service, or paid on a "productivity" basis either per hour or per new case.

To an even greater extent, the existence of psychiatric exclusions will play a role in the treatment of the psychiatric patient from the patient's own point of view. One can hope that, as a subscriber of the particular managed care plan, such a patient will know upon enrollment that a type of exclusion does exist. But even with adequate explanations by marketing representatives at the point of enrollment, people will present for diagnostic evaluation in the mental health department with issues that would then be classified as falling under an exclusion.

At that point, the clinician has several alternatives. Sometimes it may be difficult to predict the speed of improvement with the selected treatment for a particular patient. Where motivation is an important factor, additional motivation can be mobilized by telling the patient that the treatment will be started and continued for a time and then another review will be made to determine whether the response justifies further coverage under the managed care plan. I have used this approach with success, particularly with people commonly described as having personality disorders.

After the initial stages of treatment are over, the issue of termination because of an applicable psychiatric exclusion may still arise. The decision to terminate should be announced by the treating professional in a manner compatible with the therapeutic needs of the patient. This may include some reasonable extensions in time, such as allowing time to discuss the emotional implications, to consult with patient's relatives, and to clarify realistic alternatives for treatment to be continued elsewhere. Any tendency by administrators to be rigid or exacting in this area may backfire and result in legal questions of abandonment or dereliction of duty.

Soon after a patient is excluded and psychiatric treatment in the managed care plan is stopped, there may be repercussions from within the excluding agency as well as from outside sources. If the patient continues his or her general medical care in the original plan, the family physician may suddenly miss the heretofore available psychiatric consultation (even if an outside agency takes over the psychiatric treatment, it usually will not be as accessible to the primary physician). I have known cases where a primary physician would take it upon him- or herself to simply take over psychiatric care single-handedly where the terminating psychiatric provider had left it—after the patient declared that he or she was unable to find psychiatric care elsewhere in the community. Situations involving exclusions are mostly unpleasant to the primary physician, and it is therefore essential to forewarn him or her of an impending termination. On occasion, it may likewise become necessary for a psychiatric provider to see the excluded patient in an emergency, when the primary care team of the original plan is in desperate need of immediate psychiatric screening and disposition. There are no neat administrative solutions for these problems.

Following an exclusion, there may also be unpleasant calls from psychiatric providers elsewhere in the community, where the patient ended up for emergency or continued care. These providers, particularly in the public sector, may perceive the patient as being "dumped" on them, and may offer very unflattering comments on the functioning of the original plan. Handling these situations will require discretion and diplomacy in addition to the customary sharing of clinical information. Not surprisingly, psychiatric exclusions do not enhance the reputation of managed care with clinicians in other systems of care. Most often one hears accusations of patient abandonment and dereliction of duty here in an ethical rather than legal context. It is to be hoped that the managed care professionals are mindful of the very real ethical caveats inherent in these situations. With this in mind, I have made various suggestions in this chapter to fulfill this obligation—once the reality of managed care is accepted. Yet even if this obligation is realistically fulfilled, accusations will often follow because of the emotionally charged economic and political aspects of such situations.

Conclusions

It is tempting to speculate on the future of exclusions as I have discussed them in this chapter. As long as there is continued intense effort to cut the cost of medical care (and no end to such effort is in sight at this time), exclusions are likely to proliferate. An exception to such proliferation might come about through emergence of proof that under certain clinical conditions, prolonged psychiatric treatment significantly reduces the subsequent expense of *total* medical care of a defined type of patient (i.e., that the offset effect is verified in a particular context). Currently the closest case in point exists in the area of chemical dependency, where with control of addiction, medical costs may decline dramatically. Thus there is in a managed care system a need for research of this type, with clinicians remaining on the lookout for opportunities to suspend exclusions in specified cases, by an agreement of the psychiatric team and the administration.

In conclusion, the psychiatric exclusions can be seen as an unfortunate but necessary "cap" on clinical coverage in a managed care system. Formed in an arbitrary but experientially validated manner that prevents abuse, they may in fact help to secure quality service under conditions of scarcity—until such time as a more equitable and comprehensive solution is found for the totality of American health care.

References

Bonstedt T: Psychotherapy in a public psychiatric clinic: an attempt at "adjustment." Psychiatr Q 39:1–15, 1965

Bonstedt T, McSweeney JEJ: Interpretation of psychiatric exclusions in HMOs, in 1985 Group Health Proceedings. Washington, DC, Group Health Association of America, 1985, pp 97–103

Borus JF, Olendzki MC, Kessler L, et al: The "offset effect" of mental health treatment on ambulatory medical care utilization and charges. Arch Gen Psychiatry 42:573–580, 1985

Freud S: Turnings in the ways of psychoanalytic therapy (1919), in The Standard Edition of the Complete Psychological Works of Sigmund Freud, Vol 3. Translated and edited by Strachey J. London, Hogarth Press, 1953, pp 401–402

MacLeod JA, Middelman F: Wednesday afternoon clinic: a supportive care program. Arch Gen Psychiatry 6:72–81, 1962

Menninger WW, Hannah GT (eds): The Chronic Mental Patient/II. Washington, DC, American Psychiatric Press, 1987, pp 42–48

Solomon P, David J, Gordon B: Discharged state hospital patients' characteristics and use of aftercare: effect on community care. Am J Psychiatry 141:1566–1570, 1984

Weiss JMA: An editorial. Journal of Operational Psychiatry 1:1, 1970

✦ 6 ✦

Management of Quality, Utilization, and Risk

Alex R. Rodriquez, M.D.

Perhaps no issue is more relevant now than how well mental health services will be defined as efficacious, cost-effective, and essential to basic health. Furthermore, issues related to the defining, measuring, and improvement of quality outcome, utilization efficiency, and risk management have now emerged as the pinions upon which the entire super- and infrastructures of health care services will operate in a competitive market and democratic society. In this respect, the themes of quality and costs that reverberate throughout this book reflect what must be "managed" in managed care. In this chapter, I will focus on developments in what will be termed "medical quality management," encompassing the many creative or desperate efforts that have emerged and will unfold to "manage" quality, utilization, and risk in health care services. These developments are intimately related to the survival of mental health benefits and services in future American health care in general, and managed care in particular.

In the short course of 10 years, the United States has evolved from a system primarily guided by relative freedom of beneficiary choice in seeking health services and fee-for-service reimbursement according to "usual, customary, and reasonable (UCR)" rates, to one driven by managed care. Although each area of specialized care has experienced unique and common changes by force of externally directed management initiatives, no area has struggled to maintain its equilibrium under managed care with such difficulty as mental health services.

Moreover, no specialty area seems so peculiarly well prepared *and* ill prepared to accommodate to the rapid evolutions taking place in managing quality, utilization, and risk. This situation poses definite risks and opportunities for mental health services under growing managed care systems.

Other chapters in this book and numerous other commentators (Fielding 1984; Fox et al. 1984; Pollard 1983; Relman 1980; Sorkin 1986; Tavernier 1983) reflect upon the directions the United States has evolved over the past through phases in health benefits. (See Chapter 1.)

Increasing real and relative costs of health care, recession and inflation, accelerated costs due to sophisticated technology and therapeutic advances, public demands for life and health, and a number of other supply- and demand-side factors have fueled the popular view that current rates of escalations in health costs cannot be afforded and thus must be restrained (Blendon and Rogers 1983; Caulfield and Haynes 1981; Mechanic 1985). Successful efforts nationally to destigmatize mental illness, growth in numbers of mental health providers, and increased real incidence or public awareness of dysfunctions related to mental disorders have fueled costs in both private and public sectors in recent years. This has led to conclusions that such services are unaffordable, require containment and management, and are often questionably required (Rodriquez 1985, 1988, 1989b). Traditional approaches to managing these phenomena do not seem to offer much in the way of effectiveness or efficiency. The next sections outline the major current developmental directions being undertaken in mental health utilization and risk management in contemporary and future managed care activities.

Several utilization management mechanisms have been utilized in recent years in order to "contain" at best, or restrain at least, rising costs of mental health care. These approaches have been utilized in minimally managed indemnity, managed indemnity, and managed care system programs to variable degrees and in varying configurations. As such, they represent both the creative and frustrated efforts of payors to regulate the supply and demand factors that have contributed to increased utilization of mental health services (Rodriquez 1989a).

These phenomena have resulted in progressive general increases in utilization of mental health services, with some interesting epidemiologic trends:

✦ A relatively small minority of persons generate the great majority of demand for mental health services (Howard et al. 1989).

✦ Most of the variation of intensity of mental health services provided is variably but generally positively correlated to the patient's severity of illness and desire to seek treatment and to local practice habits (Knesper et al. 1988).

✦ The degree of utilization management in the setting in which the mental health service is rendered will affect the continuing utilization frequency per user, but not necessarily the number of individuals seeking services (McGuire and Fairbank 1988).

The steady progression of utilization within these epidemiologic contexts has been matched by increasing overhead and profit components in delivery systems, which collectively have ensured increased costs of mental health services over time. Benefit managers have been unnerved by a number of negative media portrayals of psychotherapy and a small number of "outlier" (high-cost, long length of stay) cases that underscore their concerns that mental health services are poorly defined and justified and equivocally effective. These cost phenomena have laid the groundwork for specific approaches for cost containment.

Utilization restraint mechanisms commonly instituted include the following (Fielding 1984; Fox et al. 1984; Wolfson and Levin 1985).

Benefit redesign and structuring.   Employers are frequently tempted to control utilization through economic disincentives to seek care, such as increased copayments and deductibles and reduced absolute benefits. Mental health benefits have traditionally lagged in parity of coverage with other health benefits, but have especially been vulnerable to limitations, given escalations in mental health benefit utilization and costs. Although increasing beneficiary-borne mental health benefit costs through increased cost shares and/or caps has been clearly demonstrated to reduce utilization (Manning et al. 1984; Tsai et al. 1987), studies have yet to account for the impact of such an approach upon mental and physical health status, disability, and social-occupational productivity. Given such uncertainties and the troubling ethical, legal, and public health ramifications of rationing, such an approach as a sole means of utilization control remains highly questionable. Restricting access and related costs through administrative policy mechanisms is achieved through a number of approaches, including the following:

✦ "Inconvenience" to beneficiaries, such as use of procedural complexity and confusing terms, slowdown of administrative processing of claims and inquiries, uneven communications, fragmentation of transactions, and other planned and untoward actions (Grumet 1989).

✦ Clinical and administrative "riders" to coverage policy that delineate conditions under which services would be provided, limited, or result in disenrollment (e.g., exclusions for chronic or custodial conditions, requirements for patient compliance as condition for eligibility; see Chapter 5).

Such approaches frequently not only result in negative beneficiary satisfaction but can also result in cost inefficiencies associated with unattended or poorly managed psychological problems, such as impairments in productivity and increased ambulatory-emergency general medical costs. Benefit managers are increasingly learning that psychiatric distress and dysfunction can express itself in many different ways and with variable costs over time, each heavily influenced by benefit structures.

Alternative reimbursement mechanisms. Reimbursement methodologies for health services have received considerable attention in recent years, as the amounts of reimbursements allowed have been shown to affect both prescription and seeking of those services (Ricardo-Campbell 1982). Prospective payment systems such as Diagnosis-Related Groups (DRGs) under Medicare have shown some promise in both reducing unnecessary costs and improving the health organization's efficiency (Ziegenfuss 1985). However, these systems are largely unreliable for controlling psychiatric cost variances (New York State Office of Mental Health 1987) and thus pose problems relative to parity and potential impact on quality outcome. Schemes such as the federal government's recent overtures to imposing resource-based relative value scales and "expenditure targets" for health services are fraught with similar risks and would certainly lead in some cases to unregulated rationing.

All such approaches, untested or imposed as singular or primary utilization controls, appear to be particularly inadequate and inequitable for utilization control for mental health services. Nevertheless, indemnity and managed care systems eventually will need to develop a cost-based psychiatric reimbursement system that would provide equitable payments for services rendered to specific patient or grouped patient categories. This will be a most difficult task, given the limitations of current pricing models and data bases. Additional problems will follow inherent resistances that should be expected from professionals and mental health delivery programs that have grown considerably under conventional market reimbursement and budgeting systems.

Alternative delivery systems. Given the cost escalations inherent in indemnified health services where the beneficiary exercises freedom of choice in selecting providers who are reimbursed by billed charges, employers are increasingly structuring benefits to steer beneficiaries to managed care programs. Such systems reduce costs by prompt identification and triage of patients to appropriate levels of care in an organized continuum of services. Mental health services are particularly focusing on utilization management by various potential user interventions (e.g., risk assessment, health education), early intervention activities for those manifesting mild signs and symptoms of mental disorders, and "alternative" levels and constructs for services (e.g., intensive focused outpatient therapies, psychiatric and substance abuse day and evening programs, community residential services, community self-help activities). Decisions about access, timing, sequencing, and "medical (psychological) necessity" of services at various "appropriate" levels are conventionally directed through professional case managers and peer reviewers who are guided by explicit administrative and clinical protocols.

Utilization review and management. Review of the medical-psychological necessity of clinical services has been a regular but variable component of health benefits management for the past 40 years. Such administrative, clinical, and financial reviews have increased in their formal structures so that now they are a standard aspect of accountability systems incorporated both within and external to treatment activities (Table 6–1). This drive to account for costs and quality of care has evolved to the point that utilization review and other related utilization management activities now constitute a major commercial enterprise and demand up to 3% of a health care facility's operating revenues. The involvement of health professionals in these activities has generated major national professional organizations (American College of Medical Quality, American Medical Peer Review

Table 6–1.   The "ideal" psychiatric review

◆ Quality and cost focus	treatments
◆ Professional mental health reviewers only	—Specified-justified treatment goals, milestones
—Specialized	—Aftercare: family, work-school, community supports
—Multidisciplinary	
◆ Consultative approach	◆ Effective benefit decision communications
◆ Prospective-concurrent focus	
◆ Direct communications: phone-based or face-to-face	—Explicit
	—Thorough
◆ Valid criteria	—Timely
—Consensus-developed (explicit)	◆ Effective appeals mechanisms
—Objective scientific (explicit and implicit)	◆ Quality control
	—Review opinions
◆ Review focused	—Reviewer knowledge and actions
—Specific dysfunctions requiring level of treatment	—Confidentiality
—Indicated evaluations and	—Communications

Association, National Association of Quality Assurance Professionals), certifying boards, and nascent residency programs.

The several hundred companies engaged in utilization review constitute a major phenomenon in health care, to a degree that the impact of utilization management initiatives is now receiving a level of national attention that will surely influence "national standards" for the conducting of utilization management activities (Committee on Utilization Management by Third Parties 1989). Providers have become progressively more upset over a number of problems associated with utilization management, including difficulties reaching persons qualified to make review determinations about clinical evaluations and treatments, secrecy of review criteria, administrative inconveniences (Grumet 1989), and perceived intrusions into the confidentiality of the therapist-patient relationship. These problems have led to provider-led efforts in many states to impose limits on utilization management through state regulation. The profound impact of such regulation upon utilization management organizations has recently led to the formation of the Utilization Review Accreditation Commission (URAC), which has established national operational standards and an accreditation program for such organizations. States are now beginning to accept URAC accreditation in lieu of setting up large enforcement agencies, but many provider organizations continue to want local controls over "external" review activities.

Although conventional utilization review has been shown to be effective in restraining selective health services utilization and costs without adversely affecting quality (Feldstein et al. 1988; Imperiale et al. 1988), consensus is growing that utilization review activities will need to achieve the following, either through regulation or other incentives:

✦ Develop objective measures of impact upon health care costs and health status outcomes over time and for specified populations.
✦ Utilize and explicitly cite in benefit determinations the professionally developed national standards and criteria for clinical evaluations and treatments; maximize peer review as a medium for reaching these determinations.
✦ Strengthen beneficiary communications and appeals and grievance processes; minimize administrative burdens of utilization review.
✦ Operationally reinforce linkages between external utilization review and direct care quality and risk management activities.

These challenges will have particular import for utilization review and its more clinically focused derivative, psychiatric case management. Although there is evidence that case management provides more effective cost and quality accountability for indemnity and managed care programs (Burton et al. 1989; Hamilton 1985; Lizanich-Aro and Goldstein 1988; Rodriquez and Lee 1986; Rodriquez and Maher 1986), not all providers are comfortable with the administrative demands and other perceived impositions associated with such reviews (Melnick and Lyter 1987). Nevertheless, such activities are so rapidly being implemented by payors that they are becoming a major aspect of clinical practice, cost containment, and quality management.

In addition to conventional internal and external utilization review, two utilization management mechanisms that have evolved in managed care systems are the "gatekeeper" system and financial "at risk" arrangements for the provider (Table 6–2). In both approaches, the modulation of the provider's clinical decision making by explicit triage procedures, benefit coverage policies, and calculable financial loss or gain serves as a basis for heightening the provider's sensitivity to costs of health services. Such approaches have also served as a focus of considerable soul-searching among professionals regarding the ethical risks of various cost management decisions in such arrangements (Englehardt and Rie 1988; Hillman et al. 1989; Levinson 1987; Povar and Moreno 1988; Reagan 1987).

Table 6–2.   The "next generation": managed-organized psychiatric services

✦ Capitated prepayment system, tied to benefit analysis	and patient-channeling influences
✦ Coverage for all levels of psychiatric care	✦ Focused case management by mental health professionals
✦ Selected institutional and individual providers	✦ Professional resources —Provider education and relations
✦ Incentive provider reimbursement, tied to quality and utilization-efficient care	—Beneficiary education and relations
✦ Rate negotiations with providers, based on market-competitive	—Client services

Risk Management in Managed Mental Health

Where the genesis of utilization review activities was predominantly a reactive process and the evolution of quality assurance has been largely proactive, risk management has been shaped from a dual perspective. Risk management activities are based in the multiple realms of law, economics, clinical science, consumer services, and management. It conceptually and operationally embraces quality process and outcome as a goal, because quality, based on effectiveness and efficiency of clinical care and service, is the "product" of care mutually desired by patient, provider, and payor. When that desired process and outcome is thwarted by circumstances that pose unnecessary and avoidable risk to the patient, adverse consequences may ensue for each party (i.e., the patient's health may be harmed or threatened, additional health or social costs may follow, and the provider may suffer economic and legal sanctions). Minimizing any circumstances that would lead to such results would thus be in the interests of each. Therefore, risk management has evolved as a process that requires a unique collaboration among clinicians, administrators, attorneys, and consumers. Given the emphasis in managed care operations on service coordination, prevention, and resource management, risk management activities have received special attention in the managed care environment.

Risk management, like quality assurance and utilization review, is an increasingly structured and regulated set of activities that requires explicit procedural program design and protocols, dedicated and expert staff, and effective infrastructure support systems, such as medical records, management information systems, and legal services

(Kraus 1986). The following are among the major components of an effective risk management system.

Legal expertise. Consultants and providers must be familiar with current legal trends and decisions that affect quality, utilization, and risk management activities, such as *Patrick v. Burget, Wickline v. California,* and *Hughes v. Blue Cross of California* (Couch 1989; Gnessin 1989; Morlock et al. 1989). Requirements for informed consent, confidentiality or privileged information, due process in peer review actions, and accurate and thorough documentation of actions and communications about medical, administrative, and related patient care matters necessitate access to current knowledge of health case law. This knowledge needs to be embodied in operational protocols related to risk areas within treatment settings and through continuous education of staff (Hiatt et al. 1989).

Monitoring of risk areas through routine identification of potential and actual risk occurrences. Dedicated risk management and quality assurance staff must work collaboratively to identify problems. A system of professional chart review of cases demonstrating failure to follow prescribed treatment may be independently developed, using readily available national professional practice standards (Chassin 1988) and other common quality-risk indicators, or commercially available occurrence screening systems that may be purchased. Monitors must generate sensitive, reliable, and valid data that allow for practical remedial interventions.

Correction of risk areas through systematic use of data. Information about potential or actual problems must be utilized to effect changes in administrative systems and practitioner behaviors that contribute to the problems. More defined protocols and credentialing sanctions are among the methods that are commonly employed. These interventions are then evaluated in the ongoing monitoring cycle. It is essential that these activities become a defined part of professional staff responsibility and that they be incorporated into the organization's quality improvement philosophy and structured quality assurance activities (Berwick 1989). These integrated and promotive activities are prominent components of the "Total Quality Management" initiatives of such organizations as the Joint Commission on the Accreditation of Healthcare Organizations. They also reflect a mega-

trend in the business community toward management through com-
munalistic commitment to quality products rather than by sanction-
driven inspection.

Risk management activities become "owned" by practicing clinicians when they are based on clearly defined practice standards and
effected through ongoing peer review and professional education. To
minimize risk and maximize optimal clinical quality outcome, clinicians require clinical and legal knowledge, organizational supports,
lines of communication, and sufficient time. When the organization
demands, defines, structures, and reinforces the total organizational
provision of highest quality care, risks are minimized and thus "managed." The combination of initiatives at the "micro" (e.g., treatment
program, institution, local professional society) and "macro" (e.g.,
state licensing and tort reform legislation, national professional practice parameters) levels should, over time, reduce the current malpractice quandary by steering treatment outcomes toward a more
predictably positive and less risky axis. Clinical risk management
should remain a major area of focus within various competing managed care programs, which may largely succeed or fail according to
their relative capacities to deliver effective, low-risk health services.

The Need for Data and Information Systems

This nation's ability to continue to afford utilization-efficient, quality
health care and to avoid rationing or apportionment decisions that are
not arbitrary or discriminatory depends upon the development of more
effective management information systems for health services. Major
investments are now being made in computer hardware and software
by payors, providers, and regulators in an effort to better understand
the clinical and cost parameters of both effectiveness and efficiency of
various treatment modalities and programs. One of the major reasons
the "medical necessity" of mental health services are so often questioned by payors is the historical lack of national professional consensus regarding what constitutes appropriate services for specific
clinical conditions and the efficacy of specific modalities and durations
of service.

Underpinning the development of any professional consensus,
upon which standards and criteria of care are based, is the scientific
evidence for outcome effectiveness, represented by convincing data
and other information. Acknowledging this relationship, reimburse-

ment systems that are tied to technology and therapeutic assessment mechanisms are turning to outcome studies as a basis for payment policies. This is placing ever-increasing pressures on individual providers and their professional associations to "prove" that their "standard" of care is appropriate and necessary.

The "New Federalism" philosophy of the Reagan and Bush administrations during the 1980s viewed medical efficacy issues as more properly being resolved in the American marketplace, rather than by federal agencies such as the National Institute of Mental Health. Professional organizations have struggled with the possible consequences of their assuming a more proactive role in establishing professional standards, such as the costs of definitive efficacy research, the lack of support for such efforts by many professional members, and the feared adverse uses of such information by litigious attorneys and cost-cutting payors. Notwithstanding these fears, professional organizations such as the American Medical Association and the American Psychiatric Association are attempting to maintain the offensive in the battle to retain adequate health benefits, by publicly stating what constitutes appropriate care (Schier 1988; Task Force on Treatments of Psychiatric Disorders 1989). Such organizations are progressively becoming involved in standards development and technology-therapeutic assessment, not only because such activities are the "right and proper" role of the professions, but also because to *not* do so would lead to further development of potentially arbitrary and conflicting standards and reimbursement policies by payors.

The growing momentum toward outcome-related standards is causing many to realize that conventional means of assessing medical evaluations and treatments will be insufficient for the larger national purpose of establishing an "outcomes management" system, consisting of multiconnected national data bases linking providers, payors, and assessment organizations (Ellwood 1988). This envisioned system is drawing increasing attention from each constituency, as the nation attempts to establish a health care system that is managed through science, information, and effective decision making and that bases any rationing policies on data-supported principles of fairness and parity.

The Future of Utilization and Risk Management

By any current logical estimation, managed care programs, in a variety that seems characteristically American, will be a dominant part of

American health care in the future (Council on Economic Affairs 1987; Winkenwerder and Ball 1988). As the major conventional focus of managed care has been accountability, this focus will be greatly broadened to include utilization and risk management (Relman 1988). This phenomenon will continue to have major ramifications for mental health services within managed care programs (Bennett 1988; Sederer and St. Clair 1989; Shadle and Christianson 1989).

Advocacy and resolution of professional issues will require both increased professional leadership and followership. Professional organizations will need to expedite the development of explicit practice parameters and ethical positions, establish strong local peer review systems, broaden professional education in clinical outcome management, remain active in lobbying for patients' rights for quality and access and for reasonable practitioner fees, and strengthen certification and licensing mechanisms. Somehow, interdisciplinary conflicts must be bridged. In a competitive marketplace where practitioners are free to practice wherever they can economically survive, this may be difficult, particularly if professional organizations see their role as primarily that of an economic guild. Increasingly, supply-side economic dynamics will be regulated by some combination of legislation and free-market competition, including the provider selection influence of managed care. In the future, practitioners will be required to demonstrate even more their capacities to provide effective care, with low risks to the patient and with utilization efficiency. Failure to do so will result in limitations in licensing and credentials and requirements for structured remediation. These regulatory initiatives will no doubt be too intrusive to many, who will choose to leave clinical practice or not enter the profession. Such a process may be advantageous both to patients and to the profession, where unskilled or unethical practitioners would be influenced to leave, or disastrous in communities that would be left with insufficient health care resources.

The positive opportunities that are possible within managed care organizations—such as preventing disease and disability, coordinating medical with mental health and social services, developing community-based comprehensive treatment systems, and strengthening the science and delivery of quality care—are currently threatened by the uncertainties of economics, the whims of politics, and the anxieties of providers, payors, and consumers. The outcome of the next epoch of health care will be determined by how well the current generation of leaders will define, measure, and promote quality. This should serve as the ultimate bottom line for future evolutions in managed care and will become a major determinant in the future of mental health services.

References

Bennett MJ: The greening of the HMO: implications for prepaid psychiatry. Am J Psychiatry 145(12):1544–1549, 1988

Berwick DM: Continuous improvement as an ideal in health care. N Engl J Med 320(1):53–56, 1989

Blendon RJ, Rogers DE: Cutting medical care costs. JAMA 250:1880–1885, 1983

Burton WN, Hoy DA, Bonin RL, et al: Quality and cost effectiveness management of mental health care. J Occup Med 31(4):363–366, 1989

Caulfield SC, Haynes PL: Health Care Costs: Private Initiatives for Containment. Washington, DC, Government Research Corporation, 1981

Chassin MR: Standards of care in medicine. Inquiry 25(4):437–450, 1988

Committee on Utilization Management by Third Parties: Controlling Costs and Changing Patient Care? The Role of Utilization Management. Washington, DC, Institute of Medicine (National Academy of Sciences), 1989

Couch JB: Legal Aspects of Medical Quality Management. Tampa, FL, American College of Physician Executives, 1989

Council on Economic Affairs: Status Report on Developments in the Health Care Industry. Washington, DC, American Psychiatric Association, 1987

Ellwood PM: Outcomes management: a technology of patient experience. N Engl J Med 318:1549–1556, 1988

Englehardt HT, Rie MA: A code of ethics for the mass marketing of health care. N Engl J Med 319(16):1086–1089, 1988

Feldstein PJ, Wickizer TM, Wheeler JRC: Private cost containment: the effects of utilization review programs on health care use and expenditures. N Engl J Med 318(20):1310–1314, 1988

Fielding JE: Corporate Health Management. Menlo Park, CA, Addison-Wesley, 1984

Fox P, Goldbeck W, Spies J: Health Care Cost Management. Ann Arbor, MI, Health Administration Press, 1984

Gnessin AM: Liability in the Managed Care Setting—Proceedings. Washington, DC, Group Health Association of America, 1989

Grumet GW: Health care rationing through inconvenience. N Engl J Med 231(9):607–611, 1989

Hamilton J (ed): Psychiatric Peer Review: Prelude and Promise. Washington, DC, American Psychiatric Press, 1985

Hiatt HH, Barnes BA, Brennan TA, et al: A study of medical injury and medical malpractice. N Engl J Med 321(7):480–484, 1989

Hillman AL, Pauly MV, Kerstein JJ: How do financial incentives affect physicians' clinical decisions and the financial performance of health maintenance organizations? N Engl J Med 321(2):86–92, 1989

Howard KI, Davidson CV, O'Mahoney MT, et al: Patterns of psychotherapy utilization. Am J Psychiatry 146(6):775–778, 1989

Imperiale TF, Siegal AP, Crede WB, et al: Preadmission screening of Medicare patients: the clinical impact of reimbursement disapproval. JAMA 259(23):3418–3421, 1988

Knesper DJ, Belcher BE, Cross JG: Variations in the intensity of psychiatric treatment across markets for mental health services in the United States. Health Serv Res 22(6):797–819, 1988

Kraus GP: Health Care Risk Management. Owings Mills, MD, National Health Publishing, 1986

Levinson DF: Financial incentives for physicians in HMOs: is there a conflict of interest? N Engl J Med 317(27):1743–1748, 1987

Lizanich-Aro S, Goldstein L: A successful approach to the start-up of a mental health case management program. Quality Assurance and Utilization Review 3(3):90–94, 1988

Manning WG, Wells KB, Duan N, et al: Cost-sharing and the use of ambulatory mental health services. Am Psychol 39:1077–1089, 1984

McGuire TG, Fairbank A:Patterns of mental health utilization over time in a fee-for-service population. Am J Public Health 78(2):134–136, 1988

Mechanic D: Cost containment and the quality of medical care: rationing strategies in an era of constrained resources. Milbank Q 63:453–475, 1985

Melnick S, Lyter L: The negative impacts of increased concurrent review of psychiatric inpatient care. Hosp Community Psychiatry 38:300–303, 1987

Morlock L, Lindgren DH, Mills DH: Malpractice, clinical risk management and quality assessment, in Providing Quality Care. Edited by Goldfield N, Nash DB. Philadelphia, PA, American College of Physicians, 1989

New York State Office of Mental Health: Report of the Alternative Reimbursement Methodologies Project. Albany, NY, New York State Office of Mental Health, 1987

Pollard MR: Competition or regulation. JAMA 249:1860–1863, 1983

Povar G, Moreno J: Hippocrates and the health maintenance organization: discussion of ethical issues. Ann Intern Med 109(5):419–424, 1988

Reagan MD: Towards full disclosure of referral restrictions and financial incentives by prepaid health plans. N Engl J Med 317(27):1729–1734, 1987

Relman AS: The new medical-industrial complex. N Engl J Med 303:963–970, 1980

Relman AS: Assessment and accountability: the third revolution in medical care. N Engl J Med 319:1220–1222, 1988

Ricardo-Campbell R: The Economics and Politics of Health. Chapel Hill, NC, University of North Carolina Press, 1982

Rodriquez AR: Current and future directions in reimbursement for psychiatric services. Gen Hosp Psychiatry 7:341–348, 1985

Rodriquez AR: The effects of contemporary economic conditions on availability and quality of mental health services, in Handbook of Quality Assurance in Mental Health. Edited by Stricker G, Rodriguez AR. New York, Plenum, 1988

Rodriquez AR: Managed care and psychiatric services. Yale Psychiatric Quarterly 11(3):11–15, 1989a

Rodriquez AR: Evolutions in utilization and quality management: a crisis for psychiatric services? Gen Hosp Psychiatry 11:256–263, 1989b

Rodriquez AR, Lee FC: The next generation of managed mental health care. Health Cost Management 4(2):1–9, 1986

Rodriquez AR, Maher JJ: Psychiatric case management offers cost, quality control. Business and Health 3(4):14–17, 1986

Schier RL: Can medicine bear the scrutiny? American Medical News, January 1, 1988, pp 1, 20

Sederer LI, St. Clair RL: Managed health care and the Massachusetts experience. Am J Psychiatry 146(9):1142–1148, 1989

Shadle M, Christianson JB: The impact of HMO development on mental health and chemical dependency services. Hosp Community Psychiatry 40(11):1145–1151, 1989

Sorkin AL: Health Care and the Changing Economic Environment. Lexington, MA, Lexington Books/DC Heath, 1986

Task Force on Treatments of Psychiatric Disorders, American Psychiatric Association: Treatments of Psychiatric Disorders, Vols I, II, III. Washington, DC, American Psychiatric Association, 1989

Tavernier G: Companies prescribe major revisions to medical benefits programs to cut soaring health care costs. Management Review 72(8):9–19, 1983

Tsai S, Reedy SM, Bernacki E: Mental health benefits redesign. Business and Health 4(6):26–29, 1987

Winkenwerder W, Ball JR: The transformation of American health care. N Engl J Med 318:317–319, 1988

Wolfson J, Levin PJ: Managing employee health benefits: a guide to cost control. Homewood, IL, Dow Jones-Irwin, 1985

Ziegenfuss JT: DRGs and Hospital Impact. New York, McGraw-Hill, 1985

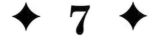

7

Setting Up Provider Networks and PPOs

Doyle Carson, M.D.

As the search for more effective health care delivery systems continues, one increasingly popular approach is the preferred provider organization (PPO). Sometimes referred to as a "laid-back cousin" of the health maintenance organization (HMO), it offers features of several different systems. In a sense, it is a compromise of extremes, incorporating features of HMOs and independent fee-for-service medical care. However, there is enormous variation among PPOs (Bloom 1987). To know about the structure of one PPO is just that—to know that single PPO.

PPOs differ from health maintenance organizations in two basic ways (Altman 1989). First, they reimburse providers on a fee-for-service basis. Second, they offer subscribers the opportunity to use a designated (preferred) provider or a nonparticipating provider. The fee-for-service feature is appealing to those providers who wish to avoid the salaried position associated with HMOs. Freedom to choose a provider is appealing to many users of health care who may have special doctor-patient relationships with nonparticipating physicians. However, as health care costs continue to escalate, PPOs attempt more stringent cost control by lowering the fees that are paid and by using stronger financial pressures to channel subscribers toward preferred providers. PPOs are more flexible than capitated programs and use approaches that influence rather than require. The degree of influence depends upon how strong the pressures have to be in order to control costs.

Historically, negotiated fee-for-service medicine is not new (Trauner 1983). At the turn of the century, many fraternal organizations were established by immigrant groups, especially in the northeastern United States, that would contract with physicians at discounted rates; the physicians obtained more patients, and members of the fraternal orders received treatment at reduced costs. There have been other historical examples of negotiated fee-for-service care, which tend to develop when large segments of the population perceive that traditional fee-for-service medicine has become so expensive as to be inaccessible.

There are several features that are present in today's PPOs. First, a group of providers is selected by the payors of care as preferable. The selection of providers to be part of a preferred network is based on a variety of factors, which include quality of care, efficiency of treatment, financial issues, willingness to participate in utilization review programs, and a compatible treatment philosophy. Patients can choose providers outside the preferred network, but financial incentives are put in place to encourage selection of preferred providers. For example, insurance payments for treatment may drop from 80% to 50% of charges if patients select an out-of-network provider. Naturally, this becomes a powerful financial tool to influence provider choice.

The importance of influencing provider choice through financial incentives cannot be overstated. Controlling provider choice is the single most important mechanism in influencing treatment and health care costs. Through such an agreement, the preferred provider receives an increased volume of referrals in return for certain agreements, which may include discount pricing, utilization review, utilization targets, and shifting the focus of care from inpatient to partial hospital, residential, and outpatient settings. In a competitive marketplace, such agreements become an important economic strategy for providers, and payors are able to influence treatment approaches and costs accordingly. The providers may be individual practitioners who agree to participate in a provider network or an organized group of providers who may market their services to a PPO. Hospitals as well as individual providers are participants in PPO networks. Providers who do not agree to participate with the goals of a PPO program are excluded from participation. Although excluding some providers limits a member's freedom of choice, this provider selection is an essential element of cost controls in managed care.

Discount Pricing

A frequent component of PPOs is a discount from usual charges. The percentage of discount varies and obviously depends on what the usual charges are. Discounts tend to be 20% lower than market rates (Curtiss 1989). Each PPO has a different approach to pricing issues. Some negotiate a flat per diem hospital rate and expect the hospital to manage all inpatient costs with that payment; others choose to establish discounted rates for each procedure. To reach agreement on the type and degree of discount, providers and payors meet in negotiating sessions prior to signing or renewing a contract. These hard-nosed business approaches to establishing charges may represent a new experience for health care providers, but it is one that is likely to continue. The provider must learn the art of negotiating prices and managing a practice with increased patient volume at a discounted per-unit price.

Payors are able to negotiate discounted rates only when there is an excess of providers. Empty professional hours or hospital beds represent the essential background that leads to negotiated rates. It is a matter of supply and demand. PPOs are an outgrowth of a pro-competitive health care policy that emerged in the 1970s after the failure of regulatory approaches to control costs. In 1973, federal legislation was passed that required employers to offer HMO plans as an alternative to indemnity insurance plans. This legislation opened the door to increased competition among health care organizations. PPOs emerged as a type of competitive organization that promoted a decrease in health care costs but, at the same time, some preservation of autonomy for the private practitioner.

In 1982, the state of California initiated selective hospital contracting in a move to control Medicaid costs. This established a model public PPO in California and was followed by private purchasers of care initiating PPO arrangements with select providers at discounted rates. PPO discount pricing is now a growing nationwide phenomenon.

Utilization Review

Some type of utilization review is usually associated with PPOs. It is the major mechanism of conveying a treatment philosophy to providers. Utilization review occurs at all levels of treatment and includes preadmission certification, concurrent hospital review, and partial hospital and outpatient concurrent review. Ordinarily, utilization review decisions are based on clinical criteria that are unique for each utilization review organization. The criteria may or may not be made available to the providers. Utilization reviewers do not make treatment decisions; they make decisions about payment of benefits. However, for most people, benefit decisions are treatment decisions. The question of who is making the treatment decision is currently of great concern to clinicians (Gurevitz 1984). Who has the liability in such decisions? Most likely there will be a series of judicial decisions in the future that will resolve these issues.

Those doing utilization review do not believe they should have any liability as they do not make treatment decisions, only decisions about payment. Also, providers who enter into contracts with a PPO do so with the full knowledge of the treatment philosophy to be used. These generally mean that patients will have only brief hospital stays. However, there are individual clinical situations that spark controversy. For example, patients with a diagnosis of borderline personality disorder are difficult to manage. Because of the impulsive and self-destructive behavior that such patients demonstrate, providers often wish to hospitalize them for extended periods of time. Utilization reviewers frequently see such patients as consuming inordinate amounts of health care resources without benefiting substantially; in fact, they fear such patients may even regress in a hospital setting. It is amazing how a provider and reviewer who have previously agreed to work together can be split in the face of such clinical material, and it is an inevitable happening in utilization review. In the face of this, an important part of a PPO structure is the presence of mechanisms to deal with utilization review tensions. Frequent dialogue, appeal mechanisms, and consultants are essential.

In today's climate, utilization review criteria primarily limit hospital stays to the resolution of acute psychiatric crises. Patients are rapidly discharged to outpatient settings for further care. Interactions between clinicians and utilization review providers may take on a tense, adversarial quality. One source of strained relations is a difference in the treatment philosophy of the professional provider and the managed care component. Some psychiatrists are more comfortable treating some clinical conditions with long-term hospital stays. It is difficult to change practice patterns. Aside from the specific clinical problems that are encountered and the difficulty in changing established practice patterns, another difficulty is that the very nature of the utilization review process diminishes a physician's autonomy—a potential cause of aggravation and demoralization. The physician has the responsibility—why not the autonomy? There is one overriding reason—the cost of health care. Rightly or wrongly, there is a widely held belief among payors of care that physician autonomy contributes to the escalation of costs. As long as health costs are rising, physician autonomy will be challenged by the utilization review process.

The most frequent source of disagreement has to do with hospital length of stay. Psychiatry is being encouraged to follow the lead of other medical specialties and shift more treatment to the outpatient level. In order for this to work, there must be excellent outpatient programs available. The utilization review emphasis should not be simply on limiting inpatient stays, but rather on emphasizing excellent outpatient alternatives.

Utilization review may be on-site or by telephone. On-site review may provide much better knowledge about patients and treatment, but telephone review is more economical and permits review in remote locations. Utilization review may be carried out by a managed care company or by an insurance company. The professionals involved are nurses, psychologists, social workers, and psychiatrists. The failure to meet and develop personal working relationships with reviewers contributes to tensions in the review process.

The utilization review industry is growing rapidly because of its effectiveness at controlling health care costs. However, acceptable standards for utilization review have not been agreed upon throughout the psychiatric field. Concerns about diminishing quality of care have led to concerns about some utilization review approaches. It is a growing and largely unregulated field; undoubtedly, state legislative approaches will add some degree of regulation. However, the fact that mental health and chemical dependency costs are being managed more effectively with utilization review means that PPOs will continue to grow.

Continuum of Care

The strong emphasis on reducing inpatient treatment requires the development of excellent and accessible outpatient, residential, and partial hospital services. Patients who were previously treated on inpatient units are being shifted to outpatient programs. Services that offer frequent and intense treatment must be in place to ensure quality patient care. The adage that patients are being discharged "quicker and sicker" is accurate in today's managed care environment.

Much organizational work must be done to develop the necessary intensity of outpatient services in a PPO. Without such outpatient services, sicker patients will quickly relapse and require readmission to the hospital. For example, the treatment of some individuals with alcoholism may be accomplished with an inpatient detoxification, followed by discharge to intense outpatient services for rehabilitation. Without accessible outpatient rehabilitation programs, the patient will resume drinking. A PPO may be a loose network of providers. In order for the program to work, there must be leadership that appropriately organizes outpatient care into integrated, intense treatment.

The recent shift in emphasizing outpatient treatment provides an opportunity for the mental health care field. For years, psychiatrists criticized the insurance industry for failing to pay for outpatient and day treatment programs. Payment mechanisms are in a state of rapid transition, and now is the time to emphasize the need for excellent outpatient programs. Outpatient services should be comprehensive and include day treatment programs, residential facilities, medication clinics, and home health care. There is a need for specialized treatment for families, children, adolescents, the elderly, and a host of specific clinical problems such as chemical dependency, schizophrenia, affective disorder, eating disorders, and others. Outpatient programs should be comprehensive and accessible. PPO clinics should be distributed throughout a metropolitan area for ready patient access. It is important that problems of public hospital deinstitutionalization be avoided with current delivery system changes. Strong support must be given to developing extensive outpatient services so that a true continuum of care can exist (Altman and Frisman 1987).

Treatment Philosophy

When a business or an insurance company contracts for utilization review services from a managed care company, it enters into an agreement for more than the individual utilization review components—it "buys into" the treatment philosophy of that particular managed care company. Differences in treatment philosophies account for the major variations among PPOs. Usually one or more professions, often psychiatrists, have developed the treatment philosophy, and they must convince purchasers of the wisdom of that particular therapeutic approach.

Although short-term hospital treatment is the centerpiece of all the programs, the treatment approaches utilized in achieving this goal may vary greatly. Examples include emphasis on medications or somatic treatments such as electroconvulsive therapy (ECT), intense outpatient individual or group psychotherapy, teaching individual skills while de-emphasizing individual psychotherapy, intense family therapy, supporting individual strengths and avoiding regressive treatment approaches, lengthy group sessions with the patient and significant others to resolve crises, self-help groups (such as Alcoholics Anonymous), or treating only patients who have positive motivation for therapy and change.

The very nature of mental illness and treatment leads to many different concepts regarding etiology and appropriate care. For every strong advocate of one particular view about mental illness, there are many who see the issues differently. Many different theories about mental illness and treatment are being played out with current utilization review approaches. Sometimes the lack of a consistent approach by a utilization review firm may leave providers bewildered. Even with a consistent philosophy, there may be a clash in beliefs that causes tension. For example, a utilization review approach emphasizing family therapy as the major treatment modality will have an abrasive interface with providers who rely on individual psychotherapy as the major therapeutic approach. Values regarding treatment philosophy should be thoroughly explored before establishing an agreement between payor and provider.

Effectiveness of Cost Containment and Treatment

With the enormous growth of PPOs, questions are naturally being raised regarding their effectiveness. Those questions are directed at both cost containment and treatment outcome. Concerns about rising mental health and chemical dependency treatment costs have been the driving force behind development of PPOs. Indications are that costs are being more effectively managed with PPOs (Altman 1989). Representatives from corporations are expressing satisfaction, and increasing numbers of businesses are moving into PPOs.

What about effectiveness of treatment and quality of care? This is much more difficult to measure. There are strong advocates and critics of managed care in general and PPOs in particular. There is much yet to learn, and research is desperately needed in this area. Many questions need answers:

1. When inpatient stays are shortened, how are long- and short-term outcomes affected?
2. Do some patients need more hospital care?
3. How do we identify which patients are helped and which are harmed by these evolving treatment approaches?
4. Which outpatient treatments are most effective for which patients?

There are many opportunities to do valuable research in the managed care field. Varying opinions about effectiveness exist in the literature. Additional information is needed.

Businesses have a vital interest in the outcome of this research. Although cost has been the driving force behind the growth of PPOs, there is a genuine interest on the part of payors that effective care be available. Otherwise, benefits for mental health and chemical dependency treatment would have been eliminated. Payors wish to balance cost with effectiveness. The mental health field needs to develop more data about effectiveness to help answer these questions.

Flexibility

One reason for the appeal and growth of PPOs is the flexibility that is available (Bloom 1987). Payors perceive that traditional indemnity insurance approaches lead to overutilization of mental health and chemical dependency services. The incentives are rigidly on the side of overutilization of the most intense services. This leads to problems of cost. Some payors perceive that HMOs have strong financial incentives to provide less care. They are perceived as being locked into a rigid underutilization of services, and this leads to problems of quality. The PPO is an outgrowth of concerns about rigidity of overutilization and underutilization and is perceived as a compromise. Although the care is managed with utilization review, the providers are not as driven by financial incentives to provide less treatment. There is the perception that greater flexibility is available to meet varying patient needs.

Problems

Each type of delivery system has problems inherent to itself. PPOs are no exception. They include:

1. *Provider knowledge and cooperation.* Because a PPO may be loosely organized with a widely dispersed group of professionals, problems may develop in attracting individuals with knowledge to do this type of care and in gaining their cooperation. Orientation programs and special efforts to develop a professional alliance with them is essential.

2. *Inexperienced utilization reviewers.* Because utilization review is an essential component of PPOs, it is critical that knowledgeable reviewers be available. The rapid growth of the utilization review field has led to a shortage of experienced reviewers. This can create serious problems for a PPO. Intense efforts at developing educational programs for reviewers is a must.

3. *Provider shopping.* Managed care firms will inevitably have some problems in working with providers. They must develop an approach to resolving such problems. Two very different methods have emerged for resolving difficulties. The first approach involves resolution of differences by dialogue and negotiation. The relationship between the managed care firm and the provider is characterized by a long-standing association with regular and frequent meetings to resolve problems. It is a relationship where a partnership develops, characterized by occasional meetings of considerable intensity where serious problems are solved. The other approach is characterized by terminating contractual relationships rather than resolving differences through negotiation. Inevitably, this involves shopping from provider to provider when differences develop. Such PPOs are not likely to survive in the long run, for they will not develop a loyal, experienced, dependable pool of providers.

4. *Failure to inform employees.* As businesses face the problem of escalating mental health and chemical dependency costs, they turn more and more to managed care approaches such as PPOs. They contract with managed care companies and providers to utilize

hospital care for treatment of acute crises and to rapidly shift to outpatient treatment for further care. Unfortunately, more often than not, they fail to tell their employees of this change in treatment approach. It is left up to the provider to communicate this change in treatment philosophy. Families and patients are so angry to learn that the approach to treatment is different than what they believe they have been told that valuable time and resources are spent dealing with that issue before attention can be turned to treatment of the acute psychiatric episode. Businesses need to inform their employees of the changes in treatment philosophy that occur with the development of a PPO.

5. *Confidentiality issues.* Confidentiality issues are important in treatment of people with mental illness. Utilization review brings in new professionals who learn about patients. Is this ethical? Should this be tolerated? Is there a choice? This issue will continue to be a difficult one.

Conclusion

For many years, patients and doctors have met to evaluate symptoms, make a diagnosis, and develop a plan of treatment. The payor of care—the business or insurance company—passively accepted that process and paid the bill. That process is undergoing drastic changes. Payors are no longer willing to passively pay the bill; they are demanding to be active participants in the process. Managed care is best defined as the active involvement of the payor in the doctor-patient relationship. PPOs are one type of delivery system where the payor has some input into the doctor-patient relationship, treatment decisions, and the cost and quality of care.

References

Altman LS: Preferred provider organizations: a historical perspective, legal considerations, and special issues. ALMACAN, March 1989, p 22

Altman LS, Frisman LK: Preferred provider organizations and mental health care. Hosp Community Psychiatry 38:360, 1987

Bloom J: HMOs. Tuscon, AZ, The Body Press, 1987

Curtiss FR: Managed health care: managed costs? Personnel Journal, June 1989, p 80

Gurevitz H: Psychiatry and preferred provider organizations. Psychiatric Annals 14:348, 1984

Trauner JB: Preferred Provider Organizations: The California Experiment. San Francisco, CA, University of California at San Francisco, Institute of Health Policy Studies, 1983

✦ 8 ✦

Capitation and Management of Mental Health in the Public Sector

Haroutun M. Babigian, M.D.
Sylvia K. Reed, Ph.D.

Care for seriously and persistently mentally ill patients has tended to be fragmented for a variety of reasons. In the long course of chronic illness, a patient has ample opportunity to be brought or to choose to go to a variety of agencies for care. If patients are too disorganized or paranoid to reveal their treatment experience, there may be no way for a treatment center to know of prior outcomes or problems. It is also not unusual for patients to drop out of care when they are feeling better or to stop taking medications that have unpleasant side effects, only to end up in crisis a short time later.

In caring for seriously and persistently mentally ill individuals, the goal is typically not to attempt to cure, but to bring the patient to an optimum level of functioning and quality of life and to prevent relapse. These challenges are as much social or rehabilitative as medical in nature. Until the late 1980s, case management was not reimbursed under Medicaid, and many social and rehabilitative programs are still not covered under insurance. Most local programs were oriented toward acute patients who were not dependent upon public sector support. Progressive programs often "failed" these patients, as they were unable to fulfill model patient roles. Frustrated families shopped among independent programs, finding few viable options outside of the state psychiatric facility.

The fee-for-service health system, which was the primary mode of health care reimbursement until the 1980s, is predicated on the assumption that the patient assumes major responsibility for maintaining continuity and consistency of care. Thus a fee-for-service delivery system may not be ideal for maintaining continuity of care among less sophisticated users. This may not be problematic for acute care, but if the patient has a chronic condition and is often psychotic or disorganized, it can be disastrous. The current health maintenance organization (HMO) health coverage option is organized to deliver acute care and has also not dealt particularly well with chronic conditions. HMOs do not always provide the full range of services needed for management of chronic disability. In addition, high costs may force agencies to limit care, thereby requiring patients or their families to advocate for needed services.

Mental health care planners in recent years have encouraged use of capitation as an appropriate method of financing and managing care of people with serious and persistent mental illness (Lehman 1987; Sharfstein 1982). This emphasis has led to the development of several early capitation model programs throughout the United States, in Arizona (Santiago 1987; Santiago and Berren 1989), Washington, DC (Harris and Bergman 1988), Rhode Island (Christianson and Linehan 1989; Mauch 1989), and South Carolina. One of the early experimental capitation programs was initiated in Rochester, New York, with enrollment beginning in November 1987. Mechanic and Aiken (1989a, 1989b) summarize these capitation programs and discuss the potentials and difficulties of using capitation plans to care for chronically mentally ill individuals. In the same volume, Schlesinger (1989) reviews some of the considerable obstacles to capitation implementation and viability, and potentially troubling incentives, which balance the generally positive theoretical value of capitation.

Rochester and Surrounding Area

The counties of Monroe and Livingston in New York, which include the city of Rochester and its suburbs, implemented a mental health demonstration project involving a capitation program for seriously and persistently mentally ill people. As part of the 5-year demonstration, which began officially in 1987, both counties and the state delegate many of their planning and funding responsibilities to a local membership corporation: Integrated Mental Health, Inc. (IMH). This corporation assumes management of the publicly funded mental health system and coordination of involved parties toward resolution

of system issues. The demonstration was the result of a complex negotiation between the New York State Office of Mental Health (OMH),
the counties, the United Way, and provider agencies. All parties were
motivated to improve system coordination and integration, with a special focus on the coordination between the state hospital and the community providers. The provider agencies were primarily motivated to
stabilize public funding to allow for greater efficiency and effectiveness and to develop more rational methods for community mental
health planning and integration. OMH was primarily motivated to improve community services to seriously and persistently mentally ill
patients and to facilitate further reduction of the number of inpatient
beds in the area psychiatric center.

The Mental Health Care System of Monroe and Livingston Counties

Monroe County, with a population of approximately 725,000, is served
by four hospital-based community mental health centers (CMHC).
Eleven other agencies also receive public funding to provide specialized rehabilitation, clinical, residential, and social programming. A
handful of other agencies provide mental health services but do not
receive public funding and are not directly represented through the
IMH corporation. Livingston County is a rural county of 55,000 persons, and it receives mental health care from a county counseling service. Both counties are served by the state-operated Rochester
Psychiatric Center (RPC), a 500-bed facility with a variety of ancillary
clinical and rehabilitation services. Other than RPC and the relatively
limited county services, all provider agencies are private, not-for-
profit agencies.

In spite of the relative richness of services for mentally ill people in
the Rochester community, there were a number of significant gaps in
the system of care available to seriously ill patients before the demonstration. These system deficits included the following:

1. Lack of continuity of care as patients moved from one agency or
   program to another;
2. Lack of aggressive follow-up and management of patients to prevent their dropping out of care;
3. Lack of available community programs to treat patients in crisis,
   resulting in a tendency to overhospitalize;

4. Lack of appropriate community residential placements;
5. Lack of education and support for family members and significant others of individuals with persistent mental illness; and
6. Lack of training programs for treatment of seriously mentally ill people.

The CMHCs were planned to assume responsibility for this population but funding was not made available to sustain service programs needed by this underinsured group. The state Community Support Services (CSS) financing stream was designed to fill this gap but was not viewed positively by providers because of its tendency to fragment programs and discriminate against persons in need who did not meet CSS criteria. All CMHCs had personnel and programs for care of seriously and persistently mentally ill patients. However, there were limited resources dedicated to these programs, and it was very difficult to maintain continuity of care if the patient needed inpatient treatment or dropped out of care.

Capitation and Chronic Mental Illness

The concept of having a flexible sum of money designated for the care of specific seriously and persistently mentally ill patients has considerable promise (Babigian and Reed 1987a; Lehman 1987). The most fundamental reason that deinstitutionalization did not result in effective community programs for long-term care was the lack of appropriate, flexible funding following patients into their community settings. Capitation addresses this need in several ways:

+ It involves enrollment of specific patients, thereby designating responsibility for their care.
+ It attaches funds to the patient, facilitating development of treatment plans unique to specific patient needs.
+ It presses the mental health system to maintain a more active follow-up of seriously and persistently mentally ill patients, who otherwise may drop out of contact with services.
+ It creates incentives for providers to minimize expensive hospitalization of capitated patients and to manage mentally ill individuals in the least restrictive environment.

Assuming sufficient funding of a capitation program, these features overcome many of the hurdles associated with maintaining seriously and persistently mentally ill individuals in community settings. Although a high proportion of the Monroe County work force is enrolled in HMOs for their health care, the Monroe-Livingston demonstration did not elect to use existing HMO programs to demonstrate a capitation program for chronically mentally ill people. General health HMOs are designed to enroll and address the needs of relatively healthy individuals and to monitor and limit service delivery. Capitation programs for seriously and persistently mentally ill people must be designed to enroll the sickest individuals and to ensure adequate provision of medical and special services to avoid deterioration of fragile patients. The annualized capitation rate for mental health for an HMO population of members who did not have mental illness would be less than $100, whereas the annual mental health treatment capitation rate *alone* for a seriously and persistently mentally ill population would exceed $10,000. Placing these two groups in the same capitation pool would lead to strong incentives to shed or underserve the costly, chronically ill members.

Capitation Payments System

The Capitation Payments System (CPS) was developed as a model capitation program. Eligibility for CPS was defined in terms of utilization of state inpatient and outpatient services in the past 3 years. Utilization was used as the basis for enrollment not because it is an ideal method for defining chronicity, but because it served as a fiscal yardstick for the state, which hoped to finance the project ultimately through savings in reduced psychiatric center expenditures. Eligibility was determined at four levels, with different capitation rates and levels of care required as shown in Table 8–1.

Five CMHCs were designated as Lead Agencies that could enroll patients in CPS. Each Lead Agency receives prospective quarterly payments based on their proposed enrollment plan, with adjustments made to the next quarterly payment. Initially, there were fairly large discrepancies between enrollment plans and actual enrollments, but agencies were able to project enrollments more accurately as they gained experience with the program. Capitation rates were initially established based on negotiated "average" treatment plans, which

Table 8–1. Capitation groups, care, and rates

Group	Eligibility	Care	Capitation ($/Pt/Yr)
Continuous	> 270 days inpatient in past 3 years (RPC)	All care: room, board, health and mental health, clothing, allowances	39,000
Intermittent	> 30 continuous or 45 total days and < 270 days inpatient 3 years	Coordinate care, provide all ambulatory mental health care	13,000
Outpatient	> 25 outpatient visits at RPC in 3 years	Coordinate care, provide all ambulatory mental health care	5,000
Intermittent with outpatient	Eligible as outpatient and as intermittent	Coordinate care, provide all ambulatory mental health care	18,000

were then costed at community average rates. Other aspects of the CPS program are described elsewhere (Babigian and Marshall 1989; Babigian and Reed 1987b).

There are actually two levels of capitation involved, with the responsibility for the continuous group including everything required for community living (health, social support, physical necessities, etc.). The other three capitation rates do not require any provisions besides coordination and ambulatory mental health care. Unfortunately, lead agencies are not required to cover psychiatric hospitalization of these rate groups, leaving a perverse incentive to hospitalize. This is being closely monitored but has not yet surfaced as a major problem.

Enrollment officially began on 1 November 1987, though very few patients were enrolled before 1988. During the $2\frac{1}{2}$ years of enrollment (November 1987 through June 1990), 650 individuals were enrolled, of whom 91 were disenrolled, leaving a balance of 559 enrolled patients (Table 8–2). The 91 disenrollments included 30 patients who were readmitted to long-term care, 23 patients who left the area, 11 patients who opted for disenrollment, 8 patients who died (5 were suicides), 11

Table 8–2. November 1987 through June 1990 enrollment in CPS

Category	Enrollments	Termination	Balance
Continuous	245	41	204
Intermittent	226	40	186
Outpatient	179	10	169
Total	650	91	559

patients who abridged their treatment plans, and 6 patients who were lost to contact. In addition, two patients were disenrolled because they had improved sufficiently and did not require managed care. CPS patients can be disenrolled through IMH only for one of the reasons noted, and only with acceptable explanation of the circumstances. For a patient to be disenrolled for readmission to long-term care, the state psychiatric facility must agree that long-term hospitalization is appropriate.

Over the 5-year demonstration, total enrollment was originally planned to reach approximately 1,800 patients. Subsequent state fiscal problems have resulted in a slowdown of enrollments. In the development of the CPS program, it was noted that the utilization criteria for eligibility for CPS would have to be replaced with a functional definition to avoid erosion of the eligible population in need of such a program. This is especially true in view of the typically lower service utilization patterns of seriously and persistently mentally ill young adults in the deinstitutionalization era. To avoid a new institutionalized generation, young chronic patients have not been kept indefinitely in the hospital. Instead, they developed patterns of repetitive hospitalization while maintaining some ties to the community. Many of these younger patients have developed problems with substance abuse, and some are quite resistant to any type of treatment.

CPS Program Evolution

New programs developed within CPS Lead Agencies are quite variable, as no guidelines or requirements were dictated other than for quality assurance. Each CMHC has designated clinical staff to work with CPS patients and has established comprehensive continuing treatment programs. Some patients were continued with prior non-CPS therapists in accordance with patient preferences. Organization of personnel around treatment is quite variable. The three dominant individual treatment approaches are:

1. Intensive case management in which a single highly trained therapist (master's level) manages all aspects of patient care;
2. Therapist–case manager teams in which the therapist is the team leader conducting predominantly office-based therapy, and the case manager performs advocacy and active mobile support; and

3. Larger treatment teams, permitting continuity of care in the event of vacations or staff turnover.

Intensive case management bypasses the problems in communication that often beset the therapist–case manager team, but leaves the patient with relative strangers in the event of vacations or turnover. Larger teams are better for maintaining continuity of familiar staff but can result in distributed responsibility and communication problems. It has generally been assumed that it is best not to change therapeutic personnel on teams that deal with fragile patients. However, one program has gone to a transitional model, with one team specializing in preparing the patient to leave the hospital, one team helping the patient adjust to the community, and one team for long-term community support. All CPS teams reported an increased empowerment of case managers to spend money on behalf of the patient. Numerous examples can be cited in which purchase of commodities on behalf of patients has been instrumental in maintaining patients outside the hospital. CPS agencies have purchased furniture, food, pots and pans, dishes, clothing, cable TV, and telephones, and have rented motel rooms and financed down payments for apartments. One agency developed an arrangement for its CPS patients to use a designated pharmacy on a credit basis.

Initially, relatively high levels of staff turnover were experienced in several of the programs. One program lost almost all of its staff in making the transition from a traditional model to intensive case management, as many therapists found the change in roles not to their liking. On the other hand, some therapists find it very satisfying to be free of fixed direct service requirements and to be allowed to provide support to their patients as needed.

This type of capitation requires quite a lot of administration—both within the enrolling agency to monitor expenditures and patient progress, and within the managing entity to oversee enrollments and disenrollments, to manage and distribute funds, and to monitor quality assurance. The CPS lead agencies have added several components:

1. An ability to track and report costs associated with individual patients including units of service provided and services and commodities purchased;
2. An ability to be a payor or purchaser of services including extensive contract development with other agencies, and an ability to

process bills linked with the patient/services data base; and
3. An ability to monitor patient progress and quality assurance indicators by specific patient.

Unexpected Developments

Placements. When the project was in the late planning stages, there was concern that there would not be enough community residence beds to support the projected levels of CPS enrollments. CPS Lead Agency staff were concerned that there would not be sufficient supervision available in less structured living settings, although most patients do not wish to go to another "institutional" setting, even a community residence. Inasmuch as patients must agree to participate in CPS, including participation in treatment planning, lead agencies were predisposed to respect patient desires. As a result, many seriously ill patients were placed in apartment settings at their request, with other options as backups if the preferred setting didn't work out. Surprisingly, many of these patients did much better than expected, encouraging further placements in less restrictive settings that had other support mechanisms available such as case management, psychosocial clubs, and volunteer friends.

Rate categories. Although it was not expected that patient utilization history was an ideal mechanism for selecting and bracketing patients for capitation, there were sufficient indicators to suggest that the higher utilizers were indeed generally sicker than lower utilizers. So far it has turned out that the continuous patients cost more than the intermittent patients, who in turn cost more than the outpatients. However, the differences between the groups are not as large as anticipated by the rate differences and are partly explained by different care requirements. The outpatient population has cost a good deal more than expected due to its heavy use of day program services. This group has evidently stayed out of the hospital only through an intensive, albeit appropriate, use of services. CPS Lead Agencies have found that these high levels of services must be continued to maintain the patients in the community. In contrast, some of the long-stay inpatients have been able to adjust to community living with an appropriate residential placement and limited support services. Although there is relatively large variation within groups on cost, the average costs to maintain the various capitation groups are closer to each other than expected. Ironically, our preliminary efforts to detail cost to society led to remarkably close average annual costs for intermittent and continuous patients at approximately $35,000 (in 1988 dollars).

Capitation Issues in the Care of Chronically Ill Patients

Funding and provision of care for seriously and persistently mentally ill individuals shares many of the same difficulties as programs of care for other types of chronic illness. An adequate program of care for chronically disabled persons cannot separate health from living support and maintenance issues. Patients with inadequate living conditions, little or no social support, frequent victimizations, malnutrition, or other life quality deficits will experience more frequent or more severe illness. A major problem with all types of chronic care in the past has been the lack of awareness or interest of the various service disciplines in working together to coordinate the full range of services needed by these individuals. Dollars have been spent through unrelated funding streams to provide limited pieces of the needed array of services, with little attention to what has been provided by other sectors. This disjointed approach results in some patients deteriorating because of unmet needs or incompatible treatments.

Similarly, physicians and other health professionals experience frustration with poor results and inability to coordinate medical and psychosocial care with environmental and social services. Ultimately, this creates disinterest and neglect and is not conducive to appropriate training of professionals in the care of chronically ill patients. Much of chronic care is funded through tax dollars, as costs are often quite high and patients are usually impoverished after an extended period of chronic disability. With adequate coordination and focused provision of appropriate services, the same tax dollars could buy a great deal more than they do now in overall patient health and quality of life. What is needed is the collaborative efforts of all related disciplines and service sectors working together to provide the full range of services needed by any specified group of chronically disabled patients. This type of coordination is quite difficult in our current organization of service delivery. Capitation may serve as an appropriate unifying principle by assigning responsibility and funding to a single entity to ensure adequate service delivery. However, for capitation to work it must be able to bring together the currently disparate funding streams into a stable capitation fund and to assign an appropriate group to assume responsibility and accountability for total care.

It is our sense that the appropriate locus of responsibility lies either with those groups who specialize in the root cause of the disability (e.g., Alzheimer's disease) or with umbrella agencies that specialize in the management of chronic care and are able to draw on a wide variety of needed resources for different types of disability. The ideal is probably to have the specialty sector coordinate care and either develop or buy a broad range of supportive services. It should be noted that this is a significant departure from the traditional mode of operation of the specialty sectors, which have operated as office-based health care providers. Most HMOs currently in operation are targeted toward health care of reasonably healthy populations, and though they may occasionally provide health care to patients with chronic illness, they are not designed to cope with the range of supportive services needed to manage people with chronic disabilities. HMOs do not routinely have relationships with social services and housing providers needed for care of disabled individuals, and incentive systems in HMOs do not match the demands of caring for chronically disabled patients.

Issues for Resolution

CPS designers had to resolve and negotiate a number of difficult issues to effect a viable program. We will try to summarize them briefly.

Who pays?   Inasmuch as the seriously and persistently mentally ill population lacks insurance and tends to be impoverished, the responsibility shifts among state, county, and federal programs. In the past century the lion's share has belonged to the state but shifted somewhat with deinstitutionalization to nationally funded entitlement programs. Maintaining continuity and adequate levels of funding is probably the greatest challenge for a capitation program of this type. The need to bring funding streams together and to avoid duplicate payment (e.g., capitation payment plus Medicaid payment) can lead to a variety of tortuous mechanisms. The prospective CPS capitation payments are provided by the state, but revenues are collected as available and subtracted from future payments. Because Medicaid reimbursement mechanisms were already in place, CPS planners decided to make retroactive adjustments to the state CPS funding and continue to collect Medicaid and entitlement revenues.

It is important in funding a capitation program that adequate dollars be provided to do the job responsibly. There may be opportunities to save tax dollars or to use them more effectively through capitation programs for chronic illness, but to view them only as an opportunity for economizing is penny-wise and pound-foolish.

Who gets enrolled? Eligibility for enrollment could be defined many different ways based on utilization of services (as in CPS), diagnosis or level of functioning, current inpatient status, homelessness, Social Security Insurance (SSI) eligibility, or some combination of these or other criteria. Procedures for enrollment must also be determined. Disenrollment is an even more difficult area in terms of developing appropriate guidelines and procedures. It is necessary to preserve patient rights and develop oversight mechanisms to avoid unfair practices. CPS allows disenrollments at patient request or at the Lead Agency request in the event that the patient is unable to tolerate community living or refuses to cooperate with the treatment plan. Patients are also disenrolled if they leave the area or are lost to contact.

At what capitation rate? The capitation rate should be linked to the package of services to be provided. The CPS program has four different capitation rates and two levels of service requirement (ambulatory mental health services for intermittent and outpatient groups, and total care for continuous patients). Because of the disparities between initial capitation rates and actual CPS costs, rates were revised in 1990 to bridge the gaps and allow for enrollment of larger numbers of patients. Actual 1989 average group costs and revised rates are shown in Table 8–3.

Table 8–3. Actual group costs and revised rates

Group	Actual 1989 CPS group expense	New group CPS rate
Continuous	$22,000	$28,004
Intermittent	$11,400	$15,653
Outpatient	$ 8,750	$11,672

How should programs be developed?   Program development can be complicated in a capitated environment. In CPS it was necessary to provide funds to the Lead Agencies to develop programs and have at least a minimal functional unit in place before patient enrollment began. These start-up funds were provided by the state and were used to create continuing treatment programs and to allow basic staffing to be established prior to enrollment. Further program developments are funded in one of the following ways. CPS Lead Agencies may sponsor new programs through purchase of services or through accrued "profits" in the CPS program. Because the capitation was adequately funded, agencies have accumulated some unspent capitation dollars. Some of this money has been spent to enroll additional patients in capitation programs as well as strengthening crisis care options and other programs. CPS lead agencies provided CPS funding for additional staffing for a volunteer friendship agency. Other funds may be designated to fill system gaps such as crisis residence, respite care, residential services for more seriously impaired individuals, and work programs.

How is it working?   The general impression reported by staff of CPS agencies is that capitation is an excellent mechanism for managing care for seriously and persistently mentally ill individuals, chiefly because of the flexibility it allows. We have been fortunate to have included an experimental evaluation of the CPS program that will provide definitive answers about impacts of CPS on clinical indicators, quality of life, and overall costs of care. The evaluation, funded by NIMH, provides baseline and follow-up (1 year and 2 years) information regarding 422 patients who met the continuous or intermittent eligibility requirements for CPS. Eligible patients were pre-randomized to experimental (60%) or control (40%) groups, and only experimental patients were posted to the eligibility roster. Experimental study patients may or may not be enrolled in CPS, depending on patient and agency choice. The experimental protocol includes indices of demographics, social functioning, clinical issues, general functioning, family burden, quality of life, service utilization, and overall costs. Baseline assessments have been completed and show no differences between experimental and control groups on any important measures. The second year of follow-up was completed by the end of 1990. Provisional findings indicate as predicted that the experimental group is using fewer hospitalization resources than the control group.

Where do we go from here? There is obviously a long way to go before this project and others are able to provide all the needed answers for the design of alternative methods of financing and caring for seriously and persistently mentally ill individuals in the least restrictive environments. However, early indications are that capitation has a promising place in bringing together the available resources to make necessary improvements in this care.

References

Babigian, HM, Marshall PE: Rochester: a comprehensive capitation experiment. New Dir Ment Health Serv 43:43–54, 1989

Babigian HM, Reed SK: Capitation payment systems for the chronically mentally ill. Psychiatric Annals 17:599–602, 1987a

Babigian HM, Reed SK: An experimental model capitation payment system for the chronically mentally ill. Psychiatric Annals 17:604–609, 1987b

Christianson JB, Linehan MS: Capitated payments for mental health care: the Rhode Island programs. Community Ment Health J 25(2):121–131, 1989

Harris M, Bergman HC: Capitation financing for the mentally ill: a case management approach. Hosp Community Psychiatry 39(1):68–72, 1988

Lehman AF: Capitation payment and mental health care: a review of the opportunities and risks. Hosp Community Psychiatry 38(1):31–38, 1987

Mauch D: Rhode Island: an early effort at managed care. New Dir Ment Health Serv 43:55–64, 1989

Mechanic D, Aiken AH (eds): Paying for services: promises and pitfalls of capitation. New Dir Ment Health Serv 43:1–116, 1989a

Mechanic D, Aiken AH: Capitation in mental health: potentials and cautions. New Dir Ment Health Serv 43:5–18, 1989b

Santiago JM: Reforming a system of care: the Arizona experiment. Hosp Community Psychiatry 38(3):270–273, 1987

Santiago JM, Berren MR: Arizona: struggles and resistance in implementing capitation. New Dir Ment Health Serv 43:87–96, 1989

Schlesinger M: Striking a balance: capitation, the mentally ill, and public policy. New Dir Ment Health Serv 43:97–115, 1989

Sharfstein SS: Medicaid cutbacks and block grants: crisis or opportunity for community mental health? Am J Psychiatry 139:466–470, 1982

✦ 9 ✦

Managing a Mental Health Department in a Staff Model HMO

Kathleen Schneider-Braus, M.D.

anaging mental health care in a health maintenance organization (HMO) is a relatively new task to administrators. Although staff model HMOs have been in existence since the 1940s, mental health benefits were not typically included in the health care coverage until it was federally mandated in 1973 (Bennett 1988). Since that time, the sharply rising costs of mental health care and chemical dependency treatment has moved managed health care systems to examine *who* provides this care and *how*. Currently HMOs obtain their mental health services by 1) contracting for them under capitation agreements, 2) purchasing them through discounted fee-for-service arrangements with or without gatekeepers, or 3) maintaining an internal mental health department. In this chapter, I discuss the philosophical and practical issues pertinent to those intending to manage a staff model mental health department. The importance of purpose and mission, role of the director, designing a spectrum of services, staffing patterns, utilization and gatekeeping, centralization versus decentralization, medical records, and patient service are addressed, based on my experience in managing a mental health department (which includes chemical dependency services) in a midwestern, member-owned, not-for-profit staff model HMO serving 300,000 members.

Purpose and Mission

The most essential task in a staff model mental health department is the establishment of purpose and mission. The *purpose* of any "managed care" mental health department is to provide comprehensive mental health care to a given population in a cost-effective manner. However, it is the *mission* of the department that reflects the organization's values (e.g., profit versus nonprofit; preventive care versus a pure medical mission of serving those who are ill). These values are generally determined by the Board of Directors, who speak for the members or stockholders.

In addition to the overall organizational values, in a staff model the collective professional values of the clinicians influence the mission of the mental health department. This is perhaps the primary distinction between a staff model HMO and an Independent Practitioners Association (IPA) model. In a successful staff model department there exists an alignment of values between the professional caregivers and the insuring organization. This means that each provider incorporates the value of efficiency in his or her treatment planning. Practically speaking, in situations for which more than one type of treatment is proven effective or when research is lacking, the least costly treatment is chosen. The insuring organization, on the other hand, is guided by its staff's professional values as it designs benefits, staffs its departments, and funds treatment programs.

Cost offset studies (Longobardi 1981; Mumford et al. 1984; Shemo 1985) have demonstrated that providing mental health services reduces the amount of general medical utilization and proves to be cost-effective overall. Yet insurers remain reluctant to provide readily accessible, high-quality mental health services because of the enormous rise in utilization and cost of those services in recent years (Gelber 1989).

Managing the cost of health care is frequently confused with the management of health care itself. Managing costs requires attention to funding mechanisms (capitation, copayments) and methods of limiting utilization. Management of the health care involves the appropriate intervention with each patient by the professional best equipped to manage each case wisely and efficiently. A well-managed staff model department is composed of many health care providers efficiently managing the day-to-day care of the members, and a small number of administrators monitoring health care costs and passing this information on to the providers. If the challenge of managing mental health care is ever to be met, it requires the administrators of cost and deliverers of care to collaborate on solving the problems. A staff model department offers a unique opportunity for bringing these two groups to common ground.

The Role of the Director

The director of a mental health department is responsible for the distillation of the departmental mission from the organizational and professional missions. He or she is typically answerable to the Board of Directors through a medical director and/or a chief executive officer. It is the responsibility of the director to ensure that the needs of clients/patients, providers, and clerical staff—everyone who functions within the department—are taken into account (Greenblatt 1972).

There are many practical reasons for a department to be headed by a clinician. It is the department head's responsibility to develop the mission for the department that is compatible with the ethics of mental health professionals (Povar and Moreno 1988). It is the leadership role, more than any other, which requires that the department head be a clinician.

Having a clinician in charge of management is also practical. In the course of treatment there are times in which a therapist assumes the role of advocate for an individual patient (Schneider-Braus 1987). Many mentally ill individuals have treatment needs that do not adhere to the contracted benefits. These instances require a careful balancing of the needs of the individual member with the needs of the whole membership. Shifting benefits between outpatient and inpatient, utilizing special in-home services, or working with institutions that have treatment provided by research grant funds may be the best clinical course for the patient and, in the long run, the least costly to the organization. If these decisions are made by nonclinician administrators, the short-term financial values may overshadow the therapeutic needs. In such a system, therapists would quickly become demoralized as they attempted to provide low-cost but low-quality care. Many such settings develop an adversarial relationship between those members of the department managing the cost versus those members of the department managing the care.

As the director of a mental health department, the clinician-administrator assumes many roles in addition to that of leader and manager. These include educating managers and benefits officers, acting as liaison to employee assistance programs (EAPs) and the HMO's primary care departments, and consulting to HMO sales and marketing departments as benefits are designed (Anderson 1981). All of these require the balancing of clinical and managerial principles.

Although it is essential to recruit talented clinician-administrators, they are sorely lacking in the marketplace (Levinson and Klerman 1966). One such department head lamented that administrators viewed him as a second-class manager because he was a physician, and his peer physicians viewed him as a second-class doctor because he had become an administrator. Clinicians demonstrating interest and talent in management will benefit from some formal training in the field of administration. An organization can make an important investment in its future success by offering such training.

Any large mental health department will probably benefit from having a management team answerable to the director. Competent clinicians with managerial skills can assume a great deal of the day-to-day running of the department and the direct supervisory responsibility of the provider staff. This provides help to the director as he or she focuses on the tasks of leadership, planning, and networking in the greater organization.

Spectrum of Clinical Services

It is important as a first step to establish a conceptual framework that describes and links the services necessary for the patient population. Generally speaking, a mental health department serves two populations—*mentally ill* and *mentally healthy*—with four sets of services: adult mental health, child and family mental health, chemical health, and medical consultation. There is overlap in these populations and services, but it is most helpful to deal with the overlap as the exception rather than the rule. Presented with this overview, purchasers of health care generally breathe a sigh of relief. Although the complexities of the human mind and soul are endless, it is necessary to use a practical framework that guides management strategies.

Differentiating people who are mentally ill from those who are mentally healthy is not typically done. Medically speaking, the mentally ill "patient" suffers from mental/emotional illness, abuses alcohol or other substances, or experiences physical manifestations of emotional problems. When providers document mental illness for reimbursement from insurers, it is often defined broadly (e.g., anyone with a DSM-III-R diagnosis [American Psychiatric Association 1987]). Within a staff model, no such pressure for reimbursement exists, and a more practical definition can be chosen. For instance, mentally ill patients are those who will probably experience morbidity or mortality without some form of health care intervention. This may be suicide, parasuicide, or loss of functioning in the work/school or family environment. It seems clear that health insurance is as necessary to this population as to those suffering from heart, lung, or kidney diseases.

Examples of mental illness in adulthood are affective disorder, schizophrenia, borderline personality disorder, anxiety disorder, and obsessive/compulsive disorder. The treatments are generally prescriptive in nature and require multidisciplinary efforts and a higher degree of case management than treatment for people who are mentally healthy. Treatment strategies include judicious use of hospitalization, day treatment (Sharfstein 1985) or intensive outpatient programs, medication, and supportive ongoing therapy (Sabin 1978) for coping with a chronic illness.

A practical definition for the mentally healthy client is an individual who is experiencing normal emotional pain when facing a difficult developmental step (e.g., puberty or mid-life crisis), a significant life trauma/change, or a problematic interpersonal relationship. Without intervention, the individual will probably cope with the problem and tolerate the pain. Adults who are mentally healthy generally suffer from self-limiting emotional distress. Analogous to any medical self-limiting illness, it is the role of the health care practitioner to assess the situation, give reassurance and advice, normalize the person's suffering, give him or her a reasonable time frame over which to expect improvement, and instruct the person to return if the problem worsens. Brief, problem-focused, and strategic interventions prove most useful.

Research conducted at Kaiser Permanente in California looked at 200 patients who were seen for only one visit and never returned for follow-up sessions. The therapists thought these clients were either resistant, not motivated, not ready for treatment, or lacking in insight. They were not viewed as "good candidates for therapy." These clients were surveyed and asked to rate themselves on a 7-point scale. Seventy-five percent reported being a 6 (improved) or a 7 (much improved). Further, they considered the one-visit therapist "their" therapist with intentions of returning if the need arose (Talmon 1990). This "single-session therapy" research challenges many theoretical models that view "more as better" and equates early patient termination with treatment failure.

At present many models of brief psychotherapy demonstrate effectiveness (Budman and Gurman 1988; DeShazer et al. 1986; Weakland et al. 1974). EAPs, health education classes, and community support groups are ideally suited to these healthy populations. Mentally healthy individuals do not usually require evaluation by a psychiatrist or multidisciplinary team staffing. There is little need for case management, as the client remains in charge of managing his or her own life choices, rather than following careful prescriptions. Marital discord, including divorce, mid-life issues, and adjustment disorders, are some of the most common complaints in the adult group.

There exists a group of patients seeking treatment who fall between illness and wellness. These include people with underlying chronic but not severe psychological problems. Although not obviously dysfunctional, with effective psychotherapy these clients become more successful in their relationships and workplace. Many of these members specifically request long-term psychotherapy in order to develop improved self-esteem or a better understanding of their family-of-origin dynamics. For this population, psychotherapeutic models that are goal-oriented and problem-focused, but respect the significance of the therapeutic relationship, are useful (Austad et al. 1988; Bennett and Wisneski 1979; Kisch and Makover 1990). Defining this group as mentally ill rather than mentally healthy needs to be done within the context of the mission of the department.

For children and adolescents, mental illness is less common and less frequently requires restrictive, intensive hospital services. Exceptions to this are depressive and psychotic disorders in which safety is a major concern. Adolescents with adjustment disorders who pose a suicidal risk generally require a brief hospitalization, with a rapid return of the child to the family setting. Any situation in which the treatment plan includes the child returning to the home requires intensive family therapy focusing on strengthening the parents' ability to take charge of the situation (Neilans 1985). Removing a troubled child from the home for a lengthy hospital stay may exacerbate the parents' loss of confidence in their ability to competently rear their child. Day treatment is a useful mechanism of offering the intensive family treatment while maintaining the child within the home. Vigorous work with schools and social agencies is a necessary ingredient to successful treatment.

Examples of mentally healthy family problems are adjustment disorder without suicide risk, parent-child problems, difficulties associated with normal developmental stages of childhood, and marital problems. Working collaboratively with the departments of pediatrics and family practice is helpful to develop health education classes and community resource lists. Reassurance and brief, strategic, problem-focused therapy solves the majority of these problems (DeShazer and Molnar 1984).

The *chemically ill* population includes those patients abusing alcohol and other substances. The treatment spectrum ranges from intensive inpatient to supportive outpatient services. The *chemically healthy* population requires services including preventive and outreach programs in the schools and work settings. Codependent family members seek help in developing skills for managing family problems resulting from chemical abuse. Again, educational and community support groups, reassurance, and brief problem-focused therapies are most useful.

A final category of services are those requested by the medical physicians. Mentally ill patients present with somatization disorders and chronic pain; these patients require vigorous case management, and sometimes hospitalization and medication (or detoxification from medication). A rehabilitation model that focuses not on cure but on managing the illness is useful (see Chapter 23). The mentally healthy population are those people with minor somatic worries who would benefit from stress management, health education, and managing or changing their life-styles. Brief, problem-focused, educational orientations are appropriate.

Utilization and Gatekeeping

Epidemiological data point to a prevalence rate of 15.4% and greater for DSM-III-R diagnoses in the population (Regier et al. 1988). The disruption of the nuclear family, the high number of homeless and poor, the reduced emphasis on community structures, and the increased use of substances in the population all suggest an ever-increasing need for mental health services. The unknown long-term effects of substance abuse by pregnant women on their unborn children exemplifies the escalating mental health needs of our population. The overall trend toward destigmatization of mental illness and the many scientific breakthroughs that bring hope to people with emotional ills further increase the trend toward increased utilization of these services. As early as 1976, the Community Health Care Plan of New Haven, Connecticut, reported 11.2% of its membership using mental health services. "Emotional problem visits" account for 8.3% of the total health care visits within the plan (Kisch 1988). Utilization figures range from 3%–10% in HMOs across the country depending on size, age of the HMO, and benefits provided (Feldman 1986).

Gatekeeping for mental health services is an issue that generates debate. As an effort to control utilization, many plans require patients to obtain a referral from a primary physician for mental health care. Research demonstrates reduced use of specialty services, not specifically mental health, when a gatekeeping system is in place (Martin et al. 1989). This research challenges mental health cost offset studies (Longobardi 1981; Mumford et al. 1984; Shemo 1985). Many departments find gatekeeping does not reduce mental health utilization (Feldman 1986). Rather, busy primary physicians experience an added burden by the gatekeeping responsibility. The physicians receive requests from patients who have chosen them to provide care but have never actually been seen by them. In these situations, which happen frequently, a physician's choices are to bring the patient in for an evaluation for which the doctor has little time or inclination, or to rubber-stamp the referral. This system is also troublesome to members who require a high degree of confidentiality. This is especially problematic for an HMO's own employees. In these instances, gatekeeping discourages not only referrals but also appropriate care.

Several years ago, my plan changed from a gatekeeper system to a self-referral system. The dramatic increase in utilization that was anticipated and feared did not materialize. The change was well received by members and physicians. However, it was quickly discovered that some mechanism for screening and triage was necessary for these intakes. The department developed an Intake Coordination Team of psychiatric nurses who screened all requests and assigned intakes based on urgency and specialty need. The team allowed the department to provide a therapeutic posture from the first telephone contact with the member. The nurses also served as liaisons with the primary physician when it was clinically indicated. This system also helped the managers to determine the need for intake availability and staffing patterns throughout the department. The 1-year evaluation of this system showed it to be a significant improvement over the primary care gatekeeping model.

There is ever-increasing pressure in the marketplace for mental health departments to reduce costs. The trend of employer groups to "carve out" mental health services from the overall delivery of health care threatens the continuity of care offered in a staff model HMO. Consultants have suggested that if mental health costs are greater than 10% of the overall medical expenditures, a purchaser of health insurance ought to consider seeking services elsewhere (Gelber 1989). This places deliverers of mental health care in direct financial competition with one another. There is a strong temptation to design copayments, gatekeeping, and even treatment philosophies to discourage utilization of mental health services in an effort to decrease costs for the department. But, in the greater analysis, allowing utilization of mental health services and managing the care efficiently will be most cost-effective for the entire HMO.

Staffing and Productivity

Staffing patterns and ratios vary from plan to plan. Scientific study has not established the optimal number of professionals required to treat a given population. The most significant variable affecting staffing ratios is the level of contracted benefit provided by the HMO. This is frequently dictated by state law, which mandates the level of coverage for mental health services. For example, Minnesota requires HMOs to provide all members who have a DSM-III-R diagnosis with up to 30 inpatient days and up to 20 outpatient visits per year. For patients with serious or persistent illness, up to 40 outpatient visits per year is mandated. No exclusions for chronicity are allowed. Because state mandates vary so widely and change so rapidly, each practitioner needs to be familiar with his or her own state regulations.

Several articles have addressed the issue of "productivity" in detail (Boaz 1988; Craig and Patterson 1981; Taubman 1986). The productivity issue plagues most managers, because it demonstrates the lack of incentive for face-to-face treatment of patients built into the staff model. Fee-for-service practice is criticized for providing a financial incentive to create treatment strategies that increase face-to-face utilization. In contrast, the capitated IPA models of HMOs are criticized for providing a financial disincentive to treat, thereby perhaps compromising the quality of care rendered. The staff model removes the financial incentive in either direction of care, freeing the clinician to determine a treatment plan based on clinical need. Actually, there is a subtle *disincentive* to treat based on *marginal* time, because the fee for an additional face-to-face patient does not increase a professional's salary.

In everyday practice, time becomes equated with money. It is every manager's most challenging task to inspire and direct clinicians to fill their schedules with direct service when supervision, research, team consultation, and teaching are frequently strong interests among the staff. One staff member recently described the HMO's employee benefit package to include health insurance, 3 weeks of vacation, 2 weeks of sick leave, and a 10% cancel/fail rate! Policing schedules and looking over productivity statistics are energy-demanding and frequently less than effective. It is extremely helpful to return to the underlying shared mission of every member of the department—to provide members with quality care in a cost-effective manner—and then promote professional responsibility to that mission. It is important to set fair and realistic expectations about a staff member's individual direct patient contact based on clinical years of experience, amount of clinical supervision required, and time allotted for "extra projects" (e.g., participating in research or quality assurance reviews).

Clinicians need to be aware of the trends toward "total carveouts," which threaten the staff model philosophy of care and increase the demand for efficiency. It is helpful to supply providers with information regarding the financial efficiency of the department on a regular basis and in understandable language. Defining a department's costs in dollars "per member per month" demonstrates the clear relationship between services rendered and premiums paid. It is also useful for nonprofit HMOs to do a profitability study. A comparison between the actual cost of an HMO office visit with the fee-for-service charges in the community generates no definitive conclusions, but it gives the HMO staff a useful perspective. If cost-per-visit is higher than community fees, the staff will understand the need to see more patients in order to remain competitive in the marketplace. Staff members will be more inclined to make good time management decisions if they understand the larger perspective on these health care cost issues.

Little has been written on the number of intakes clinicians perform weekly. Members of my department do 3 to 6 per week; some clinicians with a brief model of treatment do as many as 12 or more per week. In addition to new intakes, every clinician needs to absorb intakes for former patients who resurface for more services. One study found 27% of the overall number of intakes to be returning clients (Siddall et al. 1988). Thus, providers who have been in practice for many years may be overwhelmed with clinical work if required to do four new intakes per week. Some adjustment needs to be made to offer new staff the greater share of intakes.

Another variable affecting the number of scheduled intakes is the fluctuation in seasonal demand. My HMO routinely experiences peak demand in January because of the sales of new member contracts and a renewal of benefits for all members. Similarly, October and April are high months for utilization, probably reflecting seasonal variations in mood disorders. Summer and the early fall months are periods of low demand, and it is useful to schedule training seminars, off-site planning retreats, and special research projects during these times. Coordinating staff vacations with seasonal variation is another useful way to optimize staff time. Because few guidelines exist on this issue, it is probably most useful to collect data over time on the demand for services and create staffing patterns tailored to the specific HMO's needs.

Lest all of this sound simplistic or easy, it is important to point out the many complexities involved in staffing a department. If a director has the luxury of building a department "from scratch," more important than the staffing ratios is the hiring of staff whose attitudes and training are a good fit. Ideally, a staff member embraces the concept of managed mental health care and is experienced in a variety of treatment modalities. He or she should not be wedded to a particular theory but should instead practice treatment strategies that have been shown to work and documented in the clinical research literature. The individual should show a high degree of flexibility in working with an interdisciplinary team and eagerly pursue the development of innovative treatment strategies and programs that are cost-effective and of high quality.

The scarcity of psychiatrists makes recruiting them extremely difficult. The HMO setting is still perceived as a second-rate practice that is stereotyped as psychiatrists in small back offices writing prescriptions and signing off on charts. Perceptions of the staff model are influenced strongly by the far more prevalent IPA models. The practice styles in the two models are so different that it is perhaps a misnomer to refer to both of them as health maintenance organizations. Recruiting good staff takes time and a commitment to not settle for whomever might be available and looking for work. The mission and purpose must be clear up front. Quality professionals want to be sure that the department's values are in harmony with their own professional goals. Developing a teaching relationship with medical and professional schools is helpful; research, publications, and presentations at professional meetings are all useful tactics.

Most departments come already made with a culture, history, and theoretical belief system that may be far from ideal. Making changes in the attitudes of an HMO's existing staff is frequently essential and nearly always the greatest challenge in leadership. Autocratically declaring the mission of the department and making policies and procedures for staff to follow is generally not a good solution. Morale problems, staff burnout, and passive resistance can result in reduced productivity. Instead, taking the time to have the mission come directly from the staff will bring the greatest long-term results. One staff member describes the mission as the compass: whenever a problem surfaces, he just checks the compass, and 9 times out of 10 he is able to discover a workable solution. Frequently, institutions have thick, outdated policy and procedure manuals that are created by managers and rarely used, even by new staff who generally get oriented to their new surroundings through word of mouth. The goal of the leader is to have a word-of-mouth culture where the mission of managing health care is discussed in exciting and imaginative terms.

Centralized Versus Decentralized Services

A major consideration for clinic location is the desired degree of integration of mental health services with medical care. In a large HMO with several medical clinics, a centralized department of mental health allows for easier psychiatric coverage and greater programming flexibility, because all the services are at one site. However, it may be less accessible to members.

Offering full mental health services within each medical clinic has the advantage of being readily accessible to members and physicians requesting consultation. Proponents of this integrated system quote studies that show that because 53% of the mental health care is delivered by the primary physicians (Kisch 1988), having the services on-site places the specialists where they are available to the generalists. In a model of decentralized services, each site has a limited number of mental health providers and frequently only a part-time psychiatrist. It is difficult to offer full psychiatric emergency services, a day treatment program, intensive group programs for eating disorders or domestic violence, and health education courses in small multiclinic sites.

A combined model includes a main centralized mental health department that offers full psychiatric services and the potential for treatment programs. In addition, a mental health care coordinator in each medical clinic provides on-site consultation for primary physicians and initial assessments for all patients. Coordinators provide a very limited number of crisis management sessions and, when indicated, facilitate appropriate access to the mental health department. The coordinator performs the very useful therapeutic task of "pre-therapy therapy" (i.e., focusing the patient on the goals of treatment, problem solving, or learning to manage his or her chronic mental illness). Many of the high-utilizing patients with somatization disorders can be managed in the medical setting with a multidisciplinary team approach.

This model is somewhat analogous to an EAP in the work setting. Limited services are provided directly within the medical clinic; more extensive treatment requires the patient to access the central mental health department. Many IPA organizations already use such a model. Frequently these coordinators also perform prior authorization, gatekeeping, and case management as part of their responsibility. In a staff model HMO the coordinator does not perform utilization review duties, because the mental health department receiving the referrals already manages the treatment in a cost-efficient manner.

Mental Health Records

Generally, having a single medical chart for each patient provides the highest degree of integrated care in a staff model HMO. However, mental health and chemical dependency records frequently require a higher degree of confidentiality than do general medical records. At times outside agencies, employers, or the legal system access medical charts. If mental health records are inadvertently released, a patient's employment or child custody may be jeopardized. For this reason it becomes advisable to keep all mental health records separated from medical records. At the same time, the primary physician needs access to much of this information. If a patient is in treatment for chemical abuse or a depressive disorder, this vital information guides the primary physician's pharmacological treatment strategies. The issue is further complicated by the trend toward computerized medical records. Developing policies that take into account both the member's need for confidentiality and the physician's need for information is a major challenge.

Patient Service

On a busy day in a prepaid staff model mental health department, it becomes easy to overlook the impact patient service has on quality care. There was a time that an HMO offered significant cost savings in premiums to individuals and employers. Members were more tolerant of long check-in lines or delays in phone service because they knew it represented a financial savings to them. In today's marketplace, because indemnity and prepaid carriers have competitive premiums and competent staff, the major difference between plans can be the quality of patient service. Some service factors considered important by patients include a customer-oriented clerical staff, nicely kept facilities, and prompt access to care. Also helpful are patient service specialists who will listen and respond to concerns or complaints respectfully and promptly. It is necessary to have a mechanism for patients to obtain second opinions. An appeal process for members who wish to have their particular treatment requests heard and evaluated is advisable; settling these issues directly with patients is superior to having members contact state agencies with their requests and complaints. Much of the patient service needs of the HMO will be dictated by the overall mission of the organization.

Conclusion

A well-run staff model mental health department is a cohesive clinician group in which the mental health needs of a patient population are served within a culture emphasizing efficiency as well as quality.

Mental health care traditionally has been focused on the dyadic relationship between caregiver and client. This has fostered the therapist's role as patient-advocate in an attempt to help the patient solve life problems. At times the advocate relationship included overstating diagnoses for the purpose of obtaining as many health care dollars as possible from third-party payors. This was done on the premise that insurance generally shortchanged the patient in the mental health arena in favor of medical coverage (Flinn et al. 1987). It is this collusion against the insurers that has resulted in insurance companies' mistrust of the mental health professional community. Insurers who manage mental health services without trust in their providers require additional costly administrative services such as surveillance mechanisms (including preadmission screening and concurrent review) and maintenance of confidential information regarding admission criteria.

The field of managed mental health care is young and will continue to evolve. The purchasers of health care, the insurers, and government agencies are all sure to influence the direction of mental health care. Patients needing service will most likely never be strong enough as a consumer group to reverse the trends of cost-cutting. Turning back the clock to a time when health care funding was based solely on the practitioner's treatment recommendations is *not* within the mental health profession's power. If management of mental health care is left to those institutions whose values are based on financial concerns, the result will be a product that is limited and of poor quality. What *is* available to mental health professionals is the opportunity of joining together with financial managers to meet the challenge of providing high-quality, cost-effective mental health services.

References

American Psychiatric Association: Diagnostic and Statistical Manual of Mental Disorders, 3rd Edition, Revised. Washington, DC, American Psychiatric Association, 1987

Anderson RO: Negotiating with the partners: a role of the HMO mental health director. Hosp Community Psychiatry 32(8):547–549, 1981

Austad CS, DeStafano L, Kisch J: The health maintenance organization, II: implications for psychotherapy. Psychotherapy 25(3):449–454, 1988

Bennett MJ: The greening of the HMO: implications for prepaid psychiatry. Am J Psychiatry 145:1544–1549, 1988

Bennett MJ, Wisneski MJ: Continuous psychotherapy within an HMO. Am J Psychiatry 136(10):1283–1287, 1979

Boaz JP: Delivering Mental Health Care: A Guide for HMOs. Chicago, IL, Pluribus Press, 1988, pp 101–104

Budman SH, Gurman AS: Theory and Practice of Brief Psychotherapy. New York, Guilford, 1988

Craig TJ, Patterson D: Productivity of mental health professionals in a prepaid health plan. Am J Psychiatry 138(4):498–501, 1981

DeShazer S, Molnar A: Four useful interventions in brief family therapy. Journal of Marital and Family Therapy 10(3):297–304, 1984

DeShazer S, Berg IK, Lipchik E, et al: Brief therapy: focused solution development. Fam Process 25:207–220, 1986

Feldman S: Mental health in health maintenance organizations: a report. Administration in Mental Health 13(3):165–179, 1986

Flinn DE, McMahon TC, Collins MF: Health maintenance organizations and their implications for psychiatry. Hosp Community Psychiatry 38(3):255–263, 1987

Gelber S: Efficient MHSA care focuses on plan design, not bottom line. Managed Care 2:1–4, 1989

Greenblatt M: Administrative psychiatry. Am J Psychiatry 129(4):373–386, 1972

Kisch J: The health maintenance organization, I: historical perspective and current status. Psychotherapy 25(3):441–448, 1988

Kisch J, Makover RB: Psychotherapy in the HMO. HMO Practice 4(1):24–29, 1990

Levinson DJ, Klerman GL: The clinician-executive. Paper presented at the International Seminar on Evaluation of Community Mental Health Programs, National Institute of Mental Health, Grant MH-25,264-02, May 1966

Longobardi PG: The impact of a brief psychological intervention on medical care utilization in an Army health care setting. Med Care 19(6):665–671, 1981

Martin DP, Diehr P, Price KF, et al: Effect of a gatekeeper plan on health services use and charges: a randomized trial. Am J Public Health 79(12):1628–1632, 1989

Mumford E, Schlesinger HJ, Glass GV, et al: A new look at evidence about reduced cost of medical utilization following mental health treatment. Am J Psychiatry 141:1145–1158, 1984

Neilans TH: Brief therapy in a health maintenance organization, in Handbook of Adolescents and Family Therapy. Edited by Pravder Mirkin M, Koman S. New York, Gardner Press, 1985, pp 55–67

Povar G, Moreno J: Hippocrates and the health maintenance organization: a discussion of ethical issues. Ann Intern Med 109:419–424, 1988

Regier DA, Boyd JH, Burke JD, et al: Qne-month prevalence of mental disorders in the United States. Arch Gen Psychiatry 45:977–986, 1988

Sabin JE: Research findings on chronic mental illness: a model for continuing care in the health maintenance organization. Compr Psychiatry 19(1):83–95, 1978

Schneider-Braus K: A practical guide to HMO psychiatry. Hosp Community Psychiatry 38(8):876–879, 1987

Sharfstein SS: Financial incentives for alternatives to hospital care. Psychiatr Clin North Am 8(3):449–460, 1985

Shemo JPD: Cost-effectiveness of providing mental health services: the offset effect. Intl J Psychiatry Med 15(1), 1985

Siddall LB, Haffey NA, Feinman JA: Intermittent brief psychotherapy in an HMO setting. Am J Psychotherapy 42(1):96–106, 1988

Talmon M: Single Session Therapy. San Francisco, CA, Jossey-Bass, 1990

Taubman S: Developing productivity in mental health organizations. Administration in Mental Health 13(4):260–274, 1986

Weakland JH, Fisch R, Watzlawick P, et al: Brief therapy: focused problem resolution. Fam Process 13(2):141–166, 1974

✦ 10 ✦

Measuring Quality of Care and Quality Maintenance

S. Alan Savitz, M.D.

I n this chapter, I explore ways of measuring and improving the quality of care in a managed mental health care system. Improvement of quality goes beyond measurement of quality alone; it includes identifying problems in the care and in the system of delivery and taking steps to improve the deficiencies. Also, it requires an assumption by management that problems do exist. In the first section, I attempt to define quality of care; the rest of the section then looks at quality in the context of managed care, explores the special problems of mental health, and compares cost and quality concerns. The second section discusses ways of measuring quality of mental health care in a managed care system, and the third section presents methods of improving and maintaining the quality of the care. A plan is presented for quality improvement process in a mental health organization, focusing on some approaches to improvement of care.

Defining Quality of Care

An understanding of quality in health care depends on a usable definition. Donabedian has defined quality care by focusing on objectives: "Once we know the objectives of care, we can define care of the highest quality as that which has the greatest likelihood of achieving these objectives with the most efficient use of resources" (Donabedian 1983). Brook and Lohr base quality on the "difference between efficacy ('what a technology *could* do') and effectiveness ('performance under ordinary conditions by the average practitioner for the typical patient') that can be attributed to care providers" (Brook and Lohr 1985, p. 712). They compare a technologic ideal to the human reality. Steffen proposes that "the highest quality medical care is that care that best achieves legitimate medical and non-medical goals. . . . These goals are set by the patient with the help of his physician" (Steffen 1988, p. 61).

From several viewpoints (Brook and Lohr 1985; Donabedian 1983; Steffen 1988; Vuori 1987), quality is the degree to which the delivered health care reaches objectives, especially those of the patient, within the limitations of technology, the patient's status and environment, and available resources. The objectives may aim toward the ideal but must be stated carefully and be measurable.

Managed Care and Quality

Managed health care was accused of having lowered quality in order to be cost-effective (Ellwood and Paul 1986). Fee-for-service practice in this country had been the gold standard for quality. However, research has revealed that prepaid managed care systems deliver care that is equal to or better than fee-for-service practice (Ware et al. 1986). Of more importance, a managed care organization has a potential structural advantage for providing quality care. A managed care system is organized to control the manner in which care is delivered. There is at minimum a structure that selects providers and monitors the care delivered by those providers. There is the opportunity for this structure to be organized and managed to deliver high-quality care. It need not be hindered by the independent and unmanaged nature of fee-for-service care.

A staff model and an Independent Practitioners Association (IPA) model impact differently on quality. A staff model health maintenance organization (HMO) usually has a small number of providers who can be directly monitored and supervised. They often work together and, therefore, tend to develop a collegial relationship that leads to shared common values. These clinicians depend on the organization for most of their income. In an IPA, the provider panel is almost always larger and more extensive than in a staff model, which allows easy access and more choice for enrollees. However, the IPA panel is inherently more diffuse. The providers are scattered geographically, apart from the plan management, and are likely to have more diverse values. The volume of referrals to a provider has several repercussions for quality. The provider learns to be comfortable with a system when he or she regularly interacts with it. Occasional cases do not encourage this. Review of a provider's work is more reliable when there is a significant number of cases to evaluate. When the volume of subscribers referred to a provider does not have an impact on the provider's practice and income, there may be less reason for the provider to comply with standards.

Cost Versus Quality

Managed health care systems have been accused of underfunding mental health and chemical dependency treatment. A certain level of funding is required to provide appropriate benefits (Sharfstein et al. 1988). Quality cannot be provided with inadequate resources; however, more may not be better. Efficiency can lead to better care. Whenever "unnecessary services" are avoided, there is improvement in care because the risks associated with those services are eliminated. "One of the social costs of excessive stays in certain hospital programs is the 'social breakdown syndrome' in which patients experience a decline in their social and community coping skills" (Caton and Gralnick 1987, p. 861). Quality includes a cost-versus-benefit determination (Wyszewianski et al. 1987). There are indications that benefits of mental health "treatment fall off as the number of contact hours increases" (Knesper et al. 1987, p. 230). However, excluding necessary procedures will decrease quality. When there are several approaches to treatment and they vary in outcome and cost, it is a difficult choice (Wyszewianski et al. 1987).

One can avoid concerns about cost and aim at the "greatest improvement in health; this is a 'maximalist' specification of quality" (Donabedian 1988, p. 1745). However, there are large variations in the lengths and intensity of treatment without significant differences in outcome. And there are questions about which treatment method to select and which mental disorders are responsive to which treatments. Substituting less costly methods often causes concern about quality among practitioners. However, with many disorders there is evidence that using lower cost procedures or personnel improves outcome (i.e., intensive ambulatory care or partial hospitalization instead of inpatient care).

Quality care is efficient care. Evaluation and treatment at the right time can avoid costly long-term care or the need for a more restrictive level of care. Correct assessment and appropriate referrals require skilled providers who might be costly, but accurate diagnosis and treatment planning leads to productive therapy and prevents the waste of unnecessary, inappropriate care.

Mental Health

In mental health more than in other medical care, a disorder may have symptoms that are sporadic and outcomes that are unpredictable with or without treatment. There are wide variations from therapist to therapist and even within the practice of an individual provider. The therapist's personality or attitudinal stance may have more of an impact than his or her theoretical orientation and can often influence clinical decisions. The organization should determine a clinical direction with clearly delineated clinical policies. This consistent set of clinical values allows the provider to know what is expected and to be able to choose, and it allows the organization to be properly selective.

Measuring Quality in Managed Systems

Structure, Process, Outcome

The three-part classification of Donabedian—structure, process, and outcome—is generally accepted as a means of categorizing aspects of health care delivery for quality assessment (Donabedian 1966). Structure traditionally has involved the evaluation of the facility and system in terms of equipment, space, clinical records, financial management, organizational design, method of quality assurance, staffing patterns, and staff credentials.

Process evaluates how care is given to patients and what is done by patients. It includes access of care, diagnostic process, referral, treatment, and patient compliance. It identifies the availability of all the appropriate components of mental health care (i.e., partial hospitalization, family services, ambulatory programs, etc.) that provide effective treatment. In using process as a criterion of quality, there is a presumption that a particular intervention carried out properly will bring about predictable results. This often does not apply.

Outcome indicates the effect of the process on the patient's health status, including his or her subjective feelings. Outcome of care appears attractive as an index of quality, because it seems to indicate what benefit the patient received from all aspects of treatment and it is reasonable to expect quality care to produce positive results. However, the entire process would have to be assessed to determine which contributions brought about the observed outcome, distinguishing the input of the provider from the nature of the disorder and the patient's characteristics. In general, despite the provider's input, the severity of a patient's illness largely determines the outcome (Knesper et al. 1987). Outcomes of treatment include patient satisfaction as well as changes in the patient's mental status, interpersonal functioning, and social performance.

Provider Performance Review

Traditionally, a review process focuses on the performance of the provider. Donabedian (1983) separates performance into two elements: technical and interpersonal. In psychiatric treatment the technical and interpersonal performance are often ignored, because reliable and measurable standards have yet to be developed. At present, patient satisfaction surveys offer a useful approach to measurement of provider performance, although limited by differences in practice type and mix of patients.

Standards

Quality assessment traditionally requires measurement of something compared to a standard. A standard could state, for example, that no more than 30% of clinical records will lack a treatment plan; that 90% of all patients who are being medicated with lithium carbonate will be evaluated in person at least once every 2 months; or that 95% of patients will be offered an appointment within 3 working days. By their very nature, standards for treatment cause disputes among providers. It is essential to involve providers at every step in setting standards. Imposed standards or the perception of standards being imposed will not improve quality. A control system can exist only when most of the providers subscribe and adhere to the standards of practice without coercion. In effect, most providers should not notice an impact by a control system because they will have internalized the standards as values governing their behavior. Standards also require input from experts who indicate what ought to be done as well as recognizing what is done in everyday practice. Idealized standards are unattainable and can lead to a sense of failure. When standards are set low to act as a floor, they could unintentionally become the prevailing level of care. As care improves in response to meaningful and measurable standards, the standards can be raised and quality can be improved further. However, clinicians may fear this continual raising of standards and view the process as a manipulative effort by management, especially if standards were externally imposed.

"Tracers"

A generally accepted method to review medical care today is the "tracer method" (Kessner et al. 1973). A set of standards for diagnosis, treatment, and follow-up is established for a group of common discrete disorders, and the care provided is compared to the standards. This becomes an indicator of the quality of care of the providers and system and reflects the interaction of providers, patients, and the organization. For instance, available standards for the use of psychotropic medications could be developed into "tracer method" review to evaluate psychiatrists.

Patient Satisfaction

An outcome of care that is frequently ignored is patient satisfaction. Although patients may be unsure of the quality of the technical care being provided, they are able to judge the interpersonal aspect of the care. A dissatisfied patient is unlikely to participate or comply with care. This affects the process, and technical skill alone does not compensate (Donabedian 1983). Patient satisfaction indicates the degree to which the patient's goals were met (Steffen 1988). Vuori believes that patient satisfaction is a paramount measure of quality but is undervalued because professionals as a group do not appreciate the opinions of patients. He notes that for a patient with a chronic medical disease, the patient's view of the experience of the care may be the only measure of the value (Vuori 1987). Mental health outcomes often can be perceived in a similar manner. The patient's "subjective" view of the care may be the most objective data available. Patients consistently report less positive outcomes than providers (Fiester 1979). Outcome criteria should include both therapist and patient input. In a managed care system, data concerning the patient's view of care can be obtained from surveys of patients involved in treatment as well as covered enrollees at random. Patients who go outside of the health plan to receive treatment or discontinue treatment early can be surveyed. Patient complaints should be given serious attention and monitored.

Claims Review

Claims processing, when part of a computerized management information system, can be utilized for quality review in an IPA model. All the needed elements are included on the claim form: the diagnoses (DSM-III-R; American Psychiatric Association 1987) and the procedures (CPT-4; American Medical Association 1992). Claims data can pick up signal events that might indicate poor quality, which would be followed up by peer review of the entire process of care. Some of these signal criteria are:

1. Repeat admission to an intensive level of care;
2. Admission to an intensive level of care following outpatient care;
3. Return to treatment after termination;
4. Lack of aftercare in the treatment of chemical dependency; and
5. Providers with high hospital admission rates.

Data elements could be added that would provide additional information (e.g., the name and dosage of psychotropic medication or the form of psychotherapy [behavioral, cognitive, etc.]). If the appropriate treatment for a specified disorder is a series of procedures, criteria can be developed for a treatment protocol. The claims data will indicate whether the appropriate procedures have been performed for that disorder. Because claims review is computer based, large numbers of patients can be tracked with little staff time. Automated review has limitations; it can be used to indicate utilization of services and simple outcomes, but it cannot determine provider performance.

Quality Improvement

Berwick (1989) has studied quality management in industry in order to develop analogous techniques in health care. He believes that quality improvement in health care today is self-defeating, because it emphasizes searching out "bad apples," thereby intimidating providers and making them defensive. He suggests an alternative, which he calls "the theory of continuous improvement" (p. 54). It is based in large part on the work of one of the major figures in industrial quality control, W. Edwards Deming. Deming's approach was to improve each step in a manufacturing process rather than to weed out products or services that did not meet standards or to engender complaints after the products or services had been received by the customer.

The emphasis on improvement of the system and process rather than finding defects shifts the focus of quality control onto management rather than the worker. Leadership, clear values, attainable goals, careful training of workers, and an environment that encourages improvement are management issues. This system presumes that people want to do their best and in the right environment will change their behavior in order to improve the quality of their output. Deming stresses the cost-effectiveness of this approach. Inspection requires "redoing." Changes that improve the process reduce the defects and the cost (Walton 1986). In mental health, poor care can lead to institutionalization or destabilization and subsequent costly long-term care. Traditional health care quality assurance programs have been unable to resolve identified problems, because the focus has been on the individual case and not on the system (McAninch 1984).

Each managed care organization should develop a process that seeks to provide data on its performance and initiates improvements in quality of care based on that data. Quality improvement is owed the commitment and priority of top management and requires the same energy as financial management. The organization must develop a management system and an environment in which quality improvement is highly valued, well-funded, and rewarded.

The Quality Improvement Process

The senior management should establish a set of values for the organization that makes explicit the goals and importance of quality of care and service. Objectives for the quality improvement process should be specific with measurable expectations over a given time frame. A member of senior management should be responsible for the implementation. Adequate support staff is required to allow clinicians to focus on the areas where their input is most valuable, such as problem identification, interpretation of the data, and remedial action. In large organizations the process should occur in smaller units to facilitate greater involvement of clinicians and other staff. Committees should be given the responsibility to search out problems, to establish standards, to revise existing criteria, and to create mechanisms for change in the policies and procedures—all with the goal of improving care. All levels of professional and nonclinical personnel should be represented. The members of the committees must be educated about the methodology of quality improvement. The members should rotate on an infrequent basis so that an effective "culture" for the committee develops. These committees should be linked, because so many problems cross departmental lines. A single quality improvement support staff working with the committees helps the integration process.

Problem identification.   The first step in quality improvement is to identify existing problems. The problems should reflect "what" and not "who" is wrong and emphasize the process of delivery of care. One method of problem identification is to select a common diagnosis and to review the average length of treatment and patterns of care for patients with that diagnosis; wide variations may indicate problems. Another method involves patient complaints and patterns in patient satisfaction forms. Random brief telephone interviews or random review of the medical records can lead to problem identification. An organized discussion by a group of clinicians can also lead to a problem list. The problem list should be prioritized, resulting in a small number of issues that seriously affect the quality of care. Finally, the problem should be worded in such a way that standards can be established and remedial action taken.

Establishing standards.   The problem should be quantified by establishing easily documented measurable standards. Because there are limited scientific data to substantiate the effectiveness of practice patterns, it is necessary to try for consensus on standards. Therapeutic techniques that are generally accepted as being effective and as having good outcomes should be selected. The committee should discuss and then ratify the standards.

Data collection.   Whenever possible, data should be readily available from an existing process and the collection should be as unobtrusive to clinicians as possible. Sometimes the data collection will be in two stages: the support staff utilizing explicit screening standards to determine which records will be reviewed, and clinicians or experts using implicit standards. Confidentiality of the patient record must always remain and be considered when deciding on a data source.

Remedial action. After the data have been examined, analyzed by the staff, and presented to the committee, an action plan aimed at the problem should be developed. The recommended changes in procedure should be seen by the clinicians and other personnel as having specific rewards in improved care. The improvement process should be directed to the process of care, not to the individual, so as not to be perceived as either threatening or punitive.

Monitoring and follow-up. It is necessary to provide continuous monitoring to determine whether change has occurred and is producing the desired effect and that the process is improving over time. In those cases when further improvements are required, the process should begin again, and new changes should be implemented and carefully monitored.

Senior management should be given regular updates of the entire process and standards, data, and actions taken. The results should then be carefully documented and made part of the organizational record. Interdepartmental meetings provide insight into shared problems and are needed to monitor actions that involve multiple departments.

Changing Clinician Behavior

Changing clinician behavior is essential to improve quality, but it can be difficult. If an action seems imposed, it will be seen as an attack on a clinician's autonomy and will be resisted; if compliance with the action is entirely voluntary, it may be ignored. Participation by a large number of clinicians in a quality improvement program may be the best way to achieve change. The criteria and standards should be developed by clinicians and affect areas they acknowledge as important to care. When a feedback mechanism informs a clinician about his or her performance, the focus should be on a pattern of care rather than on a single case. In health care, education alone is often not enough. A system of feedback coupled with incentives and frequent reminders may produce change. Feedback from an audit that is clear and meaningful to a clinician is more likely to affect behavior than education alone (Ramirez et al. 1987). Reminders of simple tasks (e.g., lithium level monitoring) can lead to more comprehensive care. Although on-going continuous monitoring with feedback is difficult and time-con-suming, it is effective (Studnicki and Stevens 1984). In a recent study a group of physicians given audit and feedback were no different from a control group, but physicians educated by "local opinion leaders" showed significant change (Lomas et al. 1991, p. 2207).

Provider Credentialing

One method of maintaining quality in a managed care organization is to permit only competent providers to participate. The criteria for be-coming and remaining a participating provider should be carefully de-veloped, clear, and uncomplicated so that the criteria will be utilized. In a delivery system there is an additional issue regarding providers with widely varying theoretical assumptions and practice patterns. There should be less concern about which training credential a clini-cian has than where his or her practice values coincide with those of the plan. The term "privilege delineation" refers to the process by which participating providers are given access to perform certain pro-cedures for members. The granting of specific privileges usually re-quires that the provider give evidence of competence in the ability to perform a procedure or in the management of a disorder. In a man-aged care system that restricts enrollees to a limited panel of provid-ers, it is important that participating providers not attempt care beyond their capacity. Certainly inpatient care as well as other areas such as chemical dependency treatment, hypnotherapy, electroconvul-sive therapy, and psychological testing could require privileging.

The credentials of each participating provider must be reviewed and updated on a regular basis. Courts have found that hospitals are not just a structure in which providers practice (Gilbert 1984). Simi-larly, a managed care organization is not isolated from provider com-petence. The organization should use the results of provider performance review to proactively determine the competence of its providers rather than be confronted by the results of incompetence. Ongoing education of providers may be required from the organization to ensure that the providers have the skills needed to deliver the care that the organization espouses.

Access

For a long time, prepaid plans excluded coverage of treatment; later, they were seen as building barriers to care (Bennett 1988). There may be a "tension created by a system in which initiation of care is facilitated for the client, while the provider has an incentive to limit subsequent utilization" (Wyszewianski et al. 1982, p. 536). Yet, a managed care system with its limited populations is in an excellent position to inform and educate members in order to enhance access to services. Ideally, a quality managed care system should attempt to bring all those who would respond to treatment to the appropriate services.

Accessibility is a quality indicator that measures the receipt of needed care in a timely fashion, and it is an area that often requires improvement. Obvious standards relate to location, staffing, and hours of available services. Subpopulations (e.g., the elderly or the non-English-speaking) have special requirements. Accessibility requires the availability of all levels of care so that the least restrictive level of care appropriate can be utilized. Measurement of access can be by patient satisfaction surveys, which elicit information about whether care was obtained in an appropriate and timely fashion. Random surveys can identify managed care members who did not receive services although an attempt was made or did not seek care because of lack of knowledge or negative perceptions about the services. Prevalence rates of mental illness are high (15.4%; Regier et al. 1988), which indicates that only a percentage of those in need seek and obtain care. Utilization of mental health services would thus be a measure of access. Primary care physicians who serve as gatekeepers often have limited diagnostic and referral skills, do not recognize mental disorders, and are unaware of treatment options (Gottlieb and Olfson 1987). Changing the system of access could allow direct access of members to a mental health clinician. Another option would be to educate the primary care physician about mental disorders and create an incentive to refer when appropriate.

Assessment and Referral Process

In a managed care system that should provide better linkages than the fee-for-service sector, the assessment and referral process is an important area that is likely to need careful planning. Appropriate intervention and treatment depends on an accurate diagnosis and a well-thought-out treatment plan. The diagnostic process makes the patient's confused concerns and symptoms clear and meaningful—issues that are often presented in a chaotic manner by a patient under great stress. Although DSM-III-R has been an improvement, there are still few hard criteria for most diagnoses. The skill and judgment of the provider are crucial. Appropriate treatment is not determined by the diagnosis alone. Even a specific diagnosis does not lead to a single treatment path. Again, the system depends on the judgment of a provider. When a patient is evaluated, the provider who does the evaluation usually becomes the provider of treatment. Most providers tend to be comfortable with and use only one or two modalities of treatment regardless of the patient's diagnosis or need. Also, the provider's self-interest is a contributing factor in determining treatment.

To properly manage care, a special gatekeeper is needed, one who will expedite access to care. This professional should have an eclectic orientation, be skilled in assessment, know community resources, and be experienced in chemical dependency treatment. This clinician is expected to make an accurate diagnosis, develop a treatment plan appropriate for the specific patient and problem, and provide a brief therapeutic intervention or make an appropriate referral. All of this should be undistorted by the provider's therapeutic bias, limitations, or self-interest. The separation of assessment and treatment is likely to lead to information that has validity and accuracy and can be depended upon for quality review.

Treatment Plan Review

The treatment plan rather than the entire clinical record can be the basic data source for review. The commonly used data base—medical records—is often not a good basis upon which to evaluate quality (Drude and Nelson 1982). Review based on diagnosis alone often does not lead to useful information or feedback for providers. The use of the treatment plan as documentation for review can be helpful to providers, because it includes the strategic thinking of the therapist and the qualifying circumstances of the case. When the evaluation is separate from the treatment, a provisional treatment plan from the evaluator can be compared by the reviewer with the treatment provider's treatment plan. This leads to a level of validation that would otherwise be unavailable. The treatment plan and the measurable goals that are mutually agreed upon between patient and provider can be the criteria for assessing the provider's performance and the outcome of an individual case.

Conclusion

A managed care organization has a structural advantage for providing quality care compared with the independent and unmanaged nature of fee-for-service practice. It can provide controls in the form of measurable and meaningful standards, data collection, a quality improvement process that includes the involvement of providers and enrollees, and a system for taking remedial action. The patient's view of the care is especially important because of the lack of consensus of outcome criteria. Building into the organization structural elements that create an environment for quality care and ensure its delivery is more useful than attempting to monitor providers and force them to change. Easy access for members provides appropriate and early treatment. Selecting providers with excellent technical and interpersonal skills who agree with the organization's values concerning quality makes quality maintenance easier. The separation of the assessment and referral process from treatment will lead to information that is accurate and can be used for review. The treatment plan rather than the clinical record is the best available data source.

There are limitations to quality measurement and improvement. The process can elucidate defects without being able to bring changes that will improve the situation. Education of providers can be ineffective. However, whatever the limitations, it is a necessary process. Some may argue that quality concerns add an additional cost to a health care system that is already too costly. However, when used effectively, a program for increasing quality will enhance the efficiency of the system. Especially where a diagnosis does not indicate severity or a single treatment path, an orientation to quality care with careful treatment planning may well eliminate unnecessary procedures. The science of quality measurement and improvement for health care is just developing and brings special difficulties. There is no single technique or simple approach; a wide variety of techniques that include provider and patient measurements and focus on the structure of the delivery system and its management may be the most productive. Improvement of the quality of care is a challenge to which managed care organizations today are in a unique position to respond.

References

American Medical Association: Physicians' Current Procedural Terminology, 4th Edition. Chicago, IL, American Medical Association, 1992

American Psychiatric Association: Diagnostic and Statistical Manual of Mental Disorders, 3rd Edition, Revised. Washington, DC, American Psychiatric Association, 1987

Bennett MJ: The greening of the HMO: implications for prepaid psychiatry. Am J Psychiatry 145:1544–1549, 1988

Berwick DM: Continuous improvement as an ideal in health care. N Engl J Med 320:53–56, 1989

Brook RH, Lohr K: Efficacy, effectiveness, variations and quality: boundary-crossing research. Med Care 23:710–722, 1985

Caton CLM, Gralnick A: A review of issues surrounding length of psychiatric hospitalization. Hosp Community Psychiatry 38:858–863, 1987

Donabedian A: Evaluating the quality of medical care. Milbank Q 44:166–203, 1966

Donabedian A: The quality of care in a health maintenance organization: a personal view. Inquiry 20:218–222, 1983

Donabedian A: The quality of care—how can it be assessed? JAMA 260:1743–1748, 1988

Drude JP, Nelson RA: Quality assurance: a challenge for community centers. Professional Psychology 13:85–89, 1982

Ellwood PM Jr, Paul BA: But what about quality? Health Affairs 5:135–140, 1986

Fiester AR: Goal attainment and satisfaction scores for CMHC clients. Am J Community Psychol 7:181–188, 1979

Gilbert B: Relating quality assurance to credentials and privileges. QRB 130–135, 1984

Gottlieb JF, Olfson M: Current referral practices of care providers. Hosp Community Psychiatry 38:1171–1181, 1987

Kessner DM, Kalk CE, Singer J: Assessing health quality—the case for tracers. N Engl J Med 288:189–194, 1973

Knesper DJ, Belcher BE, Cross JG: Preliminary production functions describing change in status. Med Care 25:222–237, 1987

Lomas J, Enkin M, Anderson GM, et al: Opinion leaders vs. audit and feedback to implement practice guidelines. JAMA 265:2202–2207, 1991

McAninch M: Quality assurance in the residential and outpatient setting. QRB 10:181–185, 1984

Ramirez LF, McCormick RA, Hull A, et al: The effect of computerized utilization review on patterns of psychiatric inpatient care. Hosp Community Psychiatry 38:977–982, 1987

Regier DA, Boyd JH, Burke JD, et al: One-month prevalence of mental disorders in the United States. Arch Gen Psychiatry 45:977–986, 1988

Sharfstein SS, Krizay J, Muszynski IL: Defining and pricing psychiatric care "products." Hosp Community Psychiatry 39:372–375, 1988

Steffen GE: Quality medical care. JAMA 260:56–61, 1988

Studnicki J, Stevens CE: The impact of a cybernetic control system on inappropriate admissions. QRB 10:304–311, 1984

Vuori H: Patient satisfaction—an attribute or indicator of the quality of care? QRB 13:106–108, 1987

Walton M: The Deming Management Method. New York, Dodd, Mead & Company, 1986

Ware JE Jr, Brook RH, Rogers WH, et al: Comparison of health outcomes at a health maintenance organization with those of fee-for-service care. Lancet 1(8488):10–22, 1986

Wyszewianski L, Wheeler JRC, Donabedian A: Market-oriented cost containment strategies and quality of care. Health and Society 60:518–550, 1982

Wyszewianski L, Thomas JW, Friedman BA: Case-based payment and the control of quality and efficiency in hospitals. Inquiry 24:17–25, 1987

✦ 11 ✦

Legal Issues
in Managed Mental Health

Jeffrey Becker, Esq.
Linda Tiano, Esq.
Sharon Marshall, Esq.

A s with health care in general, a number of factors have affected the delivery of mental health services in recent years. First, the costs of mental health services have spiraled at the same time that there has been a dramatic rise in the utilization of such services. This development has caused many payors, including commercial insurance companies and self-insured employers, to reevaluate the scope of the mental health services that they cover. Second, mental health coverage under most traditional plans tends to be inadequate. This is due to a variety of factors, including the tradition and preponderance of using long-term therapy to deal with many mental health problems. Third, mental health providers as well as insurers who offer mental health coverage are looking for a variety of novel approaches to improve their share of the mental health market. Many of these approaches fall under the term "managed" mental health, which has become an increasingly more attractive option to patients, employers, insurers, and providers.

"Managed" mental health often refers to a mental health program wherein a third party reviews and/or oversees the cost and/or quality of services provided. Managed mental health may take a variety of forms. A company may simply impose utilization review and/or case management procedures upon existing benefits (e.g., requiring providers to obtain authorization before rendering certain services to subscribers). Alternatively, or in addition, a company may require or provide incentives for the use of a restricted panel of providers or restricted number of contracted hospitals or treatment programs. Subscribers may be invited to pay smaller deductibles or copayments if they use certain providers. Further, a company may establish a comprehensive managed mental health program (MMHP), which may be either offered directly to employers or sold to insurers and health maintenance organizations (HMOs) as part of, or in conjunction with, a health benefits plan.

Numerous legal and ethical issues arise in connection with "managing" mental health care. The scope of this chapter does not permit an exhaustive discussion of all of the issues; rather, we will focus on five major issues: 1) state laws relating to MMHPs, 2) confidentiality issues, 3) risk management, 4) selection of providers, and 5) the impact of rules relating to "affiliated service groups." Each subject will be discussed separately.

Establishment of a Managed Mental Health Program

Business of Insurance

The degree and type of state regulation to which an MMHP may be subject is contingent in part upon whether the entity assumes an "insurance risk." For example, if an entity accepts a capitated fee (i.e., a fixed payment per subscriber to cover the cost of all mental health care services, regardless of the amount of services being used), the entity may have accepted an "insurance risk" and therefore be engaged in the business of insurance (1). Most state insurance laws prohibit an entity from engaging in the business of insurance without an appropriate license or exemption therefrom (2).

In some states, an entity that accepts a capitated fee for mental health care and otherwise meets the definition of an HMO may be able to obtain a license as a single-service HMO—that is, an HMO that provides or arranges for the provision of only one type of health care services (i.e., mental health [3]). In most cases, however, the HMO laws require an HMO to provide or arrange for "comprehensive health services" in exchange for a prepaid fixed premium (4). Comprehensive health services include all necessary hospital services, medical services, and other health-related services, including but not limited to preventive services. Therefore, in states that require comprehensive health services to be provided, a plan that offers only mental health care services will not qualify as an HMO.

In some states, an MMHP may be organized as a preferred provider organization (PPO [5]). A PPO is an affiliation or combination of otherwise independent health care providers that offers services to employers or third-party payors, for an agreed-upon fee that may be at a discount from the providers' usual fees or pursuant to some other contractual arrangement. In exchange, the payor typically offers the preferred providers a more certain patient pool and prompt payment. PPOs are designed to provide enrollees with an incentive to use the preferred providers. These incentives can take the form of exclusive arrangements whereby the preferred provider must be used to obtain coverage. It may also take the form of an economic incentive to use the participating providers, such as waivers of deductibles or copayments, or coverage of a greater percentage of the cost of the services.

Unlike an HMO, a PPO generally is not at risk for the cost of services rendered. However, some state PPO laws permit the PPO to retain some risk (i.e., to participate in the financial gains or losses of a plan based upon actual versus anticipated expenditures and utilization [6]). Even in these few states, risk-taking will only be permitted if the PPO is able to demonstrate to the satisfaction of the appropriate regulatory authorities that it will be able, *inter alia,* to provide its subscribers with covered services that meet acceptable standards of care.

In states that have not enacted any legislation designed to regulate or authorize single-service HMOs or the operation of PPOs, the ability of an entity to operate an MMHP that undertakes an insurance risk is extremely limited. This is primarily because a conventional insurance license to provide indemnity coverage does not necessarily permit the insurer to manage care. Further, in most states, the laws governing nonprofit hospital, medical, and health service corporations—under which Blue Cross/Blue Shield companies are organized—while permitting more involvement in the management of care than a commercial carrier, generally only authorizes an entity to cover comprehensive health services, similar to HMOs, as described previously. These determinations can only be made on a state-by-state basis.

Freedom of Choice Laws

Many states have enacted "freedom of choice" statutes that prohibit an insurance plan from requiring that a health care service be rendered by a particular health care provider (7). In a state that has adopted such a "freedom of choice" law, an MMHP that is part of an insurance plan may not be able to limit its subscribers to utilizing only a restricted list of providers or a certain discipline of providers. Moreover, some states mandate that if an insurance policy provides for reimbursement for diagnosis and treatment of mental, nervous, or emotional disorders or ailments, an insured individual must be entitled to reimbursement for such services whether performed by a physician or a psychologist if such services are within the lawful scope of the practitioner's practice (8). These provisions may not apply, however, to a plan operated by a self-insured employer that is covered by the Employee Retirement Income Security Act (9) or to programs operated by HMOs. In these situations, certain clinical professional groups have been excluded from providing services to these members.

Unauthorized Practice of a Profession

In the absence of a statutory exception, state laws generally prohibit an unlicensed person or entity from engaging in the practice of a profession or employing a licensed professional to provide professional services (10). The premise underlying this prohibition is that only professionally trained, qualified, and licensed persons should be responsible for rendering health care services to patients. Generally, HMOs and state-regulated PPOs are permitted by state law to employ or contract with professionals to render services. Additionally, an entity organized as a professional corporation or association may employ or contract with professionals to render services, although such an entity may be limited to professionals of a single type (e.g., physicians, psychologists, or social workers [11]). More recently, some state laws have permitted professionals practicing similar professions to own and be employed by professional corporations or associations (12).

An MMHP that is not regulated under state law as an HMO or a PPO or organized as a professional corporation or association may be engaged in the unauthorized practice of a profession if it employs or contracts with professionals to render mental health services. In order to not violate this prohibition, the MMHP cannot be responsible in any way for the provision of care. Instead, the MMHP must confine its activities to the provision of nonmedical administrative services. In addition, all advertising and public documents distributed by the MMHP should clearly state that the providers, and not the program, render and are solely responsible for providing mental health services to subscribers. In short, these laws make difficult the unrestricted operation of small group clinical practices serving a population of referral mental health patients. It is imperative to know the regulations as they are applied to individual states.

Confidentiality Issues

In general, the same rules governing confidentiality of medical records apply in the context of managed mental health care that otherwise apply to the provision of mental services. A brief discussion of these confidentiality issues follows.

Medical Records

Health care providers have ethical and legal obligations to maintain the confidentiality of medical records and medical information (13). A breach of the duty of confidentiality can subject a provider to liability to a patient (14). In addition, physicians and other professionals may be found to be engaging in professional misconduct by improperly releasing confidential information (15). Statutes and accrediting bodies impose similar obligations on health care facilities. For example, some state health codes require that facilities keep medical information confidential (16). The improper disclosure of medical information may jeopardize a provider's license or accreditation. This duty of confidentiality is limited, however, where the interests of society or the patient require it to be (17).

Courts are more likely to find a duty on the part of a mental health provider to keep mental health records confidential than they are to find a duty on the part of other providers with respect to non–mental health records. This is because of the uniquely private nature of the psychotherapeutic relationship. Consequently, courts are more likely to impose liability for improper release of those records (18).

Privilege

The doctor-patient privilege permits a physician to refuse to disclose information arising from the doctor-patient relationship when the preservation of the confidentiality of that information is critical to the success of the relationship. In order for a communication to be privileged, it must have been spoken or documented in the context of a doctor-patient relationship (19). In addition, in many states, the communication must be necessary for treatment (20). Generally, a further condition of the privilege is that the information be given in confidence to the health care provider (21).

As noted previously, psychiatric records have been recognized as needing special protection, because the material may be quite personal or may concern third parties. Consequently, some states have enacted statutes that deem all communications to psychiatrists and psychologists as privileged (22).

Nonphysician Providers

Many states have privilege statutes that apply only to certain types of practitioners, usually physicians. In those states, it is possible that the privilege will not be applied to communications between patients and other types of health care practitioners (23). This may be significant for MMHPs that use primarily nonphysician providers.

In contrast, other states have extended their privilege statutes to include other health care professionals, such as psychologists, psychotherapists, social workers, nurses, and rape counselors (24). In still other states, the privilege has been extended through the courts rather than legislation. For example, certain courts, in interpreting state laws, have extended the privilege to communications to psychotherapists, even if they are not physicians, primarily because of the highly sensitive nature of the treatment (25).

Exceptions

The patient's right to have medical information kept confidential is not absolute. There are a number of circumstances in which medical information may or must be released, even without patient authorization. The following is a brief description of some of these exceptions.

Subpoena. A health care provider may be required to disclose medical information without patient authorization pursuant to a subpoena, which is a document that mandates production of documents or witnesses in court.

Waiver of the doctor-patient privilege. The doctor-patient privilege belongs to and may be waived by the patient. If a patient is incompetent to waive the privilege, a court will determine who is the appropriate surrogate (26).

Reporting child abuse. Virtually every U.S. state and territory has enacted statutes requiring health care providers to report instances of suspected child abuse (27). Federal law also requires that states that wish to receive federal funds for child abuse programs adopt laws mandating the reporting of child abuse (28). Only the information needed to fulfill the reporting responsibility should be disclosed (29).

"Duty to warn": the *Tarasoff* decision. Under certain circumstances, a mental health care provider must warn a third party of a patient's intent to harm that party. The seminal case on the obligation of a mental health care provider to report a patient's intent to harm another is *Tarasoff v. Regents of the University of California* (30). In *Tarasoff,* the patient, Prosenjit Poddar, confided to a university psychologist his intention to kill Tatiana Tarasoff. Although the psychologist had Poddar briefly detained by the campus police, they soon released him without disclosing the potential danger to Tarasoff, and no further action was taken to treat or detain Poddar. Two months later, Poddar killed Tarasoff. Tarasoff's parents then sued the university, claiming, among other things, that the university was liable for "failure to warn" their daughter. The *Tarasoff* court concluded that, to the extent disclosure is necessary to avert danger to others, disclosure is required (31). Thus, a psychotherapist must warn a potential victim whom he believes or reasonably should believe is in danger of being harmed by a patient. This "duty to warn" has been specifically adopted in other jurisdictions, such as New Jersey (32) and Nebraska (33) and approved in dicta by an appellate court in New York (34).

Mental health care providers must carefully weigh, on a case-by-case basis, the risks of notifying a potential victim of harm at the hands of a patient against the risks of not doing so. Where the risk of bodily harm appears imminent, a mental health care provider should notify the intended victim, but the disclosure should be limited to only that information necessary to protect that individual.

Quality Assurance Records

Most states that regulate MMHPs require that the licensed entity maintain records of its quality assurance activities. These records are usually considered confidential. The public policy consideration underlying this confidentiality is the societal interest in encouraging health care facilities to provide or arrange for services that meet acceptable standards of care. This position has been recognized by courts (35) and by statutes (36) that prohibit attempts to compel disclosure. Generally, to the extent that quality assurance records are confidential, they are confidential only if they are necessary to the peer review process and used exclusively for that purpose (37).

The Health Care Quality Improvement Act of 1986 (38) (discussed in further detail in a later section of this chapter) provides generally that all reports of a medical peer review committee under the Act relating to the restriction or termination of a physician's clinical privileges are confidential with certain exceptions (39).

Risk Management

Risk management refers to the identification and minimization of risks in order to reduce liability exposure. This is an ongoing process that every MMHP should undertake in order to afford itself maximum protection should claims be brought by subscribers, providers, and others. For example, in an HMO or PPO, the credentials of providers should be carefully examined and periodically reevaluated, and directors of programs that include restrictions on access to care should consider incorporating a quality assurance program in order to eliminate or minimize any adverse consequences.

Financial Incentives Regarding Treatment

One area of potential liability for an MMHP is a cost-containment mechanism that uses financial incentives that are claimed to have affected treatment decisions. The theory is that the MMHP may be liable for an injury to a patient if the injury can be attributed to a denial of treatment or the provision of inappropriate treatment as a consequence of a defective cost-containment mechanism (40; see, e.g., *Wilson v. Blue Cross of Southern California, et al.* [41] and *Wickline v. State* [42], discussed in further detail below).

Utilization Review Procedures

MMHPs may use a variety of utilization review procedures that identify and minimize inappropriate use of services and facilities, including mandatory preauthorization for elective admissions, review of length of stay, and monitoring of laboratory and other tests. *Wilson* and *Wickline* cited *supra,* are the leading cases dealing with the issues of whether a third-party payor may be liable to a patient as a result of its utilization review activities.

Patient Wickline was being treated for circulatory problems in her legs. Her hospitalization and treatment were covered by Medi-Cal (California's Medicaid program), which required precertification for hospital admission and assigned an approved length of stay for the admission. Any extension of the approved length of stay had to be authorized. Medi-Cal approved Wickline's surgery and authorized a 10-day length of stay. Before she was discharged, Wickline's treating physician requested an 8-day extension due to complications after the original surgery. The Medi-Cal reviewer approved only a 4-day extension. The treating physician discharged Wickline to her home when the 4-day extension period expired without appealing the reviewer's decision. Nine days after discharge, Wickline was readmitted to the hospital, and eventually her leg had to be amputated to the hip. Wickline brought an action alleging that her injuries were caused by Medi-Cal's negligence in failing to authorize the full 8-day extension. A jury awarded her $500,000.

The Court of Appeals reversed the jury verdict, reasoning that the decision to discharge Wickline was made by the attending physician. The court held that Medi-Cal was not a party to the medical decision and, therefore, could not be held liable. The decision was based upon a number of factors including the treating physician's failure to appeal the reduction of the extension or to seek a new extension upon its expiration. Nevertheless, the court stated that third-party payors could be held liable for "defects in the design or implementation of cost-containment mechanisms" that result in the denial of medically necessary services (43). The decision clearly recognizes that negligent utilization review decisions may result in denial of needed treatment, thereby causing injury to the patient and potential liability for the payor or other entity responsible for the utilization review decision.

On the other hand, in *Wilson,* a patient was admitted to a hospital diagnosed as suffering from major depression, drug dependency, and anorexia. His treating physician recommended 3 to 4 weeks of inpatient care in a hospital. After 10 days, the patient's insurance company, through its review agent, announced that it would not pay for any further hospital care. Because neither the patient nor his family could afford to pay for any further inpatient hospital care, the patient was discharged. Twenty days after discharge, the patient committed suicide. The patient's estate sued the insurance companies, the review organization that was under contract to the insurers, and a physician who was an employee of the review organization.

The trial court granted a motion for summary judgment brought by the defendants; the Court of Appeals, however, remanded the case for trial and indicated that the conduct of the insurance companies and the review agent may have been a "substantial factor" in causing the patient's death. The court indicated that if it were, the insurance company and review organization could be considered responsible for the harm that occurred to the patient. The court added that since there was testimony directly indicating that the sole reason the patient left the hospital was because he had no other funds to pay for hospitalization, there was evidence that the decision of the agent was a substantial factor causing the harm. The court rejected the claim that, as in *Wickline,* the physician must pursue avenues of appeal when insurance benefits are denied. The court indicated in this regard that the insurer had only an informal policy of allowing reconsideration and, moreover, that the defendant had not proven that such a reconsideration request would have been granted. This case was therefore remanded for trial.

This case clearly indicates that MMHPs may have a duty of care to the patients who are enrolled with respect to their utilization review programs. It is, therefore, essential that any utilization review program implemented in connection with an MMHP comply with industry standards, including having a formal appeals policy that is known to both the patients and the providers.

Risk-Sharing Arrangements

MMHPs may have arrangements with their providers that include risk-sharing mechanisms. For example, MMHPs may use "withholds," whereby a portion of the amount otherwise payable to a provider either on a capitated or fee-for-service basis is put aside in a reserve fund, to be used in the event of budget overruns for specified services (e.g., specialist services and hospital services). One of the first cases to analyze the relationship between "withholds" and the quality of care delivered was *Bush v. Drake* (44).

In *Bush,* the plaintiff, an HMO enrollee, alleged that the physician compensation system was improper and the proximate cause of her injury. The patient in question was treated for vaginal bleeding. After several months of treatment, her symptoms were not arrested. She was referred to a specialist who performed some tests and advised the patient to return in a month if the symptoms persisted. The symptoms persisted, but her primary care physician refused to authorize a second referral to the specialist. Neither physician performed a Pap smear.

The patient was later diagnosed as having cervical cancer. She claimed that a Pap smear would have revealed the condition earlier. She also claimed that, pursuant to the physician compensation system, only the primary care physician could perform Pap smears, for which he did not receive additional reimbursement. Accordingly, she claimed that the compensation system provided the physicians with financial disincentives to properly treat, refer, and hospitalize patients, and this contributed to her improper treatment and delay of diagnosis (45). The court held that, if proven, such allegations were sufficient to state a cause of action.

Cases such as these could arise, for example, if a treating psychiatrist is at risk for hospital expenses and refused to hospitalize a patient who later harms him- or herself or another person.

Breach of Contract

An MMHP may be liable under contract theories as well as under negligence theories. Typically, a contract exists between the patient and a third-party payor to pay for medically necessary services. Hence, an improper review decision that results in nonpayment is a direct breach of contract. The measure of damages for breach of contract is all damages reasonably foreseeable from that breach (46). Because it is foreseeable that denying authorization of treatment may result in the patient forgoing medical services, the third-party payor may, depending on the circumstances, be potentially liable for injury or death caused to the patient (47).

For example, if a patient requests admission to an inpatient facility for detoxification and the request is denied because it is believed that the detoxification program can be properly conducted on an outpatient basis, and during the course of treatment the patient overdoses on drugs and dies, the estate may claim that the plan breached its contractual obligation to provide appropriate care. The patient's estate will, of course, argue that inpatient care was the appropriate course of treatment.

Selection of Providers

Many MMHPs use a panel of "participating" or "preferred" providers. It is essential that these providers be determined qualified and competent both initially and on an ongoing basis. This may be accomplished by implementing a quality assurance program that sets standards for credentialing and periodic recredentialing. When a provider fails to satisfy the standards set by an MMHP, the program should take appropriate action including, but not limited to, termination or suspension of the provider's right to participate therein. Failure to take necessary action could result in the MMHP's being held liable for the negligence of its providers.

Patient Actions

An MMHP may be liable under a variety of theories for the injury of a patient as a consequence of a participating provider's malpractice. When an MMHP employs its providers, liability may be based on the doctrine of "respondeat superior" (48), which assumes that an employer directs the actions of its employees and consequently is vicariously responsible for the results of such actions. This type of action would apply only to an MMHP that directly employs providers and would not typically apply to most PPOs.

Recently, a number of courts have considered expanding the scope of an entity's potential liability to include the malpractice of independent contractor providers under the theories of corporate negligence and ostensible agency. These are discussed later in this chapter.

Corporate Negligence

An MMHP may be directly responsible for the negligence of a contracting provider under the corporate negligence theory. The entity, as a corporation, may have been negligent itself in contracting with the physician, or in failing to terminate the contract, and this failure may then be construed as the direct cause of the harm to the patient, even though the actual negligent act is committed by the physician subsequently.

It is well established that hospitals have a duty to their patients to properly credential and supervise physicians (49). In *Harrell v. Total Health Care, Inc.* (50), this duty was expanded to HMOs. The court in that case indicated that, by listing physicians and then requiring patients to use only those listed physicians to obtain coverage, there is an unreasonable risk of harm to subscribers if the listed physicians are unqualified or incompetent (51). For example, a provider might not actually be licensed or may have a long history of malpractice cases that suggest that the provider is likely to harm someone again. Consequently, the court indicated that there must be a "reasonable investigation of physicians to ascertain their reputation in the medical community for competence" (52). The theory could be utilized in connection with other types of entities under similar circumstances. For example, this theory could be applied to any MMHP that contracts with providers and limits the patients to using the designated providers. It also may apply to cases where there is a strong incentive for the patient to use a contracted provider so that his or her choice has been limited in a practical if not legal sense.

Ostensible Agency

An MMHP may be found vicariously liable for the malpractice of its contracting providers under the doctrine of ostensible agency. Ostensible agency exists when one either intentionally or negligently allows another to believe that an agency relationship exists (53).

The theory of ostensible agency has been used to hold that an HMO may be responsible for the negligence of independent contractor physicians (54). For example, in *Boyd v. Albert Einstein Medical Center* (55), a woman who was an HMO member called her primary care physician and complained that she had chest pains and other symptoms. Her physician referred her to an emergency room and arranged for a specialist to meet her there. After an examination, the specialist arranged for tests to be performed at his office, in accordance with HMO policy, and sent her home. Later, the patient called with further symptoms and the physician prescribed pain medication over the phone. The patient died at home.

The court held that there was an issue of material fact regarding whether the physician, notwithstanding the fact that he was an independent contractor, was the ostensible agent of the HMO. The court indicated that the factors to be considered were whether the patient looked to the HMO, rather than the physician, for care and whether the HMO held the physician out as its employee. The factors suggesting that the physician might have been the ostensible agent of the HMO were as follows:

1. The HMO provided a limited list of physicians from which to choose;
2. Approval was required to see a specialist;
3. The HMO exercised substantial control over the care rendered; and
4. The primary care physicians were paid on a capitation basis with a withhold (56).

Provider Actions

A decision to terminate a provider's participation or an otherwise adverse decision by an MMHP regarding a provider may result in a legal challenge by the provider. Typically, the challenge is based on violation of due process (57), defamation (58), interference with the physician's contractual relationship with the patient (59), or antitrust (60).

Due Process

The "due process" clauses of the Fifth and Fourteenth Amendments to the United States Constitution prohibit deprivation by the federal government and by the state or its subdivisions of life, liberty, or property without due process of law. Many courts have held that public and private hospitals must afford physicians some form of "due process" before they deny hospital privileges (61). Some states have also enacted statutes that guarantee "due process" rights to physicians regarding staff privileges (62). The failure of other health care entities to provide a terminated physician with due process in a credentialing or recredentialing procedure also may subject the entity to liability.

Because courts are less likely to intervene if the case before them appears to have been conducted in a fair manner, it is recommended that an MMHP conduct any credentialing and recredentialing procedures as if due process were required.

Guidelines regarding what constitutes appropriate due process procedures may be gleaned from the Health Care Quality Improvement Act of 1986 (the "Act" [63]). The Act provides a "qualified" immunity for peer review actions that meet stated standards of procedural fairness. The Act provides that if a professional review action (64) of a "professional review body" is taken:

1. In the reasonable belief that the action was in furtherance of quality health care;
2. After a reasonable effort to obtain the facts of the matter;
3. After adequate notice and hearing procedures are afforded to the physician or after such other procedures as are fair to the physician under the circumstances; and
4. In the reasonable belief that the action was warranted by the facts,

then the professional review body, any person acting as a member or staff to the body, any person under contract or other formal agreement with the body, and any person who participates with or assists the body with respect to the action will not be liable under federal or state law with respect to the action, with certain exceptions (65).

The term "professional review body" means a health care entity and the governing body or any committee thereof that conducts professional review activity (66). The term "health care entity" means an entity expressly including, but not limited to, health maintenance organizations or group medical practices that provide health care services and follow a formal peer review process for the purpose of furthering quality health care (67). Therefore, the Act provides immunity from liability under state and federal law for HMOs and possibly PPOs, as well as their committees and individual committee members, when participating in peer review activities conducted in good faith and in an effort to further the quality of care provided through the entity (68).

In addition to immunity under the Act, some states confer limited immunity upon persons who participate in certain peer review functions if the action taken and recommendations made comport with "due process" standards and procedures (69). Thus, it is important, at least with respect to peer review activities that may have significant adverse consequences, such as terminating a provider with a substandard patient load, to use appropriate due process (e.g., a notice and a hearing). This may result in the inability of the provider who is the subject of the action to recover damages from the MMHP.

Defamation and Contractual Relations

An MMHP may face a potential defamation claim by a provider if the entity informs a patient that the provider rendered or proposes to render treatment that is not medically necessary.

In *Slaughter v. Friedman* (70), plaintiff Slaughter, an oral sur-
geon, brought an action against a dental insurance company and its
dental director for defamation and intentional interference with prospective advantage. In denying claims for Slaughter's services, the insurer enclosed a letter to the patients that described Slaughter's work
as "unnecessary," claimed that Slaughter had been "overcharging,"
and stated that the insurance company would report him to a dental
association for disciplinary proceedings. The letters also advised the
patients to make no further payments to Slaughter. The California
Supreme Court upheld Slaughter's right to sue for defamation; the interference claim was not before the court.

In such a case, an MMHP might have a defense of "qualified privilege." This means that the MMHP may have the legal right to disclose
certain information to its patients/members. This right applies to communications between persons who have a mutual interest in the subject matter (71). Thus, because an MMHP and the patient both have
an interest in the competency of the provider, the provision of services
to the patient, and the payment for the services, the MMHP and the
patient have a mutual interest in matters affecting the provider's competence and ability to provide services, and the MMHP may disclose
such information to the patient.

The privilege is not absolute, however, and does not apply if communication was made with malice. In the *Slaughter* case, the court
found that the pleadings sufficiently raised the issue of malice to allow
the complaint to stand (72). For these reasons, an MMHP should be
careful to limit its communications simply to the basis for its denial
decisions and should avoid unnecessary embellishments or inflamma-
tory language.

Antitrust

A full discussion of potential antitrust liabilities is beyond the scope of
this chapter (73). However, a few points are worth noting. When an
MMHP excludes a provider because of high utilization and/or professional incompetency, the entity's conduct may be subject to antitrust
challenge by the excluded provider. The general rule is that the conduct will not be *per se* (74) illegal but will be tested under the rule of
reason (75). Under the rule of reason test, the challenged activity will
be upheld where legitimate, pro-competitive interests outweigh the
potential anticompetitive effects (76).

In general, the *per se* rule will be applied only to conduct that has been deemed to be so inherently noncompetitive that there is no reason to further analyze the conduct. For example, price-fixing is considered to be *per se* illegal, and if proven, will result in liability, notwithstanding any further analysis as to the purpose or effect of price-fixing (77). Generally, the exclusion of providers has not been deemed to be *per se* illegal. So long as the defendant's market share is within reasonable bounds (78) and the defendant has a reasonable business justification for limiting the provider panel, these justifications are likely to prevail over the interests of a single provider in remaining on the panel.

For example, let us assume an MMHP determines that it only needs 5 psychiatrists on its panel, although there are 25 in the community. The MMHP may have significant utilization review requirements, referral procedures, and other rules and regulations that must be followed closely by participating providers. Furthermore, the MMHP may limit its patient/beneficiaries to participating providers, and thus must conduct a thorough credentialing process. Accordingly, the MMHP may conclude that some of the providers do not qualify, based on its credentialing requirements, and further, that the psychiatrists will be more likely to comply with the procedures, and it will be more able to monitor such compliance, if a limited number of psychiatrists participate. Although one or more of the nonparticipating psychiatrists may lose some patients as a result of this action, it is not likely to constitute an antitrust violation, so long as the particular MMHP does not have a significant market share in the community and the decision to exclude the other providers is made by persons or entities who are not themselves in competition with the excluded providers.

As long as the defendant succeeds in having the court apply the rule of reason test, the beneficial effects of limiting the provider panel to cost-effective, quality providers are likely to prevail over the interest of a single physician in remaining on the panel, at least where the defendant's market share is within reasonable bounds (78).

With respect to an exclusion of a provider for either utilization review or professional competency criteria, so long as the MMHP acts in good faith, without malice, and provides "due process" protection for the excluded provider, the entity in question may be entitled to an exemption from liability pursuant to various state statutes (79) as well as the Act (80).

Affiliated Service Groups

As indicated, many MMHPs utilize a panel of "participating" or "preferred" providers. An MMHP may contract directly with such providers. Alternatively, the providers may organize an individual or independent practice association (IPA), which contracts with an MMHP on behalf of the providers, or the program itself may be organized as a professional corporation or association (PC). Where the providers organize as an IPA or if the program is a PC, the providers should be aware of certain tax considerations, including the impact of the rules relating to "affiliated service groups" (ASGs).

Section 414(m) is one of several provisions of the Internal Revenue Code (81) designed to prevent the unequal contribution of funds to employee benefit plans, primarily in the professional corporation area, by the separate incorporation of each professional in a corporation or the formation of a separate company for nonprofessional employees. Section 414(m) provides that whenever employers enter into certain relationships with each other, they will be treated as an ASG for purposes of determining the tax qualified status of their pension, profit sharing, or certain other employee benefit plans. As a result of being deemed an ASG, all employees of the affiliated employers are thereafter aggregated and treated as if they were employed by a single employer. This is for the purpose of determining whether the employee benefit plans for each employer meet the requirements in Section 414(m)(4) that such plans not discriminate in favor of highly compensated employees.

When employers are deemed an ASG, it is necessary to establish that each of the affiliated employer's employee benefit plans is comparable to all of the other plans. If certain plans fail to meet the qualification requirements, those plans will be disqualified, resulting in unfavorable tax consequences. For example, contributions to such plans may cease to be deductible to the employer, or the employee may be required to pay tax on the sums contributed on his or her behalf at the time they are contributed by the employer.

It does not appear from the legislative history of the law that IPA-type entities were intended to be covered by the rules relating to ASGs; however, the literal language of the statute seems to suggest otherwise. Therefore, whether an MMHP's providers organize as an IPA or the MMHP is a PC, the providers should be aware of the potential risk and should structure their relationships, to the extent possible, to avoid the application of these rules.

Summary

An MMHP should be structured and operated in compliance with the laws of the state in which it will be offered. In this regard, the program may need either to be licensed as a single-service HMO or a PPO, or to otherwise avoid assuming an insurance risk. A program that is part of an insurance plan must comply with applicable "freedom of choice" laws that may prohibit the program from restricting subscribers to using a limited number of providers or a particular kind of provider to render a covered service. Further, if the MMHP is not regulated as an HMO or a PPO, it must comply with the laws regarding the unauthorized practice of a profession and should be cautious in its advertising materials and other public documents to reflect the proper relationship between the program and its providers and to stress that the responsibility for provision of treatment lies with the providers.

The MMHP must be sure to maintain the confidentiality of patient records and communications, particularly in light of the uniquely private nature of the psychotherapeutic relationship. However, at the same time, the program must be aware of the important exceptions to the confidentiality requirement, including the obligation to disclose a patient's intent to harm another.

Cost-containment measures by an MMHP constitute a valid and appropriate method for controlling the spiraling costs of mental health care. However, the use of such measures may increase an MMHP's potential liability if an injury to a patient can be attributed to a denial of treatment or the provision of inappropriate treatment as a consequence of defective cost-containment measures. The *Wickline* and *Bush* decisions set the stage for further developments in the allocation of legal responsibilities in this area. Therefore, MMHPs that employ rigorous cost-containment measures should establish equally rigorous quality assurance programs to ensure that the cost-containment measures do not negatively affect the quality of care rendered.

An MMHP could be held liable for the negligence of its "participating" or "preferred" providers based on a variety of theories, including "respondent superior," corporate negligence, and ostensible agency. Accordingly an MMHP that uses such providers should verify that they are qualified and competent initially and on an ongoing basis. In addition, MMHPs should check the sufficiency of their own malpractice coverage to ensure that they are adequately covered against liabilities that may arise.

Any decision by an MMHP that adversely affects a provider's participation therein could be the basis of a lawsuit brought by the provider. However, if the program's decision is made in good faith and in an effort to further the quality of care, and if the provider is afforded due process, a court will be less likely to intervene. Due process should include, at a minimum:

1. Not having a competitor of the provider participate in the decision-making process;
2. The right to a hearing;
3. The right to be represented at the hearing; and
4. The right to present evidence and cross-examine witnesses.

In addition, the Health Care Quality Improvement Act of 1986 and certain state statutes limit the liability exposure of MMHPs with respect to peer review activities that meet due process standards and procedures.

Finally, if the MMHP is organized as a PC or the "participating" or "preferred" providers are organized as an IPA, the providers should be aware of certain tax considerations, including the impact of the rules relating to affiliated service groups.

Notes

1. See, e.g., 7 Op. Att'y Gen. (Conn.) 10 (Nov 13, 1911) (A contract issued to individuals to cover the cost of counsel to protect them against all accident claims up to an amount not exceeding $4,000 in exchange for an annual premium of $10.00 was business of insurance); State v Blue Crest Plans, Inc., 72 A.D.2d 713, 421 N.Y.S.2d 579 (1st Dep't 1979); State v Abortion Information Agency, Inc., 37 A.D.2d 142, 145, 330 N.Y.S.2d 927, 929 (1st Dep't 1971), aff'd, 30 N.Y.2d 779, 285 N.E.2d 317, 334 N.Y.S.2d 174 (1972) (The practice of an abortion referral agency in guaranteeing its clients that a comprehensive fee would cover all expenses, even if minor complications required additional treatment, constituted unauthorized insurance); (N.Y. Ins. Law 1109(b) (McKinney 1985), but see Yale Health Plan Not Defined as Insurance, Insurance Administrative Code. AGO-25, AGO 29 (Conn. January 17, 1974); Op. Att'y Gen. (Wis.) 192 (1936); 2 Op. Att'y Gen. (Mass.) 226 (1900).
2. See, e.g., Cal. Ins. Code 700(a) (West 1979 & Supp. 1989); Conn. Gen. Stat. 38-20(a) (1989); Fla. Stat. Ann. 624.11(1) (West 1984); Mass. Gen. Laws Ann. ch. 175, 32 (1987); N.J. Stat. Ann. 17B:17-13(b).
3. Cal. Health & Safety Code 1343(a) (West 1979); N.C. Gen. Stat. 57B-1 et

seq.; Tex. Ins. Code. art. 20A.03 (1989).

4. See, e.g., Ill. Rev Stat. Ann. ch. 111 1/2 1420 (Smith Hurd 1987); Kan Stat. Ann. 40-3202(b),(e), f(1) (1986); N.Y. Pub. Health Law 4401(1) (McKinney 1985).

5. See, e.g., Cal. Ins. Code 10133(b) and (c) (West Supp. 1989); Fla. Stat. Ann. 627.6695 et seq. (Supp. 1989); Mass. Gen. Laws Ann. ch. 176I (Supp. 1989); 50 Pa. Cons. Stat. Ann. 764a et seq (Purdon Supp. 1989).

6. See, e.g., Mass. Gen. Laws Ann. ch. 1761 et seq (Supp. 1989) Mass. Reqs. Code tit 211, 51.02(12); 40 Pa. Cons. Stat. Ann. 764a et seq (Purdon Supp. 1989), 31 Pa. Code 152.2.

7. See, e.g., Conn. Gen. Stat. 38-167(9) (1989); Mo. Rev Stat. 375.936(11) (Vernon 1968 & Supp. 1989); N.C. Gen. Stat. 58-260 (1982); N.Y. Ins. Law 3216(d)(1)(I) (McKinney 1985).

8. See, e.g., N.C. Gen. Stat. 58-260 (1982); N.J. Stat. Ann. 17B:30-15 (1985 & Supp. 1989); N.Y. Ins. Law 3216(d)(1)(I) (McKinney 1985 & Supp. 1990).

9. 29 U.S.C. 1001 et seq. (1985 & Supp. 1989). According to these provisions, a self-insured company covered by ERISA is exempt from the application of state laws governing insurance.

10. See, e.g., McMurdo v Getter, 298 Mass. 363, 10 N.E.2d 139 (1937) (licensed practitioner of a profession, in the absence of a statutory exception, may not lawfully practice his profession as a servant of an unlicensed person or corporation, and, if he does so, the employer is guilty of practicing such profession without a license); 28 Op. Att'y Gen. (Conn.) 248 (1954); Conn. Gen. Stat. Ann. 20-9 (West 1989) repealed by and substituted in lieu thereof 1989 Conn. Pub. Acts 89-389, 4; Mass. Gen. Laws Ann. ch. 112, 52; Mass. Admin. Code tit. 234 2.04(3);N.J. Stat. Ann. 45:9-22 (West 1978 & Supp. 1989); N.Y. Educ. Law 6512 (McKinney 1985); 63 Pa. Cons. Stat. Ann. 129.

11. See, e.g., Conn. Gen. Stat. Ann. 33-182c (West 1987); N.Y. Bus. Corp. Law 1503(a) (McKinney 1986).

12. See, e.g., N.J. Stat. Ann. 14A:17-5 (West Supp. 1989).

13. An example of a physician's ethical obligation to maintain the confidentiality of patient information is set out in Article 9 of American Medical Association Principles of Medical Ethics, Current Opinions of the Judicial Council (1984):

> A physician may not reveal the confidences entrusted to him in the course of medical attendance, or the deficiencies he may observe in the character of patients, unless it becomes necessary in order to protect the welfare of the individual or community.

14. See, e.g., Doe v Roe, 93 Misc.2d 201, 400 N.Y.S.2d 668 (Sup. Ct. New York County 1977); Horne v Patton, 291 Ala. 701, 287 So. 2d 824 (1973).

15. See, e.g., Mississippi State Board of Psychological Examiners v Hosford, 508 So.2d 1049 (Miss. 1987) reh'g denied July 15, 1987 (Psychologist's license suspended for breaching duty of confidentiality in violation of profession ethics.); N.Y. Educ. Law 6509-6511 (McKinney 1985 & Supp. 1990); 8 N.Y.C.R.R. 29.2(b)(8) (1988).

16. See, e.g., N.J. Stat. Ann. 26:23-27 (West 1987); N.Y. Pub. Health Law 2805(g)(3) (McKinney 1985); 10 N.Y.C.R.R. 405-10(a)(5) (1989).

17. Lipari v Sears, Roebuck & Co., 497 F. Supp. 185, 193 (D. Neb. 1980), MacDonald v Clinger, 84 A.D.2d 482, 487, 446 N.Y.S.2d 801, 805 (4th Dep't 1982); McIntosh v Milano, 168 N.J. Super. 466, 490, 403 A.2d 500, 511-512 (Law. Div (1979); Tarasoff v Regents of University of California, 17 Cal. 3d 425, 131 Cal. Rptr. 14, 551 P.2d 334 (1976); Hague v Williams, 37 N.J. 328, 181 A.2d 345 (1962).

18. See, e.g., Doe v Roe, 93 Misc. 2d 201, 400 N.H.S.2d 668 (Sup. Ct. New York County 1977); Allred v State, 554 P.2d 411 (Alaska 1976).

19. Polsky v Union Mut. Stock Life Ins. Co., 80 A.D.2d 777, 436 N.Y.S.2d 744 (1st Dep't 1981); Horne v Patton, 291 Ala. 701, 287 So. 2d 824 (1973).

20. See, e.g., People v Capra, 17 N.Y.2d 670, 216 N.E.2d 610, 269 N.Y.S.2d 451 (1966) (Patient who was injured in a car accident was rushed to a hospital. In the course of treatment, the patient's socks were removed and a package of heroin fell out. The court held that the heroin was admissible and not privileged.); Nev Rev Stat. 49.225 (1986 & Supp. 1989); Wis. Stat. Ann. 905.04(2) (9175 & Supp. 1989).

21. State v Cramer, 11 Wis. 2d 553, 283 N.W. 2d 625 (1979), aff'd 98 Wis. 2d 416, 296 N.W. 2d 921 (1980), Cert. denied, 450 U.S. 924 (1981); Allred v State, 554 P.2d 411 (Alaska 1976); 8 Wigmore, Evidence 2381 (McNaughton rev 1961).

22. See, e.g., Mass. Ann. Laws ch. 233, 20B (1986 & Supp. 1989); Mont. Code Ann. 26-1-805 and 26-1-807 (1989); Wis. Stat. Ann. 905.04(2) (1975 & Supp. 1989). Information relating to drug and alcohol abuse is also afforded special protection for the same reasons. For example, the Comprehensive Alcohol Abuse and Alcoholism Prevention, Treatment and Rehabilitation Act of 1970, 42 U.S.C. 290dd-3 (Supp. 1989), and the Drug Abuse Office and Treatment Act of 1972, 42 U.S.C. 290ee-3 (Supp. 1989), prohibit the disclosure of any information regarding a patient who has been diagnosed as an alcoholic or a drug addict or has been treated for alcohol or drug abuse, with some exceptions.

23. E.g., Belichick v Belichick, 37 Ohio App. 2d 95, 307 N.E.2d 270 (1973).

24. See, e.g., Ill. Ann. Stat. ch 110, 8-802.1 (1984); Mont. Code. Ann. 26-1-806 through 810 (1983); Nev Rev Stat. 49.215, 49-290 (1981); N.Y. Civ Prac. L. & R. 4507 and 4508 (McKinney 1989); Wis. Stat. Ann. 905.04 (1975).

25. Allred v State, 554 P.2d 411 (Alaska 1976).

26. See, e.g., Mass. Gen. Laws Ann. ch. 233 20B (West Supp. 1984-85), which provides that where a patient is incompetent to waive the patient-psychiatrist privilege, a court may appoint someone to so decide on his behalf. Accord Nagle v Hooks, 296 Md. 123, 460 A.2d 40 (1983).

27. See, e.g., Conn. Gen. Stat. Ann. 17-38 a & b (West 1988 & West Cum. Supp. 1989); Md. Fam. Law Code Ann. 5-7101 et seq. (1989); N.J. Stat. Ann. 9:6-1 et seq. (West Cum. Supp. 1984-85).

28. 42 U.S.C. 5101 et seq. (1976); 45 C.F.R. 1340 (1984).

29. State v Andring, 342 N.W.2d 128, 132 (Minn. 1984) (Statements made in group therapy session remained privileged, notwithstanding child abuse

reporting requirements, because information needed to protect child was already known).

30. Tarasoff v Regents of Univ of Cal., 17 Cal. 3d 425, 131 Cal. Rptr. 14, 551 P.2d 334 (1976).

31. Id. at 442, 131 Cal. Rptr. at 27, 551 P.2d at 347.

32. McIntosh v Milano, 168 N.J. Super. 466, 490, 403 A.2d 500, 511-12 (Law Div 1979).

33. Lipari v Sears, Roebuck & Co., 497 F. Supp. 185, 193 (D. Neb. 1980).

34. MacDonald v Clinger, 84 A.D.2d 482, 487, 446 N.Y.S.2d 801, 805 (4th Dep't 1982) ("[w]here a patient may be a danger to himself or others, a physician is required to disclose to the extent necessary to protect a threatened interest."), Shaw v Glickman, 45 Md. App. 718, 415 A.2d 625 (1980).

35. Doe v Young, 95 A.D.2d 673, 463 N.Y.S.2d 460 (1st Dep't 1983); Cofone v Westerly Hosp., 504 A.2d 998 (R.I. 1986).

36. Ill. Stat. Ann. ch. 110, 8-2101 (Smith-Hurd 1988); N.Y. Educ. Law 6527(3) (McKinney Supp. 1989).

37. See, e.g., State ex rel. Fostoria Daily Review Co. v Fostoria Hosp. Ass'n, 44 Ohio St. 3d 111, 541 N.E.2d 587 (1989); Barnes v Whittington, 751 S.W.2d 493 (Tex. 1988).

38. 42 U.S.C. 11101 et seq. (1986).

39. 42 U.S.C. 11137(b)(1) (1986).

40. See, e.g., Wilson v Blue Cross of Southern California, et al., 271 Cal. Rptr. 876, 222 Cal. App. 3d 660 (1990); Wickline v State, 192 Cal. App. 3d 1630, 239 Cal. Rptr. 810 (1986); Harrell v Total Health Care, Inc., No. WD 39809 (Mo. Ct. App. Apr. 25, 1989) (Westlaw, MO-C5 database, 1989 W.L. 39311), aff'd, 781 S.W.2d 58 (Mo. 1989).

41. 271 Cal. Rptr. 876, 22 Cal. App. 3d 660 (1990).

42. Wickline v State, 192 Cal. App. 3d 1630, 239 Cal. Rptr. 810 (1986).

43. 239 Cal. Rptr. at 819.

44. Bush v Drake, No. 86-25767 (Mich. Cir. Ct. Saginaw County Apr. 27, 1989).

45. Slip op. at 2.

46. Restatement (Second) of Contracts 351.

47. Cf. Calabria v Associated Hospital Service, 459 F. Supp. 946 (S.D.N.Y. 1978), aff'd, 610 F.2d 806 (2d Cir. 1979).

48. Restatement (Second) of Agency 219. See also Sloan v Metropolitan Health Council of Indianapolis, Inc., 516 N.E.2d 1104 (Ind. Ct. App. 1987).

49. Blanton v Moses H. Cone Memorial Hosp., Inc., 319 N.C. 372, 354 S.E.2d 455, 457 (1987); Johnson v Misericordia Community Hosp., 99 Wis. 2d 708, 301 N.W.2d 156, 164 (1981); Cronic v Doud, 168 Ill. App. 3d 665, 523 N.E.2d 176 (1988); Elam v College Park, 132 Cal. App. 3d 332, 183 Cal. Rptr. 156 (1982).

50. Harrell v Total Health Care, Inc., No. WD 39809 (Mo Ct. App. Apr. 25, 1989) (Westlaw, MO-C5 data base, 1989 W.L. 39311), aff'd, 781 S.W.2d 58 (Mo. 1989).

51. Slip op. at 5.

52. Id.

53. See Restatement (Second) of Agency 8, 159 (apparent authority of agent); Quintal v Laurel Grove Hosp., 62 Cal. 2d 154, 41 Cal. Rptr. 577, 397 P.2d 161 (1964) (whether physician was ostensible agent of hospital is a jury question); Mduba v Benedictine Hosp., 52 A.D.2d 450, 384 N.Y.S.2d 527 (3d Dep't 1976) (emergency room physicians may be named agents of the hospital despite independent contractor language in their contracts).

54. Boyd v Albert Einstein Medical Center, 377 Pa. Super. 609, 547 A.2d 1229 (1988); Schleier v Kaiser Foundation Health Plan of the Mid-Atl. States, Inc., 876 F.2d 174 (D.C. Cir 1989).

55. Boyd v Albert Einstein Medical Center, 377 Pa. Super. 609, 547 A.2d 1229 (1988).

56. 547 A.2d at 1235.

57. See, e.g., Greisman v Newcomb Hosp., 40 N.J. 3389, 192 A.2d 817 (1963); Ascherman v San Francisco Medical Society, 39 Cal. App. 3d 623, 114 Cal. Rptr. 681 (1974); Bricker v Sceva Speare Memorial Hosp., 111 N.H. 276, 281 A.2d 589, cert. denied, 404 U.S. 995 (1971).

58. See, e.g., Slaughter v Friedman, 32 Cal. 3d 149, 185 Cal. Rptr. 244, 649 P.2d 886 (1982) (defamation interference with prospective economic advantage).

59. See, e.g., Teale v American Manufacturers Mut. Ins. Co., 687 S.W.2dd 218 (Mo. Ct. App. 1985) (tortious interference with doctor-patient relationship by association of anesthesiologists against group medical insurer for insurer's letters to former patients advising that claims would not be paid in full because association's charges were excessive).

60. See, e.g., Patrick v Burget, 800 F.2d 1498 (9th Cir. 1986), rev'd, 486 U.S. 94 (1988) (Oregon physicians held liable in antitrust action for initiating and participating in a peer review proceeding in order to reduce competition rather than to improve patient care. In order to be immune from federal antitrust liability under the state action doctrine, the anticompetitive conduct engaged in by private parties must be clearly articulated and affirmatively expressed as state policy and actively supervised by the state. State action doctrine does not protect physicians from antitrust liability where Oregon does not actively supervise peer review activities).

61. See, e.g., Greisman v Newcomb Hosp., 40 N.J. 389, 192 A.2d 817 (1963); Ascherman v San Francisco Medical Society, 39 Cal. App. 3d 623, 114 Cal. Rptr. 681 (1974); Bricker v Sceva Speare Memorial Hosp., 111 N.H. 276, 281 A.2d 589, cert. denied, 404 U.S. 995 (1971); Woodard v Porter Hosp., Inc., 125 Vt. 419, 217 A.2d 37 (1966); contra Monyek v Parkway Gen'l Hosp., Inc., 273 So. 2d 430 (Fal. Dist. Ct. App. 1973); Bello v South Shore Hosp., 384 Mass. 770, 429 N.E.2d 1011 (1981).

62. N.Y. Pub. Health Law 2801-b (McKinney 1985 & Supp. 1990); Va. Code Ann. 32.1-134.1 (1985).

63. 42 U.S.C. 11101 et seq. (1986).

64. The term "professional review action" means an action or recommenda-

tion of a professional review body based on the competence or professional conduct of a physician which affects the health or welfare of a patient or patients and which affects or may affect adversely the clinical privileges or membership in a professional society of a physician. 42 U.S.C. 11151(9) (1986). The term "clinical privileges" includes any circumstances pertaining to the furnishing of medical care permitted by a health care entity. 42 U.S.C. 11151(3) (1986).

65. 42 U.S.C. 11111(a)(1) & 11112(a) (1986).

66. 42 U.S.C. 11151(11) (1986).

67. 42 U.S.C. 11112(b)(1) and (2) (1986).

68. The Act requires a health care entity to report to the state licensing board the denial, revocation or other action that adversely affects a physician's clinical privileges for more than thirty days or an action which results in the surrender of clinical privileges of a physician while a physician is under investigation or in return for not conducting an investigation. 42 U.S.C. 11133(a)(1) (1986). A health care entity also may report the foregoing information pertaining to non-physicians. 42 U.S.C. 11133(a)(2) (1986). A health care entity which substantially fails to comply with the Act's requirements will lose immunity under the Act. 42 U.S.C. 11133(c)(1) (1986).

69. See, e.g., Ill Ann. Stat. C. 111, 4400-5 (Smith-Hurd 1988); N.Y. Educ. Law 6527 (5) (McKinney 1985 & Supp. 1990); Tex. Rev Civ Stat. Ann., art. 4495b, 5.06 (t) (Vernon 1988).

70. Slaughter v Friedman, 32 Cal. 3d 149, 185 Cal. Rptr. 244, 649 P.2d 996 (1982).

71. See, e.g., California Civ Code 47(3); N.Y. Educ. Law 6527(3) (McKinney 1985 & Supp. 1989).

72. Slaughter, 185 Cal. Rptr. at 249, 649 P.2d at 891. The court pointed out that defendants were only required "to inform dental patients of the basis for rejection of their claims; they were not required additionally to defame plaintiff with accusations regarding his dental practices."

73. For a discussion of antitrust and health care issues, see Kopit and Barnes, "Practical Guide to Health Care Antitrust Issues," Trustee, May, 1986; Kopit and Barnes, "Practical Antitrust Aspects of Physician Staff Privileges," Health Care Publications, Inc., 1985; Kopit, Moses and Barnes, "Antitrust Health Law, Hospital Law Manual," Aspen Systems Corporation, Inc., 1984.

74. Certain conduct that is deemed particularly egregious, such as price-fixing, is considered illegal if it is established that the conduct took place, without regard to the intent or effect of the conduct. See United States v Trenton Potteries, Co., 273 U.S. 392 (1927).

75. Under the rule of reason approach, the court applies a standard of reason to determine if conduct constitutes a restraint of trade, and examines the purpose of the arrangement, the power of the parties, and the necessary effect of their actions. See Standard Oil of N.J. v United States, 221 U.S. 1 (1911).

76. See Board of Trade of the City of Chicago v United States, 246 U.S. 231

(1918); Dos Santos v Columbus-Cuneo-Cabrini Medical Center, 684 F.2d 1346 (7th Cir. 1982) (under rule of reason analysis, hospital permitted to grant exclusive privileges where policy is grounded in ensuring quality patient care and necessary hospital services).

77. Kiefer-Stewart Co. v Joseph E. Seagram & Sons, Inc., 340 U.S. 211 (1951); United States v Socony Vacuum Oil Co., 310 U.S. 150 (1940).

78. See, generally, Northwest Wholesale Stationers, Inc. v Pacific Stationery & Printing, 472 U.S. 284 (1985) (unless an organization possesses market power or controls access to an element essential for competition, expulsion for failure to follow reasonable rules is not per se illegal); see generally Remarks of Charles F. Rule, Ass't Attorney General, U.S. Dept. of Justice, Mar. 11, 1988.

79. See, e.g., Ill. Ann. Stat. ch. 111, 4400-5 (Smith-Hurd 1988); N.Y. Educ. Law 6527(5) (McKinney 1985 & Supp. 1990); Tex. Rev Civ Stat. Ann., art. 4495b, 5.06(t) (Vernon 1988).

80. 42 U.S.C. 11101 et seq. (1986).

81. I.R.C. 414(m) (1989).

✦ 12 ✦

Mental Health Teaching and Research in Managed Care

James E. Sabin, M.D.
Jonathan F. Borus, M.D.

I n contrast to what most mental health professionals believe, the primary characteristic of mental health practice in a managed care setting is not brief treatment, benefit restrictions, or limitation of goals—but *management*. Until recently, the models of practice taught to students came largely from the indemnity supported fee-for-service (FFS) environment in which clinicians could allocate resources to each patient with little concern about total cost. In sharp contrast, managed care clinicians must apportion explicitly defined resources to contractually defined populations. This means that they must optimize the use of resources for the entire population of enrollees (the "denominator"), rather than utilizing an unlimited amount of these resources on particular patients as they present themselves for care (the "numerator"). Management, the sine qua non of health maintenance organization (HMO) practice, is the process by which clinicians seek to achieve this optimization. The accelerating national shift from FFS to managed care highlights difficult but unavoidable problems that occur at the boundaries of ethics, policy, and clinical practice. These thorny problems create unique opportunities and responsibilities for teaching and research in managed health care organizations.

The central teaching missions for managed care clinical teachers are to define the unique skills, knowledge, and attitudes required for practice under these constraints and values, and to develop teaching strategies that promote their acquisition. For managed care researchers, the central mission is to build a foundation for ethical clinical and policy decisions by evaluating the effectiveness and efficiency of different treatment alternatives. With a defined denominator population, researchers can determine rates of illness and care utilization and investigate costs and outcomes for subpopulations receiving specific types of interventions. Studies of these kinds can provide a scientific basis for treatment planning and allocation decisions.

In this chapter we will address four topics. First, we will describe the six skills uniquely important for managed care practice and distinctive in managed care clinical teaching. Second, we will present three brief examples of mental health teaching programs in managed care settings. Third, we will review four major areas of mental health research in managed care. Finally, we will offer some recommendations and speculations regarding the potential for teaching and research in managed care settings.

Teaching For Managed Care Practice

The growing demand for health care cost containment in American society will shape mental health practice in the 1990s and beyond. In this environment, clinicians of all disciplines will need new clinical management skills in order to practice—and to compete—effectively. In his discussion of "The Future Role of Psychiatrists" in *Training Psychiatrists for the '90s: Issues and Recommendations,* Melvin Sabshin, Medical Director of the American Psychiatric Association, presents a pithy characterization of the psychiatric generalist of the future:

> What is unique about psychiatry is its *integrative,* empirically based and theoretically sound spanning of psychosocial and biological approaches. . . . In the nineties . . . the generalist will most often use a mixture of combined techniques, and will be able to *titrate* each, or *move from one to the other* with a diverse age and sex-stratified sample of patients. (Sabshin 1987, p. 143; italics added).

Managed care sites provide special promise for teaching the skills Sabshin calls integration, titration, and moving from one technique to the other because these are everyday necessities for managing an HMO practice. However, to apply the clinical approaches presented in this volume in the flexible manner Sabshin prescribes, HMO clinicians have to balance and integrate tensions of focus, role, and stance in a way that current training programs rarely address. Table 12–1 contrasts the clinician's situation in FFS and managed care to show the tensions that managed care creates and identifies six indispensable skills for managing the process of integration. The distinctive contribution managed care systems can make to mental health education is to teach clinicians how to integrate these tensions. We have organized the discussion of teaching around the six skills.

Skill 1: Individual practice management. HMO clinicians are responsible not only for their current patients but also for members who will need treatment but have not yet presented for care. For the individual HMO clinician, this public health perspective of responsibility for the entire denominator population of enrollees is best symbolized by the requirement to maintain open access for a specified number of new patients. An FFS clinician, by contrast, may close access to his or her practice when the "treatment slots" are filled.

Integrating both individual patient and public health perspectives is easy to describe but hard to do. Van Buskirk and colleagues (1985) delineated a phenomenon, colloquially called "the crunch," that occurs when psychiatry residents training at an HMO find that they have precluded access for new patients by the way they have structured their commitments to current patients. Only in the turmoil created by "the crunch" were the residents able to work with supervisors to develop skills crucial to managing the conflict between the needs of their individual patients and those of the wider membership.

Skill 2: Collaborative program development. Colleagues in a managed care practice are not simply a collection of individuals work-

Table 12–1. The clinician in two settings

	Fee-for-service	Managed care	New skills required
Focus	Individual patient	Individual patient *and* public health	1. Individual practice management 2. Collaborative program development
Role	Independent professional	Independent professional *and* employee partner	3. Ethical analysis 4. Advocacy beneficence
Stance	Empathic	Empathic *and* expeditious	5. Developmental model 6. Broad repertoire of methodologies

ing under the same roof or listed in the same brochure and paid by the same insurer. They bear a collective responsibility for the current and future needs of the HMO membership. Therefore, in addition to maintaining timely access to new patients for traditional evaluation and treatment, the group of clinicians must collectively design and provide a broad array of programs to meet needs better or more efficiently addressed by specialty services such as crisis teams, stress management classes, behavior therapy, and medication groups.

Skill 3: Ethical analysis. The treatment techniques presented in the clinical sections of this volume all emphasize *choosing* a focus and clarifying the respective *responsibilities* (and, by implication, the *rights*) of therapist and patient. Although these clinical chapters explicitly address issues of clinical practice, the concepts of choice, responsibility, and rights clearly point to ethical issues as well.

HMO clinicians must manage limited resources on behalf of the entire member population. Individual patients may seek limitless resources for themselves. For optimal clinical learning, the student must experience the tensions summarized in Table 12–1 while being helped to analyze the multiple values that must be considered in making ethically appropriate clinical recommendations. What does the patient want? What is the therapist's assessment of what the patient needs? What is the benefit contract in its letter and spirit? What are the competing interests of other members?

Skill 4: Advocacy beneficence. Barry Furrow of the University of Delaware School of Law has made a valuable formulation of how managed care influences classical concepts of medical ethics (Furrow 1988). The Hippocratic activity of beneficence—providing benefit to the patient and avoiding harm—must now be done not only directly by acts of care but also indirectly by advocacy within systems of care. Organizational conservatism seeks to avoid conflict, but robust organizations know they must cultivate conflict to thrive and grow. Although a student cannot be expected to master clinical advocacy in a yearlong placement, the student must be introduced to the concept of effective advocacy and at least begin to practice some of the skills by participating in advocacy activities and studying case methods.

Skill 5: Developmental model. Being at once empathic and expeditious requires the managed care clinician to be both psychologically and methodologically flexible. Empathy and expeditiousness, while complementary, point in opposite directions. Expeditiousness involves focus, efficiency, and speed; empathy requires an open, inquiring, receptive stance that mirrors the patient's inner world (Kohut 1971; Semrad 1980). Although students typically find managing "the crunch" to be the hardest skill to learn, for experienced clinicians maintaining the stance of expeditiousness and empathy is actually the most difficult task over the course of a career. How can students best learn to integrate this particular duality?

As described by Bennett (Chapter 13) and Gould (Chapter 22), clinicians working with an adult developmental model interpret the presenting picture in terms of the patient's current adaptive need and the strengths and vulnerabilities brought to bear on that need. As with a primary care physician, the mental health clinician makes him- or herself available to the patient over time. By making focused and often brief interventions part of this long-term availability, the clinician can begin to bridge the gap between empathy and expeditiousness.

The concepts of the adult developmental model and "primary care mental health" can be taught in a classroom, but the skills and attitudes need to be honed over time. Although short block placements allow intensive practice of skills such as hypnosis or brief therapy, they do not allow learning that by definition requires extended calendar (developmental) time. Experience to date suggests that a placement of at least a full year appears to be the minimum required time needed to begin to integrate these attitudes (J. Donovan, personal communication, 1990).

Skill 6: Broad repertoire of methodologies. Although there is no established consensus regarding the range of methods that all managed care mental health clinicians should be able to apply, psychiatric residents who train at the Harvard Community Health Plan are all taught basic-level skills in brief individual psychodynamic psychotherapy, basic cognitive-behavioral therapies, basic couples and family treatment, time-sensitive forms of extended psychotherapy, diagnosis and treatment planning for chemical dependencies, and the skillful use of "homework" and self-help groups as part of treatment (Sabin et al. 1988). Having a relatively broad range of skills makes it easier for the clinician to greet the patient while asking the internal question—"Which of my skills is likeliest to be helpful to this patient?" rather than "To whom may I refer this patient?" (See also Feldman,

Chapter 14). Although at times referral will be the correct path, the student who has developed a repertoire broad enough to address the majority of clinical issues he or she encounters can with much greater ease receive the patient in an empathic stance.

Many, perhaps most, training programs offer exposure to an eclectic range of techniques. As Shader (1988) has indicated, however, although balanced exposure of students to multiple methodologies may be common, true integration of these techniques into a coherent approach to practice is relatively rare. Because managed care is most commonly built around generalist practice rather than mental health specialty services, the process of developing an integrated eclectic model and making differentiated therapeutic recommendations is especially accessible for study and practice.

Examples of HMO Mental Health Teaching

The clinical chapters in this volume demonstrate that clinical methods in managed care are relatively well developed. HMO-based clinical teaching, however, is much less developed, and the literature describing teaching programs is extremely limited. Virtually all of the teaching activity to date has been at postgraduate levels—residency, fellowship, and continuing medical education. The three programs presented here are at mature HMOs and reflect the major directions teaching activities have taken in the 1980s and 1990s.

Group Health Cooperative of Puget Sound (GHCPS)

Family practice training is very strong in Washington State, and the GHCPS mental health teaching program is distinctive in its focus on family practice. Residents from the GHCPS-based family practice residency all do an 8-week rotation in mental health, during which they undertake supervised short-term individual and family counseling and participate in group leadership for patient groups such as those for battered women or people who are chemically dependent. Many elect to do a second rotation. In addition, GHCPS takes at least six students per year from local master's-level counseling programs for yearlong placements. Finally, on an intermittent basis, PGY 4 psychiatry residents from the University of Washington do electives in liaison psychiatry at a GHCPS family practice center.

Harvard Community Health Plan (HCHP)

At its inception in 1969, HCHP defined its primary mission as excellent service to members but made explicit secondary commitments to teaching, research, and community service. Since 1981, HCHP has offered a half-time mental health fellowship to PGY 4 residents, postdoctoral psychologists, psychiatric nurse clinical specialists, and master's-level social workers with some postgraduate experience. Ten to 12 fellows per year are placed at HCHP health centers where they carry out supervised practice. A yearlong weekly seminar provides an opportunity to build a developmental model (skill 5), to develop a broad repertoire of methodologies (skill 6), and to integrate these in accord with clinical objectives and values (skill 3).

Graduates have taken leadership positions at other clinical and training programs in the Boston area and many have been hired by HCHP itself. Since 1987, HCHP has also offered an elective seminar to PGY 4 residents who are doing chief residencies in Boston but who come to the HMO to study managed care practice. Finally, between 1978 and 1989 HCHP presented four continuing medical education (CME) conferences, each drawing a national participation of more than 250. In all of these activities, HCHP has operated as a freestanding training site with no formal relationship to any academic program.

Northwest Kaiser Permanente (KP)

This program reflects the most extensive integration to date between a department of psychiatry and an HMO. Ten of 32 psychiatric beds at the University of Oregon Health Sciences Hospital are devoted to KP patients. In the course of the first 2 years of residency, all Oregon Health Sciences (OHS) residents rotate through this unit, where they are supervised by KP attending psychiatrists, all of whom have faculty appointments. The OHS program is especially strong in community and social psychiatry and, as part of basic residency training, residents study health care organization, finance, and policy. For the past 5 years, one PGY 4 resident has been placed at KP for a half-time fellowship in outpatient psychiatry. In the 1990s the two organizations anticipate that two of the eight PGY 4 residents at OHS will be placed at KP each year. Many of the KP psychiatrists have been trained at the OHS, and as a result, a common culture is evolving between the two organizations.

Research

Evaluating the services provided in the HMO and the quality of care has an especially high value for managed care systems, because the employer and governmental purchasers of health services are increasingly (and appropriately) demanding data on the effectiveness and efficiency of the care received by HMO enrollees.

In an HMO, enrollees are "members" of an organization to which they often feel a significant level of commitment. This commitment facilitates voluntary cooperation in research and evaluation efforts that have the possibility of improving care for the individual member and the membership population as a whole. Enrollees often elect to remain members of the HMO over an extended time, providing many opportunities for long-term follow-up studies and longitudinal investigations of the natural course of illness in HMOs that may not be possible in FFS settings. Because most HMOs provide the enrolled population with comprehensive health care, of which mental health care is a defined component, researchers can study the effects of utilization in one domain of care on utilization and health status in another. HMOs often have computerized record systems that include inpatient and outpatient care, thereby facilitating the definition of patient cohorts with similar disorders as the bases of studies. Clinicians who choose to work in HMOs are usually interested in studying their care system and welcome the chance to vary their work life with research. Finally, the multidisciplinary composition of the mental health component of most HMOs provides the opportunity to investigate the approaches taken by different clinical disciplines regarding patient care.

To date HMOs have been at the vanguard of research that capitalizes on the characteristics listed above. In the remainder of this section we will briefly describe four areas of HMO-based mental health research and outline some of the problems encountered in these studies.

Effectiveness of Time-Limited Individual and Group Therapies

An obvious area for investigation by an HMO concerned with efficient use of resources in providing mental health services is the exploration of the effectiveness of short-term, time-limited individual and group therapies. Offering a limited mandated mental health benefit, most HMOs have the incentive to develop innovative ways to provide helpful care within the limits of the benefit and to "stretch" the benefit in innovative ways. Studies at HCHP and elsewhere have shown that most members are satisfied with time-limited problem-focused therapeutic services; also, for many of the problems with which predominantly healthy HMO members present to the mental health department, such interventions are sufficient (Budman et al. 1988; Cummings and Duhl 1986). Innovative ways to prepare patients for individual and group psychotherapy have been used in such settings and evaluated for their helpfulness to the patient and their ability to short-cut lengthy therapy (Budman et al. 1981b). Studies of "extended" therapy in which infrequent therapeutic contacts are provided over time within the limitations of the mental health benefit have also been studied (Budman et al. 1981a). Satisfaction and improvement in time-limited individual and group therapies have been compared (Budman et al. 1988), and psychoeducational treatment groups for members with specific types of problems (e.g., those undergoing a common life stress such as separation and divorce) have been found helpful in the HMO setting (Wertlieb et al. 1982).

Screening

HMOs have been the sites of studies that screen new enrollees for symptoms of emotional distress and attempt to provide preventive interventions to decrease the prevalence of mental illness within the enrollee population. Psychiatric screening instruments (the General Health Questionnaire [GHQ], RAND Mental Health Index, etc.) have been used to identify those patients at risk for whom such an intervention might be helpful. A study at the HCHP screened 1,649 new adult enrollees using the GHQ. Enrollees with high scores on this screen were offered interpersonal counseling by primary care nurse clinicians, and those who took advantage of this counseling had a greater self-reported reduction in stress than those who did not (Berwick et al. 1987).

HMOs also provide settings in which to assess the effectiveness of mental health screening instruments for patients coming for routine medical care and to assess the effective diagnostic prowess of primary physicians for mental disorders. In a study at HCHP, general physicians' assessments of the emotional problems and mental disorders of their own patients were compared with diagnostic evaluations of these same patients by mental health clinicians using the Structured Clinical Interview for DSM-III-R (Spitzer et al., in press). The primary physicians did not recognize two-thirds of their patients who had a current DSM-III-R (American Psychiatric Association 1987) diagnosis as having any mental disorder, including those with the most frequent disorders seen in primary care practice (affective, anxiety, and substance abuse disorders). The finding that these physicians also rated themselves as confident in the assessment of their patients' emotional state led to a program in which barriers to recognizing mental disorders in the HMO were explored with the primary physicians. These physicians were taught methods to help them rapidly screen and diagnose the mental disorders most prevalent among patients in their practices (Borus et al. 1988).

Mental Health Issues in Medical Care

The linked provision of medical and mental health care in an HMO provides the opportunity and incentive to examine issues at the health/mental health interface. Members with unusually high rates of medical care utilization can be studied to determine what types of family, social, and emotional factors may contribute to frequent use of costly physician services. Fitzpatrick and Kempler (1990) studied the impact on medical utilization of a structured intervention with pain patients in the HMO setting.

The efficacy of potential psychoeducational interventions for medical symptomatology that may have emotional components also can be evaluated in the HMO setting. For example, a randomized trial of two psychoeducational treatment regimens for HCHP patients suffering from subacute low back pain found that neither added measurably to the usual clinical outcome with customary care (Berwick et al. 1989).

Offset Studies

The provision of both health and mental health services to a denominator population also makes the HMO an excellent site for "offset studies." These studies have been used to explore the effects of mental health care for patients with psychiatric problems on their general health care utilization and cost. It has been demonstrated that patients with a psychiatric disorder have twice the utilization of general medical services as those without such a disorder; however, when these patients are provided with appropriate mental health specialty care, their utilization of general health services decreases toward that of patients without a mental disorder (Jones and Vischi 1979). Although such studies have also been performed in FFS settings (Borus et al. 1985), they are most prevalent in HMOs where rates of utilization and cost are easily definable because the enrollee population is a clear denominator for the rate (Hankin et al. 1983). In an FFS setting, one never knows the denominator. As a result, one does not know whether nonutilization indicates a lack of illness or need for care or indicates instead that the patient now receives care from another provider—or even that the patient has died.

Problems in Conducting Research in the HMO

Many of the problems that arise in evaluation and research studies in an HMO are correlates of the positive characteristics of this practice setting described previously. First, there may be the tendency to mistakenly treat HMO members as a "captive audience" and expect them to cooperate routinely in research without properly requesting their assistance. In any research project in an HMO, it is important that enrollees be invited to participate as honored members rather than captured subjects. Second, in an HMO the patient flow dynamics are the opposite of those in an FFS setting. In the latter, providers want to "keep" their patients and may provide excessive service as long as it is reimbursed; in the former, where there is no incentive to the provider to see additional patients, there may be a tendency to "dump" patients onto other care providers. For example, primary physicians in an HMO may refer patients to their mental health department whom they would continue to treat themselves under FFS. Such differences in basic patient flow limit the generalizations of findings in studies undertaken in HMOs to FFS settings. Third, with a limited mental health benefit, often primarily available as time-limited or group therapy, a substantial number of patients may go outside of the HMO to receive individuated, more intensive, and/or extensive mental health care. Such extra-plan utilization can lead to faulty assumptions about the numerator in utilization, cost, and effectiveness studies of mental health care within the HMO.

Fourth, to date, most offset studies in organized managed care systems have focused almost exclusively on the utilization and cost of mental health services without correlating these with clinical outcome and patient satisfaction. Decreased utilization and cost in and of themselves are meaningless without positively correlated patient improvement (Borus 1985). Fifth, in the cost-conscious environment in which HMOs must compete, funding for research and evaluation efforts may be difficult to sustain. Not only the investigators but also the productivity-pressured clinicians asked to fill out forms or undertake specified treatment protocols must be supported for these activities. Although outside funding may also be sought, stable monies for research efforts that evaluate the effectiveness of care and elucidate ways to improve its quality must be built into the HMO's budget as a "basic cost of doing business." Finally, most HMOs are service provision systems without primary affiliations with research-oriented university medical centers. Such nonacademic HMOs may lack the in-house expertise necessary to undertake meaningful research. As we suggest below, closer linkage between HMOs and academic psychiatry and psychology departments can be mutually beneficial and a vital component of the teaching and research efforts of both institutions.

Conclusion

Ever since The Johns Hopkins University created the first integrated teaching hospital in 1893, teaching hospitals have been the center of education and research in medicine and psychiatry. With the shift toward outpatient and community treatment that is likely to dominate the next phase of medicine already well under way, teaching hospitals are no longer optimal settings for students or researchers. As organized systems with an adequate critical mass of patients, HMOs could provide a crucial new setting for teaching and research.

What we envision is not simply marginal change of the kind that has occurred to date in which HMOs become the sites of clinical rotations or occasional research, but the creation of a new kind of institution, modeled on the concept of the teaching hospital—the "teaching HMO"—that integrates service, teaching, and research. Although we cannot predict how the teaching HMO will be structured, experience to date allows specification of three steps that must be taken for these new creations to be conceived, gestated, and born (Moore 1990).

1. Historically HMOs have evolved in an atmosphere of conflict with organized medicine and academia (Mayer and Mayer 1985). For the well-being of both Academic Medical Centers (AMCs) and HMOs, this puerile form of town/gown conflict must cease. Constructive exploration of win/win collaborations between managed care and academic psychiatry (as reflected, for example, in the authorship of this chapter) needs to occur on many fronts. For teaching HMOs to emerge, a new culture must be developed that combines the values of cost-effective care with those of academia.

2. Teams representing HMOs and AMCs need to create, study, and publicize model programs. The three examples described in this chapter demonstrate that extensive high-quality graduate education and CME can be provided in the HMO setting (HCHP), that an academic department of psychiatry and an HMO can at least begin to integrate their joint missions (KP and OHS), and that HMOs can make major contributions to the psychological and psychiatric education of primary care physicians (GHCPS). The next areas requiring most attention are how to more fully integrate the divergent missions and values of AMCs and HMOs and what combinations of AMC, HMO, and government funding will support development of the new teaching HMOs.

3. National organizations devoted to teaching and research need to create supportive links to managed care in order to foster the evolution of a culture that supports academic activity within HMOs. Training directors in psychiatry and the other mental health disciplines need to educate themselves in the realities of managed care practice and to reach out to managed care organizations. The National Institute of Mental Health can play a role in fostering research development within managed care organizations. Similarly, the Group Health Association of America, as the coordinating arm of the managed care industry, should establish a component section to review linkages to the academic world.

If these steps are carried out vigorously, by the turn of the century several true integrations of AMCs and HMOs should be well under way and the currently fanciful concept of the teaching HMO may emerge as a reality. If HMOs are to thrive as high-quality care systems, they will need the long-term infusion and retention of the best graduates of professional training programs. If HMO managed care is to be truly cost-effective rather than simply cheap, the research expertise of the AMC must be focused on the course of psychiatric illness and the impact of varied treatment interventions. If AMCs are not to become 21st-century dinosaurs, they must broaden their base of teaching and research to include HMOs. We believe that managed care and academic mental health both clearly stand to gain substantially by developing new forms of collaboration and new settings, such as the teaching HMO, in which to work together.

References

American Psychiatric Association: Diagnostic and Statistical Manual of Mental Disorders, 3rd Edition, Revised. Washington, DC, American Psychiatric Association, 1987

Berwick DM, Budman S, Damico-White J, et al: Assessment of psychological morbidity in primary care: explorations with the General Health Questionnaire. Journal of Chronic Disease 40:71s–79s, 1987

Berwick DM, Budman S, Feldstein M: No clinical effect of back schools in an HMO: a randomized prospective trial. Spine 14:338–344, 1989

Borus JF: Psychiatry and the primary care physician, in Comprehensive Textbook of Psychiatry/IV. Edited by Kaplan HI, Sadock BJ. Baltimore, MD, Williams & Wilkins, 1985, pp 1302–1308

Borus JF, Olendzki MC, Kessler L, et al: The "offset effect" of mental health treatment on ambulatory medical care utilization and charges. Arch Gen Psychiatry 42:573–580, 1985

Borus JF, Howes MJ, Devins NP, et al: Primary health care providers' recognition and diagnosis of mental disorders in their patients. Gen Hosp Psychiatry 10:317–321, 1988

Budman SH, Bennett MJ, Wisneski M: An adult developmental model of short-term group psychotherapy, in Forms of Brief Therapy. Edited by Budman SH. New York, Guilford, 1981a

Budman SH, Clifford M, Bader L, et al: Experiential pre-group preparation and screening. Group 5:19–26, 1981b

Budman SH, Demby A, Redondo JP, et al: Comparative outcome in time-limited and group psychotherapy. Int J Group Psychother 38:63–87, 1988

Cummings N, Duhl LJ: The new mental health delivery system. Psychiatric Annals 16:470–475, 1986

Fitzpatrick R, Kempler H: Integrating care for chronic pain patients. HMO Practice 4:87–93, 1990

Furrow BR: Ethics and public planning. Notre Dame Journal of Law 2:187–226, 1988

Hankin JR, Kessler LG, Goldberg ID, et al: A longitudinal study of offset in use of non-psychiatric services following specialized mental health care. Med Care 21:1099–1110, 1983

Jones KR, Vischi TR: Impact of alcohol, drug abuse, and mental health treatment on medical care utilization. Med Care 17(suppl):1–82, 1979

Kohut H: The Analysis of the Self. New York, International Universities Press, 1971

Mayer TR, Mayer GG: HMOs: origins and development. N Engl J Med 312:590–594, 1985

Moore GT: Health maintenance organizations: breaking the barriers. Acad Med 65:427–432, 1990

Sabin JE, Steinberg SM, Donovan JM: Mental health education in an HMO. HMO Practice 2:143–146, 1988

Sabshin M: The future role of psychiatrists, in Training Psychiatrists for the '90s: Issues and Recommendations. Edited by Nadelson CC, Robinowitz CB. Washington, DC, American Psychiatric Press, 1987, pp 141–146

Semrad E: The Heart of a Therapist. Edited by Rako S, Mazer H. New York, Jason Aronson, 1980

Shader RI: Balance versus integration. Seymour D. Vestermark Lecture presented at the annual meeting of the American Psychiatric Association, May 11, 1988

Spitzer RL, Williams JBW, Gibbon M, et al: The Structured Clinical Interview for DSM-III-R (SCID). Arch Gen Psychiatry (in press)

Van Buskirk D, Feldman JL, Steinberg S, et al: Teaching psychiatry in the health maintenance organization. Am J Psychiatry 142:1181–1183, 1985

Wertlieb D, Budman S, Demby A, et al: The stress of marital separation: intervention in a health maintenance organization. Psychosom Med 44:437–448, 1982

Section II:

Clinical Issues

✦ 13 ✦

The Managed Care Setting as a Framework for Clinical Practice

Michael J. Bennett, M.D.

As the name suggests, organizations that offer managed care aspire to combine medical care with modern management theory and methodology. Their ability to survive and prosper in a competitive environment requires that they market, organize, and deliver services in a manner that is both intelligible and appealing to the purchaser. In order to be appealing they must appear to offer value. Value in medical care is a combination of high quality and affordable cost. These two objectives require mechanisms to maximize efficiency without compromising technical excellence or losing the humane attitudes at the core of good medical care (Bennett 1988).

A managed care system must strive to balance the interests and priorities of three parties: the consumer (patient), the provider (clinician), and the payor (insurer). Whatever the structure of the particular managed system, it is necessary for the parties to be aware of the needs and interests of the others and thus to be prepared to modify their own. At the clinical practice level, this means that patient and provider are forced to define their activities with reference to the three-part system (a triadic, as opposed to the older, dyadic relationship) and shape their expectations accordingly. This calls for a fundamental reworking of traditional notions of health and illness, treatment and cure. In the remainder of this chapter, I will describe such a reworking as it applies to mental health outpatient practice.

The key principle underlying mental health care in a managed care system is that of optimal intervention: that the patient should receive the least extensive, intensive, intrusive, and costly intervention capable of successfully addressing the presenting problem. Such parsimony contrasts with a model common in fee-for-service practice: comprehensive, state-of-the-art care for each patient. The contrast in aims springs from the difference in context.

The ideas I will present have evolved in a closed system: a staff model health maintenance organization (HMO) with a liberal mental health basic benefit and a program that is highly integrated within the general medical setting. The program, which is described elsewhere (Budman et al. 1979), takes as its mission the provision of comprehensive mental health care to an enrolled population at an affordable cost. It emphasizes parsimony of intervention and coordination of care through balancing generalized and specialized services, and linking the various tiers of care (outpatient, partial inpatient, and inpatient) so that patients move among them in a rational manner. In the outpatient setting, clinicians function both as generalists and as specialists who consult with each other and who offer specialized forms of treatment as deemed necessary. These specialized services can be characterized as "secondary," and the generalist role as "primary" mental health care. The latter, "primary mental health care," is the core of the system.

Because specialized services are likely to be more costly than generalized services, their judicious use is a key feature of the system described. I will characterize the role and function of the primary mental health caregiver and suggest a model of psychotherapy that is consistent with it. It is my belief that such an approach is applicable to any managed care system or, more broadly, to any system that assumes continuing responsibility for a defined population with a limited budget.

Primary and Secondary Mental Health Care

Primary care, as it applies to the general medical setting, represents an attempt to preserve the values and benefits of general practice in an increasingly complex environment. Although it allows for technologically sophisticated methodology, it emphasizes the dyadic doctor-patient relationship that is at the core of all health care. Stoeckle, in his introductory chapter to *Primary Care Medicine*, defines it as follows:

Primary care is coordinated, comprehensive and personal care, available on both a first contact and continuous basis. It incorporates several tasks: medical diagnosis and treatment; psychological diagnosis and treatment; personal support of patients of all backgrounds, in all stages of illness; communication of information about diagnosis, treatment, prevention and prognosis; maintenance of patients with chronic illness; prevention of disability and disease through detection, education, persuasion and preventive treatment. (Stoeckle 1981, pp. 1–2)

The core element of primary care is an enduring relationship, in which the provider of health care may be drawn upon repeatedly over time, both to treat episodes of illness and to promote health. The concept may be applied to mental health care in the following ways. First, it is clear that patients seek to use mental health providers in much the same way that they use medical providers (or attorneys, or accountants, or car mechanics): repeatedly over time (if permitted), at times of need (Bennett 1983). Such perceived need is most likely to arise at points of life transition. This pattern stems from the fact that development is a lifelong process in which the events, challenges, and opportunities of life force repeated reworking of conflicts, introjects, historical trauma, self-esteem, and personal identity.

It has been argued by adult developmental theorists that these observations carry implications for psychotherapy (Colarusso and Nemiroff 1987). Rather than being perceived as a closed-ended process aimed at curing past hurts, psychotherapy may be structured as an intermittent process, useful at times of need and readiness, to address obstacles to development as these surface and command attention, and as the patient becomes ready developmentally to deal with them (Bennett 1984). The matter, however, is more complex. The patient who presents because of the pain of a current life impasse brings both assets and liabilities to the task of resolving it. In addition to the problem itself, he or she may bring a variety of "limiting factors" (see Figure 13–1)—for example, the presence of a major mental disorder or active substance abuse.

Whether or not such conditions are causally linked to the life impasse, their presence must be noted and their relevance to the patient's current state assessed. Such factors may require attention as a prerequisite for effective treatment of the presenting problem. Attention to limiting factors may include treatment aimed at stabilization, or it may consist only in considering how the goals of an intervention ought to be shaped or delimited by their presence. At times, specialized resources may be required in order to keep such factors from interfering with a planned focal intervention. The role of the primary mental health provider in such cases is to coordinate the care and orient it toward the resolution of the issue that caused the patient to seek help.

This insistence on the "why now," the presenting problem, usually

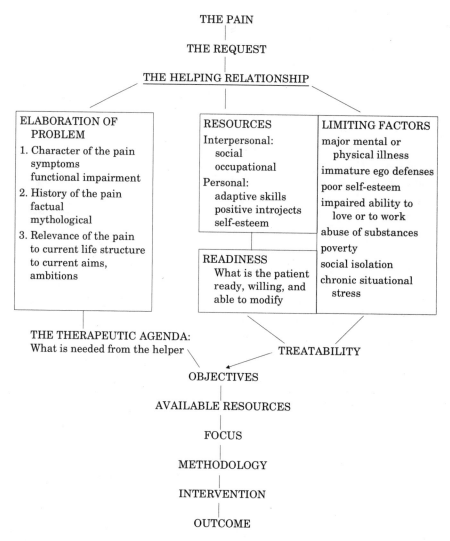

Figure 13–1. Treatment paradigm.

represents an important cultural value in the managed care system. In order to avoid superficiality, the relationship between presenting problems and psychopathology must be understood. My position can be summarized as follows. Psychopathology consists in a set of propensities that stem from the biological and psychological makeup of the individual, causing him or her to act and react in the present in a fashion shaped by biology and by sociopsychological events that took place in the past. It manifests itself, as the person moves through the life cycle, through a repeated tendency to experience one or more types of impasses that are specific to the individual. Such impasses, therefore, represent both problems in the present and active contemporary expressions of underlying developmental obstacles. Treatment holds the promise of favorably influencing underlying obstacles through *capitalizing on the energy and thrust toward health expressed by presenting agendas and motives.* In this sense, interventions may be characterized as "problem-driven" rather than exclusively "problem-centered." Although primary care services are likely to emphasize the present impasse, secondary care services are usually more attuned to underlying obstacles. Thus, coordination of the two becomes essential to both the efficiency and the healing power of an episode of care.

Care based on such a conception is likely to be brief rather than extended, discontinuous rather than continuous, and incremental rather than circumscribed. Resting on the individual's natural striving toward health, it contrasts with a model that targets psychopathology ("sickness"), which is likely to be extensive (sometimes lifelong) and highly specialized, creating a potentially avoidable dependence on the caregiver and usually incurring higher cost. When primary and secondary care are integrated with each other with the aim of solving the presenting problem, there is no contraindication to attempting a focal intervention with any patient.

Designing the Focal Intervention

When the barriers to mental health care are low, patients will seek assistance when they feel at an impasse and are in a state of pain. The initial evaluation proceeds from the patient's presenting pain and agenda (what he or she wants from the helper) to a therapeutic agenda (what he or she needs from the helper) and then to treatment objectives (what patient and therapist hope to achieve together) by identifying three separate yet overlapping sets of variables (Figure 13–1).

First, what is the character of the presenting pain, with regard to symptoms and impaired function; what are its historical roots and antecedents; and what is its relevance to the patient's current life structure and currently operative life agendas and aims? In other words, where is the patient stuck, how does he or she hurt as a result, and what is it that he or she needs the helper to do in order to become unstuck?

Second, what associated "limiting factors" exist, in the patient or in his or her life structure, that influence or limit the patient's efforts (and therefore are likely to affect the collaborative effort) to deal with the problem in question? These are factors that will color and shape the nature of the intervention and may limit what can be accomplished.

Certain limiting factors are more compelling than others. The presence of active substance abuse or suicidal depression, for example, demands an immediate shift to a secondary level of care (e.g., substance abuse program) or even a tertiary one (e.g., hospitalization). With others, such as "chronic situational stress" or "social isolation," no such shift is required, but the introduction of ancillary services (support or self-help programs, stress reduction workshops) may facilitate the focal work. When the limiting factors are related to key aspects of character structure, such as chronic problems with self-esteem or excessive reliance on immature ego defenses (splitting, projection, denial), the matter is considerably more problematic. For such patients, who may qualify for a personality disorder diagnosis, repeated courses of focal therapy may be required before any change in such features occurs. The problematic personality traits become the focus of attention to the extent that they appear in the form of specific forms of resistance in the focal work. In some instances, for example with patients who cannot establish a helping relationship or whose interpersonal behavior *has been demonstrated* to undermine focal treatment, a more extensive shift into a secondary care mode may be required: for example, longer term group or individual psychotherapy, with the specific objective(s) of mitigating the influence of the underlying factors that account for the therapeutic impasse. The use of such modes, which in the fee-for-service system have been seen as the norm, should be seen as an exceptional strategy, used only when less extensive and less costly modes prove insufficient.

An important point should be underscored: decisions to shift, either briefly or more extensively, into a secondary care mode, cannot be made on the basis of an initial assessment; rather, they can and should be made *in the course of* an intervention, as specific forms of resistance arise and prove unresponsive to simpler measures. Clearly such decisions call for constant monitoring of the course of treatment; both formal and informal review mechanisms are crucial to this issue. Monitoring, and its key place in the model described, will be discussed later in the chapter.

Third, what are the resources—personal, occupational, social, and internal—that can be drawn upon? Because change is likely to occur over time, primarily within the context of the patient's life, rather than in the office, this component is a vital element in the "inventory-ing" process that is part of planning the treatment. Associated with this is the question of the patient's readiness. In addition to wishing to make the change(s) required, the patient must be developmentally ready to do so.

The outcome of the treatment planning process is twofold: first, the establishment of a helping relationship, and second, agreement on objectives for the intervention and on the focus necessary to achieve them. The choice of methodology, which is essentially a strategic decision, follows from a consideration of the resources available, a judgment about how the patient is likely to work best, and a frank discussion with the patient.

Focal Psychotherapy and the Catalysis of Change

From this discussion it follows that the therapist's function is to facilitate or "catalyze" change, and that psychotherapy is the collaborative work of rehearsing for the necessary change (Table 13–1). Implicit in the idea of catalysis is the assumption that the patient has the capacity to grow and change. This capacity may be elicited and reinforced by life experience, *including, but not necessarily centering on,* the relationship with the therapist. It is the function of the therapist to reinforce the motives to change and mitigate the resistances as these elements manifest themselves through the clinical process. This can be achieved through strategies implemented in the therapy and through specific forms of guidance offered to the patient in regard to his or her behavior outside the office. The helper uses the patient's own life structure as much as possible in the process.

Table 13–1. Phases of a focal intervention

Phase	Location	Motive	Resistance	Agent(s)	Mode	Time Frame
establishing the helping relationship	phone or office	1. pain 2. failure of alternative resources	unwillingness or inability to accept help	patient and helper	pre-collaborative (courtship)	early in first session
reframing	phone or office	perception of impasse	commitment to mythology	helper	receptive (dependent)	late in first session
selecting a focus	office	1. readiness to collaborate with helper 2. readiness for change	1. presence of covert agendas 2. lack of readiness for change	patient and helper	collaborative	first or second session
rehearsing for change	in the office or group room; homework	1. hope for normalcy or restoration of health 2. vision of ideal self	1. felt need for the maladaptation 2. secondary gain 3. lack of hope	patient and helper	collaborative	through the intervention
implementing change: trial and error	1. outside health setting 2. occasionally office, phone	1. momentum from the therapy (optimism) 2. reinforcement by significant others 3. early success	1. pain of change (loss) 2. fear of failure 3. counterpressure by significant others 4. early failure	patient and significant others	active (independent)	after the intervention (months to years)

Source. Reprinted from Bennett 1989, p. 354. Used with permission.

The principles of the focal psychotherapeutic intervention (Bennett 1989) consist of five phases and can be characterized along six axes: where they take place, the agents involved, the nature of the relationship between or among the agents, the time frame, and most importantly, the motives supporting change and the motives opposing it.

The first phase, *establishment of a helping relationship,* is the foundation of all health care. The patient presents with pain, requesting help because other resources have failed. A negotiation follows in which the patient must be able to accept the therapist as an interested professional who can be trusted to assist him or her to address the presenting problem. For those patients who have difficulty with trust, making attachments, or maintaining the necessary boundaries, this phase may be difficult or prolonged. Adler has suggested that the most one can expect with borderline or narcissistic patients early in treatment is positive transference, as opposed to true alliance (Adler 1979). If this is true, then only a tentative or provisional resolution of this phase may be possible for some patients. Empathy, tact, limit setting (or contracting), straightforwardness, and attempts to match patients and therapists are all important in forging links with patients who have difficulties at this stage. Perhaps the most important systems issue is rapid and ready access and therapist availability. When it is feasible, a change of therapists is often preferable to a protracted struggle with negative transference.

The crucial next phase, *reframing,* is often overlooked in therapy. This function of the therapist consists of accounting for the pain in terms that are intelligible to the patient and that allow for the generation of a corrective plan of action. In overlooking the need to identify and modify the patient's existing rationale, we may underestimate the tenacity of our patients' mythologies and their commitment to them. This commitment to old beliefs is most likely to be pronounced in those with somatization patterns, fixed character problems, and chronic depressive states. Because the patient's perception of his or her impasse and the pain associated with it may counterbalance these fixed patterns, confrontation designed to highlight the pain may be useful. Some patients have difficulty accepting, even temporarily, the dependent posture required; it may be helpful in such instances to avoid unnecessary challenge, to emphasize the empowerment of reframing, and to share the control of treatment. A cognitive emphasis will sometimes buy the necessary time for the alliance to build, and with it, the patient's tolerance for sharing strong affect.

Reframing—Case Example

E. P. was a 53-year-old unemployed, unmarried woman who was referred by her internist because of a 25-year history of unremitting alcohol abuse. The referral came after one of a number of unsuccessful attempts to engage her in aftercare following detoxification. The patient had requested a psychiatrist because she was convinced that her drinking was the result of depression, which in turn was related to her dysfunctional history. She had fired her previous and only psychiatrist after their first meeting for insisting that she achieve and maintain sobriety before any attempt might be made to address her psychological problems. She had heard his position as insensitive, controlling, and rejecting. The patient indicated that she was drinking in a controlled fashion, and that she would not return if the therapist took the same stance as her previous psychiatrist.

Ms. P. was very worried about her physical health, which was deteriorating. She was ashamed of her inability to control her drinking and was guilty and chronically (but not acutely) depressed. Her assumption that depression "caused" her alcoholic dependence was based on a strong negative identification with her schizophrenic mother, whom she had failed to "save" from the ravages of her own illness. She correctly perceived that drinking sheltered her from her burdensome sense of responsibility to her mother by creating her own version of mental illness.

Rapport was established quickly by allying with the patient's pain (her fear of her own deterioration and growing "craziness"). Her sense of despair was reframed: she was demoralized (though not clinically depressed) by her early and continuing dilemma—the burden of her mother's "untreatability," with which she identified. The empathetic link enabled her to address the matter of her own "untreatability" and to ally with the therapist's dilemma as similar to her own historical one. Despite her rationalization, the patient was well aware of the nature of her addiction; a discussion of strategies to help her control her drinking was, at that point, well received and the secondary care resources were mobilized and accepted. The focal goal of treatment agreed upon was to support her attempt to achieve and maintain sobriety.

Ms. P. has been seen intermittently over 2 years. She is now 1 year sober, completing her education, and doing well. She has used Alcoholics Anonymous (AA), a self-help group program, and the therapist effectively. Recently she began to deal with her now aging parents, using the therapist as a consultant.

When there is agreement about what blocks the necessary change, *a focus* can usually be agreed upon and maintained. The literature on brief psychotherapy emphasizes this phase (Balint et al. 1972; Budman and Gurman 1988; Gustafson 1984; Malan 1976; Mann 1973). Basically the focus is the "what" of the treatment, the central content of discussion and/or exploration, deemed to be at the heart of the impasse. It is the resolution of this obstacle to necessary change, often either a conflict or an unresolved loss, that is required in order to achieve the agreed-upon objectives of treatment (resolution of the acute impasse, and mitigation of its underlying developmental source) so the patient may return to his or her normal developmental trajectory. When the patient is not ready for change, or when there are covert agendas, it may not be possible to stay with the chosen focus. It may be necessary to backtrack or start over in order to see what has been unexpressed or overlooked. The therapist may arrange a consultation, bring in a spouse or spouse equivalent, or if necessary, point out to the patient that he or she is not ready for the change required but may return when ready. Such lack of readiness may or may not be within the patient's control.

Most of psychotherapy occurring in the office involves the next phase, *rehearsal for change*. This may also involve homework, or encouragement to involve outside resources in the process, before the patient leaves the active treatment. Prompted by his or her vision of a better or ideal self and the hope for normalcy or restoration of health, the patient may be willing to take the necessary risks. Operating against this, however, is the patient's felt need for the maladaptation, reluctance to surrender whatever secondary gains it may provide, or relative lack of hope for the future. Regarding the latter, it is not unusual for covert depression or its less severe counterpart, demoralization, to make its first appearance and require specific attention at this point.

Finally, phase 5 is *trial and error*. Perhaps the major difference between brief and extended forms of psychotherapy is that, in the latter, this stage is likely to occur in the continuing presence of the therapist, whereas in the former it is not. The therapist's continuing presence in the patient's life is sometimes justified by referring to the psychoanalytic concept of the "working through," in which unconscious material is integrated into the patient's consciousness and everyday life. In fact, in most insight-oriented psychotherapy, the therapist's decision to remain in the patient's life during this phase is probably based on other factors. Given the option of return, there is usually little risk in terminating an episode of treatment at this phase.

With momentum from therapy, and especially when significant others in the patient's environment support and reinforce change, a period of high energy and increased risk-taking often follows success-ful brief intervention. The patient comes unstuck. Often, however, sig-nificant others do the opposite: undermine, sabotage, or resist change. The patient's efforts may also be undermined by early failure or fear of failure, or by reluctance to face the necessary losses. Return, often with significant others, or for a "booster shot," is common and should be provided so that the patient does not have to feel a failure. It is not uncommon for a patient who returns to have regressed to an earlier point in the sequence—for example, difficulty in trusting, or the reac-tivation of negative ideas about the self or feelings of hopelessness. These can usually be dealt with briefly and should not be misperceived as indicating a need for a secondary level of care (for example, ex-tended, continuous psychotherapy).

Monitoring Psychotherapy

One implication of the phase grid in Table 13–1 is that focal therapy ought to proceed in a more or less sequential manner, and that failure to do so may be analyzed, understood, and responded to strategically. Although this is rarely as simple as it sounds, it offers a framework for assessment and monitoring that has broad implications. As a number of authors have indicated, diagnosis alone is not a good prognosticator of the patient's ability to benefit from a focal, brief intervention (Bud-man and Gurman 1988; Malan 1976). The only test of the ability to benefit is a trial of such treatment. Because decisions to change a treatment plan, introduce secondary care elements, or shift from a pri-mary to a secondary care level have major implications for the patient and the system, they should be based on some form of objective assess-ment that takes place *during the course of* therapy, preferably at piv-otal intervals. What follows is a suggested format for such an assessment.

In the simplest focal intervention, a helping relationship will be established during (in some cases even prior to) the first session. Re-framing and agreement on a focus should occur within the first session or two. By the third or fourth session, it is usually apparent whether or not these initial steps have proceeded well and whether rehearsal for change has begun. Such a juncture should therefore be appropriate for an initial review. If the review appraises the balance between motive and resistance, it will link the failure to progress with its cause. For example, the failure to establish a helping relationship by the fourth or fifth session suggests either significant psychopathology in the patient or something quite wrong in the therapeutic dyad.

Clinical review, in its simplest form, may be conducted by the primary provider alone; however, a more structured and formal assessment mechanism should also exist, one capable of looking objectively at the patient-therapist dyad, assessing the reasons for lack of progress, and suggesting modifications in the design or conduct of the treatment. The basic review should address three questions: First, is there evidence that the patient's level of symptomatic distress and functional impairment is improving, or that the treatment focus is likely to produce such improvement in the near future? Second, is there evidence that the patient is moving toward taking appropriate and necessary action to address the life impasse that produced the need for help? Third, is the work of treatment proceeding relatively free of extreme forms of resistance: those that are likely to undermine the achievement of treatment objectives? If the answer to any of these is negative, a more formal review of the treatment plan is in order, to determine whether some significant "limiting factor" has been overlooked and must be addressed, or whether some element of the therapeutic system (the helping relationship, the chosen focus, the methodology) must be corrected or changed.

Most commonly, a therapeutic impasse at this juncture signals the need for an ancillary strategy—for example, a psychopharmacological consult, the entry of a key figure (spouse, family member, friend) into the treatment, a symptom-alleviating strategy, or self-help adjunct (AA, Al-Anon). The failure to make a clear decision to introduce such elements of secondary care into the treatment tends to produce run-on care. Paradoxically, prolonged impasses in treatment produce a pattern of overutilization that is actually undertreatment. In the absence of reassessment, however, obstructed treatment is likely to be misperceived as a demonstrated need for *more,* rather than *different,* therapy. Concurrent clinical review of the kind suggested carries the potential for enhancing efficiency and specificity (and therefore the quality of care), for educating practitioners, and for spurring the development of appropriate and necessary secondary care resources.

The phase grid is not a cookbook. Patients and therapists move backward and forward in the process, and phases overlap. It is presented as a way of conceptualizing the change process and the catalytic function of the therapist within it. This model is consistent with the primary care mental health relationship. Selective foci may involve helpers or programs other than the primary mental health provider, brought in for selected purposes (secondary care adjuncts), in the course of helping the patient proceed through the sequence (e.g., a course of medication, a group experience, stress reduction training, a course of behavioral or cognitive therapy).

Conclusion

The treatment model described in this chapter has evolved over 20 years of practice in a staff model HMO, where it is used for supervision and training of therapists new to the setting. It is shaped by ideas about adult development and by the setting's imperatives for treatment planning, conservation of resources, and sharing of responsibility with other providers and with patients themselves. It is parsimonious in both intent and design. Setting shapes values, which in turn shape practice. Managed care settings, in which responsibility to the individual patient is always balanced by responsibility for the enrolled population (future patients), are likely to have high rates of consumer demand for services. This fact, supported by epidemiological surveys on the high incidence of emotional disorder in the general population, can best be reconciled with the mandate to conserve costs by offering relatively little service to a relatively large number of people.

   In a competitive environment, cost containment and consumer satisfaction are inevitable organizational priorities. These realities filter down to the clinical level and shape the behavior of the health care provider by setting the tone for his or her relationship with the member who has become a patient. The model presented is designed to be responsive to the patient's need while conserving resources. It emphasizes early and ready (repeated, if necessary) access, responsive and tailored service, active collaboration of the patient in his or her care, and a facilitative, modest role for the health care professional. It is problem-driven (though not, as crisis intervention is, necessarily problem-centered). It rests heavily on the twin requirements of treatment planning and focality, and the principle of discontinuity in treatment within the context of an enduring, continuing relationship. Although it originated in a closed setting, it is my belief that such a model is compatible with a wide variety of clinical settings with similar missions.

References

Adler G: The myth of the alliance with borderline patients. Am J Psychiatry 136:642–645, 1979

Balint M, Orstein PH, Balint E: Focal Psychotherapy. London, Tavistock, 1972

Bennett M: Focal psychotherapy: terminable and interminable. Am J Psychother 37:365–375, 1983

Bennett M: Brief psychotherapy and adult development. Psychotherapy 21:171–177, 1984

Bennett M: The greening of the HMO: implications for prepaid psychiatry. Am J Psychiatry 145:1544–1549, 1988

Bennett M: The catalytic function in psychotherapy. Psychiatry 52:351–364, 1989

Budman S, Gurman A: The Theory and Practice of Brief Therapy. New York, Guilford, 1988

Budman S, Feldman J, Bennett M: Adult mental health services in a health maintenance organization. Am J Psychiatry 136:392–395, 1979

Colarusso C, Nemiroff M: Clinical implications of adult developmental theory. Am J Psychiatry 144:1263–1270, 1987

Gustafson P: An integration of brief dynamic psychotherapy. Am J Psychiatry 141:935–944, 1984

Malan D: The Frontier of Brief Psychotherapy. New York, Plenum, 1976

Mann J: Time Limited Psychotherapy. Cambridge, MA, Harvard University Press, 1973

Stoeckle J: Principles of primary care, in Primary Care Medicine. Edited by Goroll A, May L, Mulley A. Philadelphia, PA, JB Lippincott, 1981

✦ 14 ✦

The Managed Care Setting and the Patient-Therapist Relationship

Judith L. Feldman, M.D.

The quality of the relationship between patient and treating clinician is central to the success of any psychiatric intervention. Whatever the treatment modality, length, or ultimate goal, a helping relationship plays a major part in it.

Some of the obvious differences between fee-for-service practice and managed care practice (length of treatment, use of group treatment, prepayment, institutional setting, cost containment, utilization review) have been cited as detracting from the quality of the relationship, and thus the quality of treatment in managed settings (Sederer and St. Clair 1989). Consideration of the effects of these and other factors must necessarily lead to a general examination of the effect of any treatment setting on the therapeutic relationships within it.

Goldensohn and Haar (1974) discussed the effects on transference and countertransference of practicing in a staff model health maintenance organization (HMO). They mentioned the influence of prepayment, the duration of treatment, authority issues, and institutional transference as issues affecting the therapeutic relationship. Bennett and Feldstein surveyed patient satisfaction with mental health treatment in a staff model HMO (Bennett and Feldstein 1986). They found that patients who were highly satisfied or highly dissatisfied with their care cited the "human quality" of the therapist as the most important factor in their treatment. Patients who were unsure about satisfaction cited the modality of treatment as the most common problem in their care.

There are five major aspects of managed care practice that influence the patient-therapist relationship: payment, systems issues, regulatory issues, internal management issues, and organizational values. Examination of these factors in a managed setting provides a framework with which to examine other treatment settings—from solo, office-based practice to the state hospital. In this chapter I will discuss each of these factors as they relate to managed care practice and then present a model of the therapeutic relationship as a "family triad" of patient, therapist, and organization.

Payment

In virtually all managed settings, some mental health care is prepaid. The patient (or the employer) pays a premium, and there is a mental health "benefit" (usually 20 outpatient visits and 30 to 60 hospital days) with some copayment. These conditions immediately affect the attitude of a patient considering treatment. Some devalue the care ("I was seeing a wonderful therapist in the community, but then I joined the Plan and I guess I'll try you out because you are free"). Some feel entitled to the care, whether they need it or not ("I have some things I want to work on, and I understand I get 20 free visits here"). The way in which patients view psychiatric insurance is greatly influenced by community norms and socioeconomic class (Schneider-Braus 1987). For many, psychiatric treatment means only weekly, open-ended, exploratory psychotherapy. Others are more interested in rapid symptom relief and may not know or care how many "visits" they get. Often the therapist must educate the patient about the health care system in the midst of trying to evaluate or handle the patient's acute crisis ("I was upset *enough* about my divorce, now you're telling me you just do brief treatment!").

Payment of the clinician has an equally important influence. Mental health clinicians may be salaried (in a staff model HMO), they may be paid fee-for-service from a fixed overall capitation (in an Independent Practice Association [IPA]), or they may "own" an organization that arranges to provide service to an HMO on a capitated basis (mental health preferred provider organization [PPO]). There are often "bonuses," "withholds," or "incentives" that link payment to the financial performance of the organization, or the specific productivity of the individual clinician. Whatever the payment system, it affects attitudes and relationships. A salaried clinician has no financial incentive to overtreat. On the other hand, he or she has no financial incentive to "fit in" an extra patient in crisis or to make an extra hospital visit. If clinicians are rewarded financially for seeing more new intakes, they may resent the patients with lengthier or more difficult problems. Salaried clinicians will tend more toward a "one-class" system of care and may be totally unaware of the financial circumstances of their patients. Fee-for-service clinicians may welcome extra patients, but they are well aware of patients' ability to pay when their insurance benefit is exhausted.

In a prepaid system where there is no fee-for-service treatment, the currency of the relationship becomes time rather than money. Therapists and patients may overvalue time and use it to describe issues of commitment and caring. A free hour, for a therapist, represents not loss of income but a needed respite, so he or she is less likely to reach out to a no-show patient. Patients often become concerned about the exact length and timing of appointments. In an HMO, it is often impossible for a patient to return for an appointment on the same day and time each week. This may create some anxiety for patients, but it also lessens dependency and chances for regression. However, patients may resent a system in which they *cannot* have more treatment, even if they are willing to get an extra job to pay for it.

Systems Issues

Managed care systems can be described as more or less "closed" or "open," depending on the structure, contract, and benefit and payment system. An IPA is a fairly open system, in which a large group of primary physicians may refer to virtually any mental health practitioner in the area. Some IPAs restrict mental health providers, or close the system completely by contracting with one small mental health group for all services. A staff model HMO is a virtually completely closed system in which patients can only see HMO clinicians, often only in one particular health center. The nature of the referral system also affects relationships. In many managed systems, patients do not self-refer, but must be referred either by a primary physician or by a mental health coordinator or "gatekeeper." The referring clinician may have a fixed budget to pay the specialist (an incentive to underrefer) or may be salaried (an incentive to overrefer). If the primary physician is busy and refers without screening patients, the mental health clinician may feel "dumped on" with inappropriate referrals and may resent a particular patient for being one of too many. Conversely, if the primary physician rarely refers patients to save capitation money, the mental health clinician may feel undervalued or excluded.

The nature of the relationship with the primary physician will affect a patient's attitude and feeling about his or her future mental health clinician. Patients may feel a sense of safety that their doctor is "picking" a therapist for them, instead of leaving them to choose from a universe of unknown clinicians. However, barriers to access (phone calls, referral forms, waits for return phone calls, delays in scheduling, arbitrary appointment slots) will detract from any sense of an individualized or personal referral.

Managed systems, particularly HMOs, usually have substructures: health centers, aftercare programs, substance abuse programs, day hospitals, and so on. The configuration and interaction of these substructures has an effect on particular clinician-patient interactions. For instance, if a busy HMO clinician is aware that there are openings in a group for eating disorders, he or she will feel positive and welcoming toward a patient with an eating disorder, and might even tend to overemphasize that aspect of the patient's presenting picture because there is a handy disposition available for the patient.

In a mental health department, a patient may be cared for by many clinicians. In addition to a primary therapist, there may be crisis clinicians, on-call clinicians, hospital attending clinicians, psychopharmacologists, or case managers. This team approach may diffuse a potentially negative or intense transference, but it may also feel confusing or impersonal to a patient. There is also a danger of patients splitting, or clinicians not knowing who has primary responsibility for a case.

Another "system" is the medical record, which is often automated. The presence of an automated record, available to all other practitioners in the system, raises questions about confidentiality. Patient and therapist may conspire to omit information or use euphemistic diagnoses. The presence of the record may also contribute to making the clinician feel less "private" about the relationship with the patient. Automated records can also increase feelings of security for both patient and therapist, because needed information can be available to all parts of a system in case of emergency. Clinicians can count on backup support of on-call systems or emergency rooms that have current information about the patient's clinical condition and treatment plan.

Such availability may also curb "acting out" in manipulative patients, who are less able to make demands on covering clinicians when the current treatment plan is available in the medical record.

Regulatory Issues

State and federal regulations will affect the mental health benefit and the way in which it is delivered in any managed system within their jurisdiction. State regulations that mandate mental health benefits in HMOs and prohibit exclusions from psychiatric care put enormous pressure on an organization to give comprehensive care to its members. In states that allow exclusions, HMOs will structure their benefits accordingly (see Chapter 5). When pressed for time, clinicians may, consciously or unconsciously, attempt to put patients in categories that will exempt the HMO from providing further care. They may feel guilt over "excluding" a patient and become overzealous in treating the next patient. Some clinicians may turn into staunch patient advocates or treat patients in ways that are truly *not* covered by the HMO, and then fear reprisals from their supervisors.

The legal and legislative climate may force clinicians into defensive practice to avoid litigation. Legal issues affect all systems of care, but managed systems are becoming more vulnerable than many other settings (see Chapter 11). A clinician may feel angry or fearful at taking on a patient who is paranoid or suicidal or who demands a type of treatment that the HMO does not provide. Although the organization is urging cost containment, brief hospital stays, and outpatient alternatives, it is the clinician who is exposed in a lawsuit.

The recent cutbacks of public mental health programs that provided extended care and social services to HMO patients with serious mental illness have had an enormous effect on the comfort of clinicians who treat such patients in a managed setting. When public funding is tight, it is more difficult to welcome patients with chronic mental illness, because many necessary aspects of care (e.g., housing, legal services) are not covered by the HMO.

Internal Management Issues

The structure and mission of an organization, the dominant management style, fiscal status, rate of growth, and other characteristics have profound effects on the climate of practice and on clinician morale. Within the requirements of the law, an organization shapes a mental health benefit, plans a program, sets priorities, determines a budget, establishes policies and procedures, and rewards certain clinical behaviors and activities. For instance, one HMO may devote 5% of its budget to mental health, have a multidisciplinary department 25% of whose staff are psychiatrists, and have as a priority treating chronic illness and preventing hospitalization. Another may devote 3% of the budget to mental health, do only crisis intervention with a few in-house clinicians, and refer most patients to a panel of community practitioners. A clinician meeting a seriously ill patient would develop a very different relationship with that individual in each of these organizations.

The marketing strategy of a managed care organization also has an impact on clinician and member attitudes. An organization that is growing rapidly and marketing aggressively may promise more than it can deliver, heightening expectations of patients before they begin treatment. It is often difficult for a marketing representative to understand the intricacies of the mental health program and how it differs from community norms. Even if he or she understands it, there is rarely time to explain it fully to the employer, let alone the prospective member. Some HMO mental health departments are working actively with marketing departments to prepare patients so they are not disappointed at the actual services they receive (Rudolph Link, M.D., personal communication, November 1987).

A crucial factor is the amount of money an organization allocates to mental health services and the budgeting process involved in allocating that money. The percent of premium dollars spent by an organization on mental health varies from 2% to 15% nationally (see Chapter 3). This figure depends on the mental health benefit, state mandates, exclusions, the nature of the demand for services, and the organizational philosophy and values. A tight budget and relative understaffing will further increase the pressure on clinicians to treat patients very rapidly, and may interfere with the formation of a working therapeutic alliance. These feelings can be ameliorated by a budgeting process that is consistent, fair, and communicated openly to clinicians. Budget cuts that feel impulsive or "top-down" to clinicians are more apt to increase the wish to "fend off" patients. If clinicians are included in discussions of budgeting and priority setting, they may feel that they can discuss the reality of limitations with patients (when this is clinically appropriate). This stance can actually be quite therapeutic and can model for patients the ability to make the most of reality just as it is.

The mental health benefit itself, and how the organization interprets it, will affect relationships with patients. In a staff model HMO, outpatient utilization is limited more by available staff hours than by the benefit. Patients' perceptions of benefit limits may be important in the relationships they form with caregivers and programs.

Organizational Values

The overall values and philosophy of an organization are of utmost importance. There are certain values in particular that are most relevant to helping or hindering a therapeutic relationship.

1. *The value and priority of mental health in the overall organization.* Is it a central part of initial planning, or an "add-on" later? Do all members have a mental health benefit? How much money is spent on mental health? What physical plant houses a mental health department? The more value is placed on mental health as a service, the more valued clinicians will feel, and the better able they will be to help themselves and their patients deal with the inevitable limitations posed by a managed system.

2. *The value of the individual versus the group.* This is an ethical clash in any health care system. Do you give priority to an individual patient, or allocate resources to an entire population? A clinician in an HMO makes these decisions as a matter of daily business: "If I plan a 15-session course of treatment for Ms. Jones, am I going to have time for the other new patients I will see this week?" A mental health manager also must decide whether to emphasize access to a department for new patients or depth of treatment for the patients already there. These decisions may be made at a higher level in the organization, emphasizing access, for instance, to improve member satisfaction. However, these broad priorities have enormous influence on the attitude with which a clinician approaches a new patient.

3. *The value the organization places on training and acculturating new staff.* Managed mental health care requires a different set of skills and attitudes than fee-for-service practice (see Chapter 12). This shift is much greater for mental health than for other

branches of medicine. To the extent that an organization recognizes this and puts resources into good training, there will be an improvement in staff skills and morale, and a decrease in staff turnover.

4. *The clinical treatment philosophy.* Organizations differ greatly in their clinical mental health philosophy and priorities. Some feel that treatment of mental illness is all the organization should do and that patients with problems of living should go to family, friends, or self-help organizations. Some organizations feel that substance abuse treatment is the top priority in mental health care; others put it close to the bottom. Some believe that brief treatment is simply crisis intervention to tide patients over until they can afford long-term treatment; others believe that it is a catalyst for permanent and profound change (see Chapter 13).

Patients who "fit in" to the treatment philosophy and priorities will be more easily "welcomed" by the busy clinician. Other patients may be seen more as a problem or a nuisance. The concept of "resistance" often assumes a new twist in an HMO. In fee-for-service practice, the patient who is interested in alleviating his or her symptoms and not exploring further is seen as "resistant"; however, in an HMO, the patient who refuses to focus and set a short-term goal is seen as "resistant"!

Whatever the philosophy and values of the organization, a managed care system always serves to interject one or more extra parties into the patient-therapist dyad. In fact, doing individual treatment in a managed system is more like doing family treatment, where the other members of the family are the patient's employer, the therapist's boss, the HMO as insurance company, the marketing department, the therapist's other patients, the utilization review coordinator, and so on. Any third, fourth, or fifth party who has a financial interest in the care inevitably becomes involved in the care delivered.

These systems concerns pose interesting problems for the therapist developing an alliance with a patient. They can be diagrammed using concepts from general systems theory, to demonstrate the shifting alliances and conflicts that occur in these situations. In these examples, the triad portrayed is that of patient (P), clinician (C), and managed care organization (O). These concepts may also be used to include employer, employee assistance program (EAP), or any other "interested parties."

1. Alliance of the clinician and the patient "against" the organization:

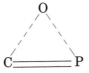

Example: A clinician, after evaluating a patient who demands weekly, open-ended treatment says, "I'd love to see you every week, but my HMO won't let me." This stance may ultimately get the therapist "in trouble" with his or her boss and will certainly lead to a false and unrealistic alliance, with the patient feeling dissatisfied with the limits, complaining to the medical director, or dropping out of the HMO. This configuration is more likely to occur in the IPA, where mental health clinicians are not employed by the organization, and where utilization management is not done by the treating clinician.

2. Alliance of the patient and the organization "against" the therapist:

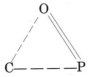

Example: The patient says, "Put me in a 28-day alcohol program tonight, or I'll call your medical director." If the organizational climate is such that a clinician does not feel free to use his or her best clinical judgment and skills because of worries about patient complaints, then there can be no alliance that has any meaning. Patients will manipulate for what they want, and no treatment can take place.

3. Alliance of the organization and the clinician "against" the patient:

Example: A busy clinician referred several patients to a group for "relationship problems." One patient complained to the chief, saying "Yes, I do have problems with relationships, but I really just wanted a few individual meetings to talk about my job." Clinicians, in an apparent identification with the organization, may begin to believe that all patients may be seen in group therapy, or given superficial advice rather than treatment. There is always a danger of being brainwashed rather than merely influenced by a powerful organizational climate. This is more likely to occur in a staff model HMO where clinicians are encouraged to identify with strong organizational norms.

4. No alliances at all; distance and animosity between and among all three parties:

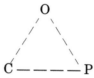

Example: A clinician, feeling burnt out, says to his or her chief, "I'm going to quit working here if they give me one more borderline patient. These patients all complain to the medical director, whatever you give them. With the workload I'm getting, I just don't have time for this." These pressures and conflicts may, at times, lead to the type of dysfunctional system where everyone is angry. This is likely to occur in an organization in rapid change or growth, which is operating with dysfunctional systems, communication, or management style. In that climate, it is very hard if not impossible to be therapeutic. Sometimes, it is necessary to share this situation with patients, although such disclosure must be done cautiously.

In this chapter, I have described five major aspects of managed care systems and their effects on the therapeutic relationships between clinicians and patients. I have also presented a model, derived from family systems theory, to describe the complex interrelationships that impinge on the patient-therapist dyad in the complex managerial and organizational climate in which patients are treated today.

References

Bennett MJ, Feldstein M: Correlates of patient satisfaction with mental health services in a health maintenance organization. Am J Prev Med 2(3):155–162, 1986

Goldensohn SS, Haar E: Transference and countertransference in a third-party payment system (HMO). Am J Psychiatry 131(3):256–260, 1974

Schneider-Braus K: A practical guide to HMO psychiatry. Hosp Community Psychiatry 38(8):876–879, 1987

Sederer L, St. Clair L: Managed health care and the Massachusetts experience. Am J Psychiatry 146(9):1142–1147, 1989

✦ 15 ✦

Models of Brief Individual and Group Psychotherapy

Simon H. Budman, Ph.D.

In recent years there has been an explosion of interest in brief psychotherapy. Books and workshops on brief treatment are available in ever-increasing numbers. Clinical psychology, social work, and psychiatry training programs have added short-term treatment seminars as an important component of their overall curricula, and entire schools of family therapy involve brief courses of treatment (e.g., DeShazer 1985; Fisch et al. 1982). Additionally, popular guides to psychotherapy (e.g., Burns 1981) and articles in the press (Turkington 1989) encourage patients to seek out clinicians who are knowledgeable about or willing to apply brief treatment principles.

This trend arises, to a large degree, from a long-standing historical interest in developing faster, more efficient modes of psychotherapeutic treatment, as well as from a growing knowledge base and greater conceptual clarity regarding the effective ingredients in psychotherapy (Bergin and Garfield 1986). However, these factors would probably be insufficient to alter service delivery patterns significantly were it not for economic factors. Previous chapters in this book have addressed such issues in depth. Suffice it to say that insurers and employer groups have a growing interest in encouraging approaches to psychotherapeutic treatment that are beneficial to clients but do not continue endlessly.

Brief Psychotherapy and Health Insurance Coverage

A major increase in public awareness and demand for outpatient mental health services for "less severe" (i.e., nonpsychotic) conditions, concern on the part of insurers regarding spiraling psychotherapy costs, and a growing array of prepaid insurance structures will all have a major impact on the provision of mental health services in this country. Over the next decade a growing percentage of psychiatrists, psychologists, social workers, family therapists, and psychiatric nurses will offer short-term, time-effective mental health services. Although in the fee-for-service sector a percentage of the population will still receive and desire long-term, ongoing, multiyear psychotherapy, the overwhelming trend will be toward brief, focused, intermittent treatment (Budman and Gurman 1988; Levin and Glasser 1988).

What is Brief Therapy?

Definitional confusion abounds as to what constitutes brief therapy, temporally speaking (Budman and Gurman 1983, 1988; Gurman 1981; Koss and Butcher 1986). Yet the identity of brief therapy must be considered before moving on to a consideration of its practice. As the term is usually used among clinicians, psychotherapy is thought to be "brief" when it is clearly a great deal shorter (in terms of number of sessions or total duration) than the ideal(ized) practice of psychoanalysis or individual psychoanalytic psychotherapy (e.g., more than one session per week over a year or more). This concept of therapeutic brevity exists, of course, in the minds of its practitioners. In the minds of most consumers of psychotherapy, quite a different state of affairs exists.

Large numbers of people seeking psychotherapy in outpatient clinic settings expect their treatment to last less than 3 months. Indeed, a very high percentage of patients terminate treatment in fewer than 12 sessions (Butcher and Koss 1978; Garfield 1989), and the median number of therapy sessions among psychotherapy outpatients in clinics is about 5 or 6 (Garfield 1986). Garfield (1986), reviewing the research on dropouts versus continuers in therapy, noted that "contrary to many traditional expectations concerning length of therapy, most clients remain in therapy for only a few interviews. . . . This pattern . . . was not the result of a deliberately planned brief psychotherapy" (p. 219). Treatments of roughly 6 to 12 visits are not (also apparently contrary to the views of many clinicians) particular to patients of lower socioeconomic status (Lorion 1973, 1974) but also occur in the general private practice of psychotherapy (Koss 1979). And although brief therapies have received most of their attention just in the last decade, the recurrent fact of the typical psychotherapy outpatient receiving fewer than 10 sessions has been noted and emphasized for decades (e.g., Matarazzo 1965; Rubinstein and Lorr 1956). By the temporal ideals of most traditionally trained psychotherapists, then, brief therapy is hardly new and was not ushered in by the emergence of HMOs, governmental cost-containing agencies, and the like. The "explosion of interest" in brief psychotherapy I referred to in the first line of this chapter has been an explosion of interest in *planned* brief therapy, that is, brief therapy "by design" versus the commonly occurring unplanned brief therapy "by default" (Gurman 1981, p. 417). This distinction is absolutely essential to keep in mind when we turn to consider the basic components of a practical model of brief treatment.

Attitudes and Brief Treatment

If brief therapy cannot be easily defined by the specific number of sessions devoted to treatment, how can it be defined? Gurman and I (Budman and Gurman 1988) have written elsewhere:

> In part, brief therapy is a state of mind of the therapist and of the patient; in part, brief therapy involves a set of limitations on service delivery system resources. The techniques of brief treatment are derived from these attitudinal and system limitation factors. (p. 10)

It is *most centrally* these attitudinal "state of mind" factors and system limitations that are the quintessential defining characteristics of brief treatment. These, in turn, lead to a number of technical treatment factors that further help in delimiting brief therapy.

The most important attitudinal distinctions between the "long-term" and "short-term" therapist that Gurman and I (Budman and Gurman 1988) have posited are shown in Table 15–1. (It should be noted that the distinctions we describe are archetypes. Many therapists who practice mostly brief treatment also see some patients for longer, continuous periods, and vice versa.)

These proposed areas of distinction between long-term and short-term therapists have been subjected to empirical examination. Bolter and Levinson (1988), in an interesting study, found that among a random sample of 222 licensed psychologists, those who preferred short-term therapy were much more likely to endorse the short-term therapist values described by Budman and Gurman (1983, 1988) than were self-described long-term therapists. This finding was maintained even when the contributions of theoretical orientation and other variables (such as years of experience and ratio of time in private practice) were controlled for. Clearly, the implications are that when one seeks to train therapists to do brief treatment at prepaid health care settings, an important primary area that must be addressed is the value system with which the therapist approaches the therapy he or she provides.

Along with the eight dominant values described below, I have recently considered one other area of value difference between brief and long-term therapists. This is the area of *patient responsibility for change.* The brief therapist makes the stated or unstated assumption that ultimately, change in psychotherapy occurs because of the patient's efforts and his or her taking responsibility for the implementation of change. This is not to indicate that the long-term therapist does not believe that the patient should be responsible for

Table 15–1. Comparative dominant values of long-term and short-term therapists

Long-Term Therapist	Short-Term Therapist
1. Seeks change in basic character.	Prefers pragmatism, parsimony, and least radical intervention, does not believe in notion of "cure."
2. Believes that significant psychological change is unlikely in everyday life.	Maintains an adult developmental perspective from which significant psychological change is viewed as inevitable.
3. Sees presenting problems as reflecting more basic pathology.	Emphasizes patient's strengths and resources.
4. Wants to "be there" as patient makes significant changes.	Accepts that many changes will occur "after therapy."
5. Sees therapy as having a "timeless" quality.	Does not accept the timelessness of some models of therapy.
6. Unconsciously recognizes the fiscal convenience.	Fiscal issues often muted, either by the nature of the therapist's practice or by the organizational structure.
7. Views psychotherapy as almost always benign and useful.	Views psychotherapy as being sometimes useful and sometimes harmful.
8. Sees patient's being in therapy as the most important part of patient's life.	Sees being in the world as more important than being in therapy.

modifying his or her life. However, it is rather easy in a long-term, ongoing treatment to lapse into a therapeutic relationship in which issues of responsibility for change or even the possibility of change itself comes to be forgotten. As Yalom (1980) writes: "Patients, often with the silent collusion of the therapist, may settle comfortably, passively and permanently into therapy, expecting little to happen or if anything is to happen, it will come from the therapist" (p. 236). Such an arrangement is virtually impossible in settings in which brief therapy is the major mode of treatment. The brief therapist assumes that given reasonable tools and input from the therapist the patient can then choose to make useful changes for him-or herself or may choose not to change. Further, positive changes may not necessarily occur at the time of a particular intervention; at times, many months or perhaps years might have to pass until the patient is prepared to use the earlier input for his or her benefit.

It is of major importance that the brief therapist make the assumption that *the patient* will ultimately make the decision to change or not to change. The therapist need not be present throughout the process for the patient to decide to use what he or she has learned in the service of therapeutic growth. Furthermore, even when therapists don't realize that patients are changing, the patients may take from each course of treatment and each therapist they see something that may be used later in their lives.

Technical Treatment Factors in Brief Therapy

The attitudes described above, as well as theory and research in brief treatment, carry with them a variety of technical implications for the practice of such therapies.

Focus in Brief Treatment

It is imperative that every model of brief treatment offer the clinician a way of focusing the therapy (Budman and Gurman 1988). Without a clear and circumscribed focus, the therapist is not able to decide how to limit his or her attention and how to set manageable goals and targets in the treatment. Brief therapies differ as to what areas are understood to be the appropriate foci of treatment. For some cognitive models of brief treatment the focus is on the internal, counterproductive conversations of the patient with himself or herself (Beck et al. 1979). For another model of short-term treatment, the focus is on the patient's interpersonal interactions (Klerman et al. 1984). In yet another approach, the patient's transferential re-creations of his or her transactional problems are emphasized (Strupp and Binder 1984). Regardless of the brief therapy model in question, it is essential that there be a means of focusing the treatment.

High Therapist Activity Level

Because the brief therapist is attempting to use time parsimoniously and with the most substantial impact, he or she must maintain a relatively high level of activity (Budman and Bennett 1983). It is unlikely that many short-term theoreticians would advocate long periods of therapist passivity while waiting for the patient to develop strong enough transference feelings or "come to the solution [him- or herself]." For the therapist to be passive and inactive would be seen by most proponents of brief therapy as being a waste of a precious commodity—therapeutic time.

Encouragement of the Patient to "Be" Outside of Therapy

This means that in a variety of ways the therapist makes use of "outside of therapy resources" and thus reduces the patient's dependence on the therapist while enhancing his or her cultivation of outside supports. Such resources are there in a more continuous way for the patient and cost less to the patient and the health care system. In encouraging the use of outside supports, the therapist makes use of homework assignments, involves significant others in the treatment process, and uses "naturally occurring therapies."

By offering the patient assignments and tasks between sessions, the therapist is aware of the fact that the majority of therapeutic work occurs not *inside* of a therapy session but *outside* in the patient's interactions. The therapeutic "homework" also keeps the therapy "alive" outside of the sessions and serves as a bridge between inside and outside therapy.

The brief therapist recognizes the value of involving the patient's significant others where and when possible in the treatment. Rather than keeping the therapy a clandestine process isolated from the patient's real world, the brief therapist sees the involvement of spouse, parents, siblings, lover, and so on as ways of expediting the process of improvement and a way of "going with the tide" of change rather than ignoring potentially facilitative aspects of the environment.

There are currently a large array of what I call "naturally occurring therapies." Programs such as Alcoholics Anonymous, Overeaters Anonymous, Toastmasters International, and so on are available to most people in this country at no cost or very low cost. These groups are structured around various problem areas and are viewed as mutual-help organizations. Patients can make use of these resources as well as using the resources of professional therapists. A unique value of these types of programs (aside from their low expense) is that many provide extremely high levels of availability to members; such availability is often well beyond the ability or the desires of most mental health professionals. There are also other natural therapies that are not in the form of an organization or group. For example, research indicates (Folkins and Sime 1981) that exercise can have a very beneficial impact upon mental state. Rather than viewing only what occurs between the therapist and the patient as therapeutic, the brief therapist can expand his or her perceptions to include a variety of endeavors on the patient's part as having a valuable impact.

Inextricability of Evaluation and Treatment

Because the realistic brief therapist recognizes that the actual number of sessions that most patients come to treatment is very low (about 3 to 6 is the norm), he or she must hit the ground running. For a therapist to assume that one will have weeks or months in which to do an evaluation *before* deciding upon a treatment plan is unlikely and, for the most part, undesirable. The brief therapist must recognize that treatment and evaluation are inextricably interrelated. Indeed, for the brief therapist, the therapeutic process begins with the first contact with the patient. By making every session count, the brief therapist attempts to use time to maximum efficiency.

Flexible Use of Interventions and Time

The brief therapist should apply an "informed eclecticism" to his or her work. This means that the therapist is minimally constricted by theoretical dogma and parochialism. It is essential that the brief therapist realize that there are useful contributions to effective therapy from various theoretical viewpoints and that different intervention techniques may offer elements that are most beneficial for particular patients. For example, certain patients may require behavioral interventions in order to most effectively modify their areas of difficulty, whereas for other types of patients examining certain aspects of the transference may be most important. Also, the inclusion of marital, group, and family modalities may broaden the therapist's armamentarium. Within HMO mental health settings, many of which function to some degree as group practices, the opportunity exists to call upon different therapists to assist in working with distinct aspects of the patient's difficulties. There may, for example, be staff members who are more interested in group therapy or behavioral therapy who can be used as resources for the other therapists at the HMO. It is extremely important that the HMO mental health department include a variety of different interests and orientations, thus allowing this type of broadly based system of resources.

Another important but often neglected area for the brief therapist is that of the flexible use of time. There is a tendency among clinicians to see time in therapy as coming in very few sizes (e.g., the 50-minute hour or the 90-minute group session). This rigid view neglects the fact that the therapist may want to use time in a variety of flexible and creative ways. Because it is clear from research evidence that it is in the first eight sessions that therapy has its greatest impact (Howard et al. 1986), it may be that it is most efficacious to see some patients "intensively" during early sessions (that is, initially use longer sessions that are spaced closely to one another) and then much less frequently in shorter sessions that are widely spaced. The scheduling of patients may differ according to the nature of the problem and issues with which the patient is dealing. However, it is most important to keep in mind that a therapist need not be locked into a rigid and unchangeable schedule of sessions.

Planned Follow-Up of Brief Therapy

Research has indicated that within a year of terminating long-term or short-term therapy, a substantial proportion of the patients who have "terminated" return for additional treatment (Budman 1990). It also appears that people who use therapeutic services tend to have numerous episodes of psychotherapy over the course of their lives (Budman and Gurman 1988; Grunebaum 1983). It may be that in the interest of efficacy and of taking a realistic perspective on the ways that people use therapy, the therapist plans a reunion with the patient at some point after the official "end" of therapy. This allows the patient to know that the therapist can be consulted at later points as the need arises and that it is not an indication of failure to return for additional treatment.

Practical Models of Brief Individual and Group Therapy

Based on many years of clinical and research work at the Harvard Community Health Plan in Boston, my colleagues and I have developed pragmatic models of brief individual and group psychotherapy. These models attempt to take into account the realities of working in a prepaid health care organization. Although it is probable that well over 100 planned brief treatment models exist, many of these approaches were conceived at academic settings or at clinics that have the luxury of being restrictive and rejecting large numbers of patients as inappropriate for brief therapy. This is certainly not the case at most HMOs or other prepaid plans where all patients must be treated as long as they are a member of the organization.

Brief Individual Therapy: An Interpersonal-Developmental-Existential Model

The brief individual therapy model that Gurman and I (Budman and Gurman 1988) developed is called Interpersonal-Developmental-Existential (I-D-E) brief treatment. In this model the patient is encouraged to view therapy as not being a complete "cure" for all of his or her problems. The patient is encouraged to use therapy as necessary and to avoid seeing the return for additional treatment as a sign of failure. Further, each episode of care can consist of relatively few sessions, because the patient is encouraged to view the therapeutic relationship as enduring even when meetings with the therapist are highly infrequent.

The I-D-E model advocates the technical intervention strategies referred to earlier. That is, the therapist, when possible, involves significant others in the treatment, is active, uses time flexibly, and so on.

Figure 15–1 presents the major treatment foci in the I-D-E model. These foci derive from the central question that the I-D-E therapist is asking himself or herself upon seeing a new patient: "Why now?" That is, of all the possible points in a person's life that he or she might choose to seek therapy, why has the patient chosen this point? The answer can usually be found in one of the major I-D-E focal areas; consciously or unconsciously, the client is most essentially dealing with one or more of the five focal areas described below.

These five focal areas—loss, developmental dysynchrony, interpersonal conflict, symptomatic focus, and personality disorder—attempt to cover the most frequent and important areas addressed by patients coming for outpatient mental health treatment.

The *loss focus* addresses the vast variety of broadly defined loss-related problems. These problems involve issues such as the death of a loved one or the loss of a relationship through separation, divorce, geographical moves, and so on. There are also a related set of loss

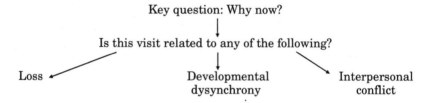

Key question: Why now?

Is this visit related to any of the following?

Loss   Developmental   Interpersonal
                dysynchrony   conflict

If the patient does not view the above focal areas as relevant, *or* if the
patient defines the symptom itself as the major issue,

Symptomatic focus

If the patient has had repeated presentations around any or all of the foci
above, without clear benefit, *or* if character issues preclude these foci
because of constant interference with the therapeutic process,

Character focus

Warning: Under circumstances of active alcohol or drug abuse, this problem
must be addressed before or simultaneously with the development
of any other focal area.

Figure 15–1. Major foci in brief therapy. Reprinted with permission from Budman and Gurman 1988.

problems that are what we call "existential losses." Such difficulties entail the loss of strongly held conceptions about the self and the world and occur when beliefs such as "I am invulnerable" ("It will happen to someone else, not to me") are challenged by a near-fatal illness.

Problems of *developmental dysynchrony* are related to the fact that most people have within themselves a sense of how they are doing in their developmental process as compared to others of approximately the same age and developmental cohort. The woman in her 40s who wishes to have children but has not been able to conceive feels dy- synchronous with her peers; the adult in his or her late 20s who has never had an intimate relationship with a lover feels "out of time" with his or her contemporaries. This sense of not being where one would like to be in one's life and/or where one feels others are is often a pressing issue for those coming into psychotherapy.

As all experienced outpatient therapists recognize, patients frequently seek treatment because they are experiencing *interpersonal conflict* with those around them. This may be the case in a family, marital, or romantic situation, or it may occur with co-workers and/or friends. In marital situations where therapists are frequently called upon to treat such conflict, the problem may very well be related to an unresolved loss for one or both partners or with a sense of developmental dysynchrony within the couple that has not been dealt with.

There may be times when a patient has no desire to deal with issues of loss, developmental dysynchrony, or interpersonal conflict (even when these issues are apparent). Such a patient might best be dealt with using a *symptomatic focus*. Under these circumstances it is the symptom itself that becomes the core of the therapy. For example, it may be impossible to try to convince a patient with severe insomnia that his or her sleep disorder is to be ignored while a series of significant losses are dealt with.

For some subset of outpatients, their maladaptive interpersonal styles may be so disruptive that any other area of focus for the therapy becomes untenable. Such patients, who usually have severe *personality disorders,* may have relationship dysfunctions so problematic that their impairments prevent them from relating effectively to the therapist. Under these circumstances the clinician is left with little option but to address the personality pathology directly.

We offer a series of algorithms for treating each of the focal areas described above (Budman and Gurman 1988). Although each of these foci has some unique facets of treatment, the overall I-D-E therapy approach makes use of the basic brief therapy principles discussed previously.

The I-D-E model of brief treatment is just one of the literally hundreds of new or relatively new approaches to planned brief psychotherapy. (For an overview of these models, see Wells and Phelps 1990 and Budman and Stone 1984.)

Time-Limited Group Psychotherapy Within the HMO

If therapy within the prepaid setting is to be provided in a high-quality, time-effective manner, a centerpiece of the treatment program must be a substantial group therapy capacity. By their very nature, time-limited groups are congruent with cost-effective models of care.

It is important that time-limited therapy groups be *integrated into an overall program of therapy* at the HMO. *Short-term groups are not a "stand-alone" program any more than individual therapy without other treatment supports is a stand-alone.* It is frequently the case that patients at the Harvard Community Health Plan are seen in a course of individual or marital therapy which then may be followed by a course of time-limited group treatment. The person may then stop treatment for some period to return again later for additional therapy. Groups can be extremely helpful to people; however, as with everything else in psychotherapy (or in life), they are not *the cure.*

Research indicates that there are not clear criteria that can help providers differentiate between who will do best in group therapy and who will do best in individual therapy (DeCarufel and Piper 1988). Therefore, a clinician can assume that with adequate preparation and information and within the context of an overall treatment program, most patients who can profit from a course of individual treatment would also be good candidates for group therapy. In one randomized trial (Budman et al. 1988), for example, we found that time-limited, 15-session group psychotherapy for young adults with intimacy problems was as effective as time-limited individual therapy. In another study on process and outcome in group therapy, we found that one of the major predictors of outcome in short-term group therapy was level of group cohesiveness (Budman et al. 1987). This finding has been replicated in a subsequent study (Budman et al. 1989) and appears to be a very robust conclusion. We have also found that in time-limited (18-

month) groups for patients with severe personality disorders, there are some major, observable within-group shifts in interaction for participants that appear to be related to outside-of-group changes (Budman et al., in press). It appears from this research that time-limited groups represent a very useful mode of therapy for a variety of different patient populations.

Central Elements of Time-Limited Group Therapy

There are a small number of pivotal elements in any successful time-limited group therapy (Budman and Bennett 1983; Budman and Gurman 1988). Although these factors may differ somewhat from one type of time-limited group to another, they are quite similar regardless of the particular group in question.

Establishment of a clear and well-defined focus.   As is true with all types of brief therapy, time-limited group treatment must be focused. A focus allows for homogeneity around a particular core area. This core area may be the fact that all members are dealing with a certain life crisis (such as having been recently bereaved), a particular developmental stage, or severe marital conflict. For a time-limited group to operate effectively, all members must have a shared set of perceptions about what is being worked upon in the group and how and why members are similar to one another. The focus in a time-limited group serves the same function that focality serves in any short-term model. It also helps a diverse group of individuals come together and begin working with one another more quickly and easily than they might under circumstances where there was not a shared commonality of aim and purpose.

Thorough screening and preparation of members.   Important aspects of all group therapies are the issues of screening and preparation (Yalom 1985). These issues are even more crucial in a time-limited group. If in open-ended group therapy a clinician finds that he or she has selected the wrong patients for the group or a number of the members are ill-prepared for the treatment, new members can be added. This is not nearly as possible when a therapist is operating under a time limit. The group may be half over by the time that the erroneous selection has become clear.

It is, therefore, most important that the short-term group therapist have procedures in place to adequately prepare the patients for the group and to screen out those patients who are inappropriate for the group or who need a different type of treatment. A variety of pregroup screening and preparation techniques for such groups have been developed (Budman and Gurman 1988). These techniques are quite useful in that they reduce dropouts (Budman and Clifford 1979), provide patients with skills in desirable group behaviors, improve patient selection, and allow the patient to make an informed decision about his or her participation in the group (Piper et al. 1979).

Need for rapid cohesion in time-limited groups.   A most important contributor to outcome in time-limited group therapy is the cohesiveness of the group (Budman et al. 1987). Cohesiveness in short-term groups is the equivalent of the therapeutic alliance in individual therapy (Budman et al. 1989). Although a therapist has an extended period of time to help build and foster cohesiveness in an open time-unlimited group, this is not the case in a short-term group. Focus and pregroup preparation contribute to the cohesiveness of a short-term group. There are also therapist intervention techniques and approaches that can help the group come together and become cohesive more quickly. For example, rather than treating members of the group individually within the group context, the skilled short-term group therapist will bring many patients into the process simultaneously. The therapist can do so by frequently "going around" in the group and asking members how they are reacting to a given event or issue in the group. He or she does so rather than simply focusing on one member at a time with little or no interaction between members. It is quite important that the time-limited group therapist understand cohesiveness and attempt to use this concept in the treatment he or she does.

Emphasis on existential and time-limit factors in a time-limited group.   As was stated previously, termination in the HMO is unlikely to be absolute as the patient remains a member and maintains a connection with other parts of the health care system. Nonetheless, when a time-limited group ends, it is unlikely that that particular group will ever again come together (except perhaps for a reunion) with the same combination of members and therapist. For this reason, the time-limited group often evokes strong feelings about the immutable passage of time and the fact that nothing lasts forever. Such groups often can act as triggers for the temporizing patient to finally take some action which he or she has been delaying for years. The group may also provoke feelings about life moving on and can thereby help the patient examine his or her life stage issues. In any case, it is most important that the therapist use the opportunity that is afforded by the time-limited nature of the group to help patients focus on existential issues.

Summary

In recent years, large numbers of people with mild to moderate psychological difficulties have been seen in the outpatient mental health departments of prepaid health care settings. To deal with this influx, mental health professionals have needed to use psychotherapeutic models that allow for brief, time-effective, and cost-effective care. Clinical and research literature indicates that such care may be relatively short-term but episodic. In many ways the mental health patient can begin to view his or her psychiatric clinician as similar to his or her primary medical care provider. That is, the psychologist, psychiatrist, or social worker may be viewed as available as needed over the life course, but not as a person who must be seen in an ongoing program of therapy.

I have discussed a number of basic principles of brief individual and group therapy in this chapter. These should be viewed as very general guidelines to such therapies. In some ways, probably the most important aspect of brief treatment within the HMO is that practitioners and administrators understand that such therapy is complex, stressful, and demanding. It is therapy that requires a set of unique skills and expertise. Strupp and his colleagues (Strupp and Butler 1989) have persuasive research data indicating that merely being an experienced psychotherapist does not make one a good brief therapist.

In order for brief therapy to be provided in a high-quality, competent manner, therapists need special training programs (Budman 1989). The next several years will, one hopes, see the implementation of such programs at HMOs throughout this country.

References

Beck AT, Rush JA, Shaw BF, et al: Cognitive Therapy of Depression. New York, Guilford, 1979

Bergin A, Garfield S (eds): Handbook of Psychotherapy and Behavior Change: An Empirical Analysis, 3rd Edition. New York, Wiley, 1986

Bolter K, Levinson H: Differences in values between short-term and long-term therapists. Paper presented at the annual meeting of the American Psychological Association, Atlanta, GA, August 1988

Budman SH: Changing silk purses into sows' ears: training experienced therapists to do brief treatment. Invited address presented at the annual meeting of the American Psychological Association, New Orleans, LA, August 1989

Budman SH: The myth of termination in brief therapy, in Brief Therapy: Myths, Methods and Metaphors. Edited by Zweig J, Gilligan S. New York, Brunner/Mazel, 1990, pp 206–218

Budman SH, Bennett MJ: Short-term group psychotherapy, in Comprehensive Group Psychotherapy, Revised Edition. Edited by Kaplan H, Sadock B. Baltimore, MD, Williams & Wilkins, 1983, pp 138–144

Budman SH, Clifford M: Short-term group therapy for couples in a health maintenance organization. Professional Psychology 10:419–429, 1979

Budman SH, Gurman AS: The practice of brief therapy. Professional Psychology 14:277–292, 1983

Budman SH, Gurman AS: Theory and Practice of Brief Therapy. New York, Guilford, 1988

Budman SH, Stone J: Advances in brief psychotherapy. Hosp Community Psychiatry 34:939–946, 1984

Budman SH, Demby A, Feldstein M, et al: Preliminary findings on a new instrument to measure cohesion in group psychotherapy. Int J Group Psychother 37:75–94, 1987

Budman SH, Demby A, Redondo JP, et al: Comparative outcome in time-limited group and individual psychotherapy. Int J Group Psychother 38:63–85, 1988

Budman SH, Soldz S, Demby A, et al: Cohesion, alliance and outcome in group psychotherapy. Psychiatry 52:339–350, 1989

Budman SH, Hoyt M, Friedman S: The First Session of Brief Therapy. New York, Guilford (in press)

Burns D: Feeling Good. New York, New American Library, 1981

Butcher JN, Koss MP: Research on brief and crisis-oriented therapies, in Handbook of Psychotherapy and Behavior Change, 2nd Edition. Edited by Garfield S, Bergin AE. New York, Wiley, 1978, pp 725–768

DeCarufel FL, Piper WE: Group psychotherapy or individual psychotherapy: Patient characteristics as predictive factors. Int J Group Psychother 38:169–188, 1988

De Shazer S: Keys to Solutions in Brief Therapy. New York, WW Norton, 1985

Fisch R, Weakland JH, Segal L: The Tactics of Change: Doing Therapy Briefly. San Francisco, CA, Jossey-Bass, 1982

Folkins CH, Sime WE: Fitness training and mental health. Am Psychol 36:373–389, 1981

Garfield SL: Research on client variables in psychotherapy, in Handbook of Psychotherapy and Behavior Change, 3rd Edition. Edited by Garfield, SL, Bergin AE. New York, Wiley, 1986, pp 213–256

Garfield SL: The Practice of Brief Psychotherapy. New York, Pergamon, 1989

Grunebaum H: A study of therapists' choice of a therapist. Am J Psychiatry 140:1336–1339, 1983

Gurman AS: Integrative marital therapy: toward the development of an interpersonal approach, in Forms of Brief Therapy. Edited by Budman SH. New York, Guilford, 1981, pp 415–467

Howard KI, Kopta SM, Krause MS, et al: The dose-effect relationship in psychotherapy. Am Psychol 41:159–164, 1986

Klerman GL, Rounsaville B, Chevron E, et al: Interpersonal Therapy of Depression. New York, Basic Books, 1984

Koss MP: Length of psychotherapy for patients seen in private practice. J Consult Clin Psychol 47:210–212, 1979

Koss MP, Butcher JN: Research on brief therapy, in Handbook of Psychotherapy and Behavior Change, 3rd Edition. Edited by Garfield SL, Bergin AE. New York, Wiley, 1986, pp 627–670

Levin BL, Glasser JH: National trends in coverage and utilization of mental health and alcohol and substance abuse services within managed health care systems. Am J Public Health 78:1222–1223, 1988

Lorion RP: Socioeconomic status and traditional treatment approaches reconsidered. Psychol Bull 79: 263–270, 1973

Lorion RP: Social class, treatment attitudes and expectations. J Consult Clin Psychol 42:520, 1974

Matarazzo J: Psychotherapeutic processes. Annu Rev Psychol 16:181–224, 1965

Piper WE, Debbane EG, Garant J, et al: Pre-training for group psychotherapy: a cognitive-experiential approach. Arch Gen Psychiatry 36:1250–1256, 1979

Rubinstein EA, Lorr M: Comparison of terminators and remainers in outpatient psychotherapy. J Clin Psychol 12:345–349, 1956

Strupp HH, Binder J: Psychotherapy in a New Key: A Guide to Time-Limited Dynamic Psychotherapy. New York, Basic Books, 1984

Strupp HH, Butler S: Report on the Vanderbilt II Project. Paper presented at the annual meeting of the Society for Psychotherapy Research, Toronto, Ontario, June 1989

Turkington C: Stop 'n' shrink: is today's short-term therapy the best choice? Self, May 1989, p 194

Wells R, Phelps PA: The brief psychotherapies: a selective overview, in Handbook of the Brief Psychotherapies. Edited by Wells RA, Giannetti VJ. New York, Plenum, 1990

Yalom ID: Existential Psychotherapy. New York, Basic Books, 1980
Yalom ID: The Theory and Practice of Group Therapy, 3rd Edition. New York,
    Basic Books, 1985

✦ 16 ✦

Managed Care and Major Mental Illness: An Overview

Steve Stelovich, M.D.

Traditionally, both the problems surrounding serious mental illness in society and the solutions to those problems have had a way of becoming narrowly focused and of haunting history, visiting it time and again in seemingly different but, in fact, surprisingly few basic forms. The rhetoric surrounding the deinstitutionalization and community mental health movement within the United States but 20 years ago sounds much like the conversation reported by Pinel's son between his father and Couthon almost 200 years ago:

> Pinel immediately led him to the section for the deranged, where the sight of the cells made a painful impression on him. He asked to interrogate all the patients. From most, he received only insults and obscene apostrophes. It was useless to prolong the interview. Turning to Pinel: "Now, citizen, are you mad yourself to seek to unchain such beasts?" Pinel replied calmly: "Citizen, I am convinced that these madmen are so intractable only because they have been deprived of air and liberty." (Foucault 1973, p. 242)

Sir Thomas More, Lord Chancellor of England; the charter founding the French Hospital General; records from prerevolutionary American colonies; much contemporary commitment legislation—all share remarkably similar language and views of mental illness. Other examples are numerous.

Guiding principles informing activities within a single psychiatric institution over long stretches of time, and a cross section of such institutions taken at a single time, reveal a surprisingly consistent set of themes regarding both the conception of madness and the techniques that are thought best employed in treating it. Hunter and Macalpine (1963), in their extracts from the "psychiatric literature" covering the years 1535 to 1860, present a multitude of variations on three basic themes: weak wills, evil influences, and bodies gone awry. In current parlance we would say that psychiatric history has been variously occupied by psychological, social, and biological conceptions of madness, each in its turn being exclusively treated and seen as fundamental.

What lessons are we to gather from this continual procession across the stage of psychiatric practice? First, biological, psychological, and social concerns *are* psychiatry's core concerns. Second, a focus upon any one, per se, is insufficient. A narrow focus leaves too many questions unanswered. If in the course of history, then, we are made to witness the recurrent failure of narrowed interest, we would do well to enlarge our scope.

A second set of issues, intimately cojoined with the aforementioned conceptions of illness and also encountered in a historical survey of psychiatric treatment, concerns the loci of care. Rothman (1971) has convincingly shown in his study *The Discovery of the Asylum* that much of the American state hospital system was founded on a belief that mental illness was predominantly a response to destructive influences, generally those arising from urban social life. The hospital or asylum, a new locus of care, was to provide an escape from such influences and to support a return to health. One hundred years later, mental illness was once again viewed as a response to destructive influence, only the influence was taken to be the hospital itself. People had become "institutionalized." Care had to be switched from the asylum to the community if progress was to be made, and deinstitutionalization was launched.

A brief sampling of historical vignettes then draws attention to two closely related sets of problems for the person interested in mental health service delivery to seriously ill patients. First, how is one to avoid the pitfall of narrowed focus—how are biological, social, and psychological concerns to be appropriately integrated? And second, what are the salient factors that should be considered in determining the locus of care? Unfortunately, though the historical approach is helpful in defining the problems, it appears to have little to offer in suggesting solutions to them. Approaches to the problems in the past appear to have been more dependent on the then-current social or political needs, on new theories being advanced, or on new and exciting discoveries than by careful evaluation of patient needs.

Today much of the impetus for exploring "new ways" to handle mental illness rests on the hope that costs may be contained; here, too, we can learn lessons from the past. John Gray (Caplan 1969), second editor of the *American Journal of Insanity* (the precursor of today's *American Journal of Psychiatry*), facing the question of establishing wards for chronic care in the United States in 1866, wrote of some of the fiscal issues we face again today. He had acknowledged the problem of high costs in an article of that same journal in 1862:

> Let us acknowledge that hereafter in the history of this nation—if indeed we can confidently anticipate a history for our distracted and debt-burdened country—public hospitals of palatial size and costly administration, for the demented and chronic insane, are out of the question.

In 1866, though, he asked in a disillusioned voice:

> What . . . are the items you would cut off or cut down? Is it in amusements you would cheapen their care? Perhaps it is in music—their ears are dull of hearing; perhaps it is in the ministrations of religion you would economize—they have no longer kind and thankful hearts, and do they need a preacher? Perhaps you will allow them no longer the visits of their friends, as they may not recognize them, and a little might be saved in attention! Is it in these you would cheapen? Perhaps it is proposed to cheapen in air? Crowding into little space without ventilation—or will you cheapen in warmth and clothing, or give them less cleanliness, that they may die off the sooner? Are you going to give them less sunshine? Oh, no! They may have an abundance of that, for you propose to turn them into the fields and make them earn their own bread. (Caplan 1969, pp. 284–285)

Current Treatment Options

A survey of current options generally available for the treatment of serious mental illness within health maintenance organizations (HMOs), unfortunately, reveals a dismal view not unlike that encountered in sampling psychiatric practices from the past. The locus of treatment is, for the most part, extraordinarily restricted. It usually consists of a choice between inpatient hospitalization or outpatient treatment—and the latter is usually limited to individual office visits. Wise (Chapter 24) has captured the essence of problems encountered in such systems through the image of a cross-country trip taken by car, but by a car with only two gears, the gear of inpatient work and the gear of outpatient work.

Even at their most robust, current hospital services seldom contain more than a rudimentary inpatient system divided between locked wards and open units. Assessment of expectable social functioning is generally restricted to the highly artificial setting of hospital activities. Passes out are generally limited, and in many areas "overnight" passes, a potential source of important diagnostic information and a setting for treatment initiatives, are not allowed at all—usually because they are not reimbursed. Day treatment programs are seldom available as genuine alternatives to hospitalization. And, structured outpatient programs are for the most part only available in the guise of self-help groups developed on the Alcoholics Anonymous model.

Shift the gaze from treatment setting to focus of concern and the view is not much improved. Seldom does one find multimodality treatment that is truly integrated and configured to patient needs.

Perhaps even more dismaying than the lack of an adequate spectrum of services or settings in which such services can be delivered is the fact that there is a virtual absence of guidelines for the differential use of services even if they were to be available. In many areas, the sole guidelines agreed upon are those of legal or social commitment regulations promulgated by state legislatures.

Finally, and perhaps most distressing of all, those few services available are seldom directed to individuals suffering from chronic mental illness. Such individuals are denied coverage because of preexisting conditions, are transferred to the public sector because they do not meet guidelines for acute or active medical conditions, or are otherwise underserved or not served at all. Indeed, though the issue is not directly discussed in this chapter on inpatient strategies, the problem of chronic mental illness raises some of the thorniest issues to face HMOs. Who and how should long-term residential care be paid for? Where is the line of demarcation to be drawn between treatment, support, and rehabilitation? Should case work—so often useful in dealing with chronic psychiatric conditions—be considered a "medical" benefit?

Despite the problems noted above, however, a growing awareness of the importance, the interrelatedness, and the complexity surrounding the issues of focus and locus of care in the psychiatry of major mental disorders appears to be developing. "Spectrum of services" and "least restrictive setting" (though this last being itself usually restricted to the narrow definition of physical environment) are phrases that are gaining increasing attention. In addition, the problems associated with the care of chronic mental illness have begun to attract some attention. Recent judicial rulings have found some psychiatric conditions—predominantly major affective disorders—to be no different from other medical conditions and thus require third-party payors to cover them fully. And, quite independently, one HMO, the Harvard Community Health Plan, in the context of its mental health redesign project has established guidelines for unbundling many serious and chronic mental disorders from their prior benefit limitations. In that HMO, such patients now have access to the basic medical aspects of treatment for their illnesses without benefit limits or increasing copays.

Options for the 1990s

If we are then to improve upon our current hospitalization practices and not simply find ourselves repeating approaches from the past, two areas, in particular, need to be considered in developing a responsible strategy for the treatment of major mental illness: 1) setting (spectrum of services), and 2) focus (biological, psychological, and social). Further, in each and between both, the problem of appropriate needs assessment and treatment matching must be solved.

Spectrum of Services

In 1963, President John F. Kennedy called for a wholly new emphasis and approach to the care for the mentally ill. In that same year, Congress passed the Community Mental Health Centers Act initially requiring the provision of five essential services in each community catchment area across the country. These included emergency care, inpatient and outpatient care, partial hospitalization, and consultation/education services. The amendment of 1975 to the Act expanded services to include screening before admission to state hospitals, follow-up care for patients discharged from hospitals, and transitional housing. In addition, the services were required to be made available to children, the geriatric population, and those suffering from alcoholism or drug abuse. The Act and the events surrounding its implementation "resulted in the largest public mental health system in the history of this country—providing access to ambulatory psychiatric care for one-half of the U.S. population and more than 50% of all reported mental health services" (Shore 1989, p. 2065).

The private psychiatric sector experienced no such broad expansion in services during this time. Increasing amounts of private reimbursement for services were being carried by third-party payors. And, as psychiatry had no recognizable guidelines for patient/therapy matching, insurance organizations generally resisted opening their benefit packages. Many feared that without such guidelines, the coverage of new services would result not in more appropriate treatment allocation, but would instead lead only to increased utilization across the board. As there was no significant reimbursement for alternative programs forthcoming, private hospitals did not diversify their services, nor were significant new ventures formed outside hospital settings.

Despite the strong push in the public sector, all did not go smoothly. Following its initial burst of success, the public community mental health movement found itself within the decade faced with major problems. Shore (1989) notes, "with these accomplishments it is ironic that the modern community mental health era is beset by a significant restriction of resources—the economic recession of the 1970s forced a review of service priorities, a phasing out of direct federal support of the community mental health centers, and a redefinition of patient populations" (p. 2065).

As hospitals have been traditionally both highly restrictive and very expensive, the managed health care movement in the United States has provided an impetus to focus on treatment in less restrictive settings for the private sector. For HMOs or other managed care systems providing mental health coverage, the search for "the least restrictive setting" has carried with it the hope that costs might be reasonably reduced. With few exceptions, however, in the private sector the only choice offered outside of hospitalization has ended to be individual or group outpatient treatment. This "least restrictive setting" certainly is less restrictive and less costly than hospitalization but all too often is clinically inappropriate to a patient's needs.

In many ways, it would seem that there could be much to gain through a marriage of the broad spectrum of services provided in a community mental health setting with the private sector's need for less restrictive treatment settings. However, beset by its own problems and with no clear guidelines in the area of appropriate patient-treatment matching, the public sector community health center movement has been unable, at least as of yet, to develop its spectrum of services for significant private sector utilization.

Nevertheless, for HMOs and the private sector in general, community mental health centers offer some important opportunities. They provide a model of comprehensive services, a spectrum of mental health services that can be adopted and modified as appropriate. In a more fully expanded form one might expect such a spectrum to include the following elaborations on the basic outline provided in the Community Mental Health Centers Act and its amendments:

> 24-hour *emergency care* providing evaluation, triage, and crisis stabilization with a capacity to hold and work with a patient up to 24+ hours;
>
> *Partial hospitalization or day treatment services* providing transition from full hospitalization, alternatives to inpatient stays, and prevention of hospitalization for persons at high risk.

A recent internal review of patients hospitalized by the Harvard Community Health Plan found that 50% of days spent on their open unit did not strictly need to be in a hospital; yet patients were unable to be discharged to home. This may argue for the development in the acute private sector of day hospital–inn combinations linked to inpatient facilities as done in the public sector by Gudeman and colleagues at the Massachusetts Mental Health Center in Boston (Gudeman et al. 1983).

> *Aftercare programs,* multimodality treatment programs configured to meet the needs of specific patient populations—patients with bipolar disorders, patients with alcoholism, patients with somatoform disorders, etc.
>
> *Case management,* providing efficient liaison and continuity of care.

For many patients, neither many visits nor multiple loci for care delivery within the spectrum of services need to be utilized. For others (generally patients with more incapacitating or complicated disorders) many visits and many sites will have to be employed. In such cases, a system that is highly differentiated can begin to contribute its own inefficiencies (e.g., referral processes, waiting times, coordination demands). Case management can ensure that patients pass smoothly into the appropriate system and level of care.

In many areas where sufficiently strong community mental health centers exist, they offer not only a model for development but the real possibility of contracting for services that can be linked to patient-treatment matching guidelines.

The possibility of working alliances between managed care systems and private mental health care organizations/hospitals in developing a spectrum of services as alternatives to traditional inpatient stays also offer potential gains to those involved (see Chapter 8).

Focus of Care

The problem of therapeutic focus is of necessity intimately tied to the concept of disorder and its causes and structure. In the realm of psychiatry, however, until recently there has been little agreement regarding either of the two. In 1980, the American Psychiatric Association (APA) issued its *Diagnostic and Statistical Manual of Mental Disorders, 3rd Edition* (DSM-III). Despite this undertaking, when Diagnosis-Related Groups (DRGs) were introduced, for good or ill, to the rest of medicine covering Medicare hospital expenditures, they were unable to be applied to the field of psychiatry. That failure spoke not only of a field that is admittedly highly complex, but of a total inability to find a common ground from which to proceed. English and colleagues, in summarizing a massive study undertaken by the APA in the early 1980s concerning DRGs and general hospital stays, stated:

> This method of analysis—looking at the coefficients of variation—gives the strongest indication that there was little commonality of resource use among the patients within a given psychiatric DRG. The psychiatric DRGs were not cohesive and did not cluster around a meaningful average and were not accurate in any particular DRG. Indeed, only 5.6% of the variance in Medicare patient length of stay was explained by the psychiatric DRGs. (English et al. 1986, p. 135)

Not everyone within the profession was pleased with this outcome. Were our treatments really so unfocused and variable that we could expect no reasonably predictable outcome, was our conception of disorder so at fault that appropriate treatment decisions could not be made, or were the suggested DRGs so far removed from either treatment or diagnosis that no meaningful matches could be made? In tackling the problem raised by earlier psychiatric DRG studies, Mezzich and Sharfstein (1985) noted, "Neither the *International Classification of Diseases, Ninth Revision, Clinical Modification* (ICD-9-CM) nor the *Diagnostic and Statistical Manual of Mental Disorders, 3rd Edition* (DSM-III) used as catalogs of mental disorder, effectively yield patient groupings that predict resource consumption" (p. 770).

Axis I and Axis II classifications have generally been used alone in attempting to define DRGs. Mezzich and Sharfstein (1985) went on to say, "One of the innovative features of DSM-III, however, is its multi-axial approach which involves the systematic description of the patient's condition along five axes. There is limited evidence that the multiaxial system in DSM-III may be useful for the prediction of resource utilization" (p. 770). In struggling with the problem of classifying patients for prospective payment systems, they comment on "the idea of using specific fields of a code to refer to different aspects of the clinical condition" (p. 770). They also speculate on the use of and revisions needed in DSM-III to improve its psychosocial axes as well as on the need to develop a composite information index or totally new axes. They conclude:

> The extended coding for indicating severity of psychiatric disorder and other direct changes in DSM-III could be made at the initial evaluation point before formal treatment is started. Such assessments would enhance prediction of clinical care utilization, improve the method of formulating psychiatric diagnoses, and ensure that data pertinent to resource consumption are routinely obtained and recorded in clinical charts. (Mezzich and Sharfstein 1985, p. 770)

They do not comment on the possibilities opened by such a system for outcome studies.

In recent work done at the Harvard Community Health Plan in Boston, Massachusetts, remarkably similar conclusions to those of Mezzich and Sharfstein (1985) have been drawn. In an extensive Mental Health Redesign Project, that HMO has focused upon a multiaxial expansion and modification of DSM-III-R (American Psychiatric Association 1987) as the foundation for prescribing appropriate patient-treatment matches. Psychological, social, and biological inputs are used to develop a comprehensive diagnosis—and let us remember that word derives from Greek stems implying "thorough understanding." Axes include the traditional Axis I and Axis II of DSM-III-R. A severity of illness scale is introduced; a modification of the global assessment scale is used to code current functioning. A change in function scale is introduced to describe the acuity or chronicity of the presentation. Social stressors and concomitant physical problems are coded and a measurement of social support systems available is included, as well as a lethality/suicidality/dangerousness scale. Finally, in view of the pervasiveness of substance abuse problems, a separate prefix is added that speaks to the type of substance, amount used, and recent use history.

With these pieces of information at hand, it is thought that solid predictions can be made regarding issues of access, intensity, and duration of treatment. Theoretically, more sophisticated matching becomes possible within the context of such a multiaxial system. The relative merit and appropriate mix of differing modalities and foci of intervention is made easier. Finally, and very importantly, a major tool is thus provided for treatment outcome studies. If treatment choices are linked to specific scale profiles, one should reasonably expect the profiles to change with the interventions prescribed (see Chapter 25).

The following is an example of the increased ability of such an assessment to match treatment to presenting patients.

> Little of substance can be suggested when one is asked what type of treatment and what setting is appropriate for a 22-year-old schizophrenic man. When, however, one adds that the young man has been actively abusing alcohol since the recent death of his mother—the only stable social support he has had—and that he has lost his job as well as his apartment and is actively psychotic with command hallucinations to kill himself, much more can be said.
>
> In the past the above information would most probably have been classified as part of the history; today it approaches the realm of diagnosis and can be quantified using a multiaxial assessment tool. In such a case, immediate and intensive intervention would be called for. Medical stabilization would be paramount and would address suicidality, possible withdrawal, and control of psychosis. Social supports from living arrangements to possible job rehabilitation may be needed and should be explored immediately if the patient is not to face a prolonged hospital stay. Finally, psychological evaluation and support concerning the patient's suicidality, his reaction to his illness, and the loss of his mother will need to be considered.
>
> Such a young man might well be treated in a few days of inpatient

hospitalization, where active suicidal concerns, the acutely debilitating aspects of his psychosis, and possible alcohol withdrawal symptoms could be addressed. He might then be followed in an active day treatment program if social supports were forthcoming and, if not, in a day hospital–inn program where a more complete stabilization could be achieved. Finally, a provider would expect the patient to need extended aftercare and might consider moving him ultimately into a treatment program designed for patients with dual diagnosis.

Summary

This review of both historical and recent psychiatric practices has focused on two significant shortcomings standing in the way of efficient service delivery to patients suffering significant mental illness outside of the public sector—a constrained spectrum of services and a narrowed focus in patient-treatment matching. Recent developments, in part arising out of the concerns of managed health organizations, have focused attention on these problems. The development of a broad spectrum of services and mechanisms for accountable patient-treatment matching is being explored and constitutes the immediate challenge to providing high-quality, cost-contained care in psychiatry. As they have not been jointly employed before, it is difficult to know whether they will be able to provide significant cost containment per se. If the answer is negative, they at least provide basic tools for outcome assessment and thus will allow work to proceed as it cannot under the present system.

References

American Psychiatric Association: Diagnostic and Statistical Manual of Mental Disorders, 3rd Edition. Washington, DC, American Psychiatric Association, 1980

American Psychiatric Association: Diagnostic and Statistical Manual of Mental Disorders, 3rd Edition, Revised. Washington, DC, American Psychiatric Association, 1987

Caplan R: Psychiatry and the Community in Nineteenth Century America. New York, Basic Books, 1969

English JT, Sharfstein SS, Sherl DJ, et al: Diagnosis-related groups and general hospital psychiatry: the APA study. Am J Psychiatry 143(2):135, 1986

Foucault M: Madness and Civilization. New York, Vantage Books, 1973

Gudeman JE, Shore HF, Dickey B: Day hospitalization in an inn instead of inpatient care for psychiatric patients. N Engl J Med 308:749, 1983

Hunter R, Macalpine I: Three Hundred Years of Psychiatry 1535–1860. New York, Oxford University Press, 1963

Mezzich JE, Sharfstein SS: Severity of illness and diagnostic formulation: classifying patients for prospective payment systems. Hosp Community Psychiatry 36(7):770–772, 1985

Rothman DJ: The Discovery of the Asylum. Boston, MA, Little, Brown, 1971

Shore JH: Community psychiatry, in Comprehensive Textbook of Psychiatry V. Edited by Kaplan H, Sadock B. Baltimore, MD, Williams & Wilkins, 1989

✦ 17 ✦

Managed Psychiatric Care for Adolescents: Problems and Possibilities

Peter Barglow, M.D.
Seeley Chandler, M.D.
Nancy Molitor, Ph.D.
Daniel Offer, M.D.

The massive expansion of managed care delivery systems over the last 5 years has posed challenging questions for those involved with the psychiatric care of adolescents and their families. Bennett and Gavalya (1982) and Friedman (1988) describe the continuum of services that can effectively be offered in outpatient staff model health maintenance organization (HMO) settings. These authors emphasize the benefits that are gained in these settings by the close relationship between the pediatrician, the child psychiatrist, and the child mental health team, and the opportunity to work closely with consultants of multiple specialties.

Historically, long-term inpatient treatment for severely disturbed adolescents has been the treatment of choice. Alternatives to such treatment have been scarce until recently. Such paucity reflects both an absence of a conceptual rationale for treatment outside a hospital and the complexities of managing a disturbed adolescent outside the confines of a controlled environment. Both Nurcombe (1989) and Harper (1989) provide conceptual frameworks for problem-focused or goal-oriented treatment with early discharge planning that facilitates shorter hospital stays. Success with early discharge also correlates with good continuity of care, effective day treatment facilities, and an umbrella of aftercare services (Herz et al. 1976, 1977). If the adolescent's fundamental acute psychopathology is reactive rather than "process," and the stressor can be quickly removed, brief hospitalization is likely to succeed (Feinstein 1980).

The extensive use of explicit stabilization goals with the aim of getting patients out of the hospital and rapidly into a safe outpatient milieu has been described by Nurcombe (1989) and has helped produce a 65% decline in average length of hospital stay over several years. Pathological family interactions may sabotage such efforts and precipitate numerous readmissions (Reibel and Herz 1976). Almost all advocates of day-care alternatives to adolescent inpatient care in a managed setting target parents for major therapeutic intervention (Cappellari 1986; Hunter et al. 1984). Fiegelman (1987) makes the same point with regard to drug-abusing adolescents. A good managed care setting needs to be effective in providing rapid, appropriate, flexible, and specific care to adolescents and their families.

With regard to its effect on the health, welfare, and mental status of young patients, research literature seems to emphasize the positive effects of partial hospitalization (Gabel et al. 1989; Kiesler 1982; Leone et al. 1986; Volovik and Zachepitskii 1984). Kiesler (1982) states that in no documented instances were the results of inpatient treatment more positive than in alternative treatment.

In the Humana Michael Reese HMO, the psychiatric benefits for all members include 30 hospital days per calendar year. Our inpatient adolescent acute treatment program differs from those previously described in the literature in that the average duration of stay is only 10 days. Every effort is made to protect the future availability of these inpatient days by maximizing and fostering the patients' opportunities to function in outpatient and everyday settings. Essential to this effort is the provision for professionally led education and support groups dedicated to identification and prevention of current and future adjustment problems and symptoms. These therapeutic activities may be attached to the HMO departments of psychiatry, health education, or pediatrics. The Department of Mental Health offers individual and family evaluation, substance abuse service, and individual and family therapy occurring once weekly, or less often, for problem-focused, time-limited interventions. Multiple high-intensity substance abuse programs are tightly linked to the other programs and treatments offered by the Mental Health team. Our program is characterized by the continuum of services provided, inpatient and outpatient treatments, with a variety of outpatient treatments designed to be safe alternatives to inpatient care.

Critics of managed care point to the limited benefits offered (e.g., 20 outpatient visits per year and 30–60 inpatient days per year). However, numerous authors have demonstrated conclusively the value and effectiveness of short-term interventions (Alpern 1956; Dulcan 1984; Phillips and Johnston 1954; Proskauer 1971, 1979; Turecki 1982). Bennett and Gavalya (1982) assert that 97% of all child patients seen in mental health need fewer than 10 sessions. Friedman (1988) states that 80% of families presenting with children with serious problems were seen for six sessions or fewer, yet had good outcomes. These authors underline the careful conservation of resources. Thoughtful, competent triage and flexible use of interventions allow resources to be allocated to longer term treatments required by the remaining few children who really need them.

More and more HMOs are finding it cost-effective to continue to manage their chronic patients in-house rather than refer them out. In treating children and adolescents, we are progressively shifting from inpatient to outpatient treatments, from a focus on pathology to a focus on strengths and resources as recommended by Phillips and Johnston (1954) and Dulcan (1984). Outpatient programs include one specialty targeting adolescents and families, and an adolescent day hospital program. The hospital is used only if a patient cannot be safely managed in these programs. As soon as the patient can again be safely managed outside of the hospital, he or she is transferred back to the outpatient Adolescent Intensive Treatment Program (AITP).

Our emphasis is on the maintenance of the child in the home, utilizing programs and services that incorporate recent advances in family therapy as well as psychopharmacological interventions for children and adolescents. We also use peer support for both parents and children. The active service interface between pediatrics and psychiatry exists in the outpatient clinics, in the Emergency Room, in the inpatient setting, and in the hospital. A tight linkage has been built up between an acute crisis-oriented, rapid stabilization inpatient Psychiatric Acute Care Unit (PACU) and the AITP, which together constitute an umbrella of intensive treatment outpatient programs. Hospitalization is recommended for those adolescents 1) who are of danger to themselves or others (suicidal, assaultive/ destructive, running away repeatedly, or engaging in prostitution); 2) who are not manageable because of the dysfunction of the family or some chronically destructive aspect of the family system; or 3) who are psychotic, unpredictable, and thus unmanageable by the family.

The Psychiatric Acute Care Unit

The inpatient PACU is a self-contained, locked unit in a general psychiatric hospital, dedicated to short-term hospital stays (less than 1 month). There are 14 total beds that are filled by patients age 11 or older. Schooling is offered beginning the second week of the hospital stay by a tutorial staff of board-certified educators. The PACU is administratively organized and staffed to interdigitate with intensive outpatient programs managed by the Humana Michael Reese Health Plan. It shares with other typical acute psychiatric care, stabilizing inpatient environments the following objectives: 1) to nullify imminent danger to an out-of-control patient or other persons from suicide or homicide; 2) to rapidly differentiate organic or drug-induced conditions from functional psychosis; and 3) to potentiate rapid psychopharmacological interventions when adolescents require this method. The PACU differs from traditional units because the therapeutic interventions of the treatment team (medical director, attending psychiatrists, social worker, nurses, psychologist, psychiatric resident) are oriented from the beginning to end of hospitalization toward the explicit goal of preparing patients smoothly to enter an outpatient service network. Spirited advocacy of the AITP to the patient's family members by the PACU's outreach social worker begins immediately at time of admission. Emphasis is placed on the advantage of converting inpatient bed days into the AITP. Funding for 1 inpatient day equals 5 days of AITP.

The adolescent is intensively observed on the unit and discussed daily by treatment members. His or her interactive skills and defensive strategies are identified. Family assessment focuses on the communication patterns and coping strategies of the adolescent and parents, and the capacity of each to accept responsibility for shared problems and to acknowledge the validity of the other's viewpoint or experience. A specific "Transition Group" focuses on the shift to the AITP specifically, in conjunction with passes for appropriate patients to visit the "hospital without walls." A patient nominated for discharge by the treating psychiatrist, after concurrence by the PACU treatment team, is immediately further evaluated for rapid placement in the AITP by a liaison psychiatric nurse. This key professional skillfully monitors the semipermeable clinical membrane that separates the "hospital with walls" and the "hospital without walls." If a patient has a trial at the AITP and his or her persisting degree of psychopathology exceeds the program's intervention capacity, a repeat hospitalization can be arranged within minutes, using the flexible informational and clinical bridge between the AITP and the PACU.

Discharge from hospital to the AITP or a less restrictive program is possible when there is a willingness for parents and children to work together. We have found that this occurs on about day 5–7 of hospitalization and is facilitated by the knowledge that the outpatient programs will continue to provide the intense 24-hour support and therapy offered by the inpatient program. Patients and parents are reassured that the inpatient program is there if needed. The awareness that *outpatient programs* are the *primary vehicles* for psychiatric interventions helps parents and adolescent accept the responsibility for the family's interactions and family function. The value of the intensive outpatient approach for the adolescent is that parents are included in a way that supports the adolescent's need to have greater responsiveness from his or her parents while also supporting the adolescent's developmental task of acknowledging and accepting responsibility for his or her actions. Factors that determine readiness for transfer to the step-down program (most frequently the day hospital, substance abuse, or intensive outpatient programs or weekly family and individual therapy) include the following:

1. The patient's safety (he or she is no longer a suicide risk, no longer at risk for running away, cutting self, etc., in the near future);
2. The parent's readiness to support outpatient treatment and engage in it as recommended;
3. Compliance with medication by the adolescent and active supervision if needed by the parents, and an explicit agreement to cooperate around the medication regimen; and
4. The capacity to handle the less restrictive environment provided by the AITP.

The Adolescent Intensive Treatment Program

As the AITP has matured and expanded to meet the needs of the more acutely ill, psychotic, and depressed adolescents, psychiatric practitioners' confidence in the program has increased, resulting in approximately 50%–70% of hospitalized adolescents being referred to the program. The remaining 30%–50% of AITP referrals come from the hospital emergency room and from urgent appointments in the outpatient clinic. Both formerly hospitalized and nonhospitalized adolescents are seen together in the AITP. The AITP, with its staff of clinical child psychologist, child psychiatrist, social worker, psychiatric nurse, and psychology intern, modulates and varies with intensity and structure of treatment for each adolescent and family by using a variety of modalities. These include the structured milieu of day hospitalization for the most acutely ill cases, the structure of a twice-weekly adolescent group therapy, a weekly parent group, and a weekly multifamily group, as well as individual, family, and marital therapy.

In addition, the program offers psychological testing, medications, and consultation with the schools and other agencies as needed. We have access to a full-service laboratory on the premises and can order CAT scans, EEGs, blood work, and drug screens on an urgent basis. Developmental specialists, including speech and language pathologists, are also available. We use the services of the hospital emergency room and the hospital unit (PACU) to treat adolescents who occasionally need a more structured 24-hour setting for their own safety. Adolescents can and do occasionally flow back and forth from the hospital to the moderately structured day hospital milieu to the less structured group and individual therapies.

Adolescents are chosen for the AITP based on behavioral and developmental criteria. These criteria usually involve assessment of the acute disturbances within the adolescent and within the family system that prevent both of them from responding to a current crisis in a thoughtful, controlled, adaptive manner. These disturbances include suicidal ideation or attempt, running away, self-mutilation, conduct explosions, and abusive violent episodes between parent and child. Occasionally we also include adolescents who have had a first psychotic break. Adolescents in the AITP range in age from 12 to 18, but younger and older adolescents are seen together. There are generally 8–12 adolescents in the AITP at one time. Groups change daily in the constituency, and adolescents flow in and out of the AITP quite rapidly. Adolescents and their families are seen in group therapy at least four times weekly while they are in the AITP. Although this level of intensity is not necessarily unique for an outpatient program, we believe that combining several different group therapies, plus the ability to modulate the structure and variety of treatment modalities, allows us to treat each adolescent and family in a unique and cost-effective manner.

Group therapies, the primary therapeutic mode in the AITP, include adolescent, parent, and multifamily groups. The Adolescent Group meets twice weekly and is led by an experienced pair of male and female cotherapists. The goal of the Adolescent Group is to increase the adolescent's impulse control while helping him or her to better identify environmental stressors and diminish the maladaptive behavior that led to the current crisis. By contrast, the focus of the mandatory weekly Parent Group (organized and led by a female therapist) is on education, emotional support, and problem solving. The goal of this group is to increase the parents' self-control and sense of efficacy while decreasing their feelings of helplessness and rage. Parents usually experience this group as nurturing, providing gratification, and increasing their patience with offspring. These attitudes enhance their commitment to the AITP.

Probably the most effective therapy group in the program is the weekly Multifamily Group. Attendance is mandatory for parents, adolescents, and targeted siblings. This group, which usually contains 15–40 members, is led by two therapists who are the leaders of the adolescents' and the parents' groups. Adolescents and parents, therefore, feel that they each have an ally in the Multifamily Group. The Multifamily Group allows each adolescent and each parent a chance to give and get feedback from other adolescents and parents without the fears of retaliation or rejection that characterize the prevalent atmosphere in almost all of the individual families.

The AITP is only a beginning intervention for the many families that demonstrate clear-cut chronic dysfunction. Aftercare planning begins as soon as the adolescent enters the AITP. Most of our AITP families are referred elsewhere upon completion of the AITP to long-term therapy or placement in the community. Every effort is made to assure linkage with a variety of referral sources in the community, including the schools, the juvenile courts, the Department of Children and Family Services, residential treatment facilities, and a variety of other community mental health agencies. However, because this aftercare treatment is considered long-term therapy and, therefore, is not covered by the HMO benefits, these referrals are at the family's expense. Efforts are made to secure the most economical and highest quality services available.

Characteristics of Humana Michael Reese Health Plan Adolescent Program

A phone follow-up evaluation of 55 (out of 90) adult care providers of patients elicited generally high approval of our intervention. A structured questionnaire was used. Seventy-one percent of parents felt that the Humana Michael Reese Health Plan helped the family, and 65% felt their child had significantly improved secondary to the program's therapeutic efforts. Through discussion of the clinical follow-up results, we came to the following conclusions.

Safe, Cost-Effective Intervention

The intervention was characterized by safety and cost-effectiveness. Our average duration of stay (10 days) is the smallest of any published study. About 70% of patients remained in the hospital less than 10 days. Less than one-third of subjects followed up had remissions. Overt negative consequences were infrequent. There were no completed suicides. Only 13% of the sample had made a suicide attempt following hospitalization, contrasted with at least 38% prior to admission. Seventy-one percent of the children were in school; 74% are still living in an intact family environment; and only 5% have been reported by their parents to have been involved in trouble with the law or juvenile court system. Only 9% were reported to be on street drugs—and fully 64% were participating in outpatient counseling at least a year following hospitalization. The costs of the program were minimal, consisting almost entirely of staff salary. We used approximately 7 hours of M.D. time, 30 hours of non-M.D. therapist time (social worker and psychologist staff), and 6 hours of psychology intern time per week. The utilization in days/1,000 HMO members/year was quite low—only 5.94 adolescent hospital days/1,000 members/year.

Program Components
Responsible for Good Outcome

I. **Rapid, accurate decision making relevant to hospitalization, discharge, or rehospitalization.** Decision-making issues included the following:

1. Immediate determination that use of substances contributed to psychic deterioration necessitates immediate use of the substance abuse treatment facility;
2. Early identification of chronicity;
3. Making a judgment that safety considerations necessitate a protective environment;
4. Routinizing a comprehensive but rapid family evaluation that can demonstrate inability to support outpatient treatment;
5. Indications that rapid neuroleptization are required; and
6. Checking hospitalization selected to be geographically near to the AITP so that inpatient care can be solidly linked to outpatient treatment.

II. A fully functioning, flexible outpatient care system for patients and families. Previous outpatient treatment programs at the Humana Michael Reese Health Plan were limited either to the usual once-weekly therapist outpatient appointments or psychiatric (M.D.) appointments for consultation and medical management. The expansion and refocusing of clinical services described above now permit rapid response to dangerously acute cases or situations that need rapid intensive focused management of home, school, and family (i.e., a recent overdose, parental abuse, or running away from home). The AITP was designed to meet this need and to offer parents support as well.

III. The early adoption of an explicit inpatient treatment plan and goals governed by the demands of limited length of stay. Our approach is fully consistent with that of Harper's (1989) Focal Inpatient Treatment Planning (FITP) principles: 1) the purpose of hospitalization is to get the patient out of the hospital; and 2) the goal of hospitalization is to produce the circumscribed minimal changes in the patient-family amalgam to permit outpatient treatment.

Nurcombe (1989) has written "seven to ten days after admission of the patient to the hospital and following multidisciplinary assessments, the clinical team should hold a diagnostic and treatment planning conference" (p. 27). We agree but replace our abbreviated 1–2 days for his recommended 7–10 days, by which time the patient should be safely admitted to the AITP. We are far more absorbed in the behavior and "manifest problem that requires the patient to be in the

hospital" than we are in DSM-III-R diagnoses (American Psychiatric
Association 1987). As a consequence, we do not aim to reach the traditional hospitalization objectives of establishment of controls and increase of psychic structure, or major shift in child-parent interactions.
We replace the hospitalization goals of Woolston's (1989) transitional
risk model striving for increased internalization, diminution of cognitive deficits, and acquisition of new defenses and adaptations, with the
modest objectives of patient safety and stabilization. More ambitious
efforts to effect personality change are initiated at the AITP and completed by therapeutic programs outside the purview of the Humana
Michael Reese Health Plan.

References

Alpern E: Short clinical services for children in a child guidance clinic. Am J
    Orthopsychiatry 26:314–325, 1956
American Psychiatric Association: Diagnostic and Statistical Manual of Men-
    tal Disorders, 3rd Edition, Revised. Washington, DC, American Psychiatric
    Association, 1987
Bennett MJ, Gavalya A: Prepaid comprehensive mental health services for
    children. Journal of the American Academy of Child Psychiatry 21(5):486–
    491, 1982
Cappellari L: The day hospital treatment facility for patients with acute psy-
    chosis. Psichiatrica Generale e dell'Eta Evolution 24(2):245–257, 1986
Dulcan MD: Brief psychotherapy with children and their families: the state of
    the art. Journal of the American Academy of Child Psychiatry 23(5):544–
    551, 1984
Feinstein SC: Developmental concepts in the quality care of adolescents. Jour-
    nal of the National Association of Private Psychiatric Hospitals 11(3):38–
    42, 1980
Fiegelman W: Day-care treatment for multiple drug abusing adolescents: so-
    cial factors linked with completing treatment. Paper presented at the Fifty-
    Seventh Annual Meeting of the Eastern Sociological Society, Boston, MA,
    May 1987
Friedman S: Child mental health in an HMO, a family systems approach.
    HMO Practice 3(2):52–59, 1988
Gabel S, Finn M, Ahmad A: Day treatment outcome with severely disturbed
    children. J Am Acad Child Adolesc Psychiatry 27(4):479–82, 1989
Harper G: Focal inpatient treatment planning. J Am Acad Child Adolesc Psy-
    chiatry 28(1):31–37, 1989

Herz M, Endicott J, Spitzer RL: Brief vs. standard hospitalization: the families. Am J Psychiatry 133:795–801, 1976

Herz M, Endicott J, Spitzer RL: Brief hospitalization: a two-year follow-up. Am J Psychiatry 137:502–507, 1977

Hunter DS, Webster CD, Christopher D: Children in day treatment: A four- to eight-year follow-up. Journal of Child Care 2(1):27–40, 1984

Kiesler CA: Mental hospitals and alternative care: noninstitutionalization as potential public policy for mental patients. Am Psychol 37:349–360, 1982

Leone P, Fitzmartin R, Stetson F, et al: A retrospective follow-up of behaviorally disordered adolescents: identifying predictors of treatment outcome. Behavioral Disorders 11(2):87–97, 1986

Nurcombe B: Goal-directed treatment planning and the principles of brief hospitalization. J Am Acad Child Adolesc Psychiatry 28(1):26–30, 1989

Phillips EL, Johnston MSH: Theoretical and clinical aspects of short-term parent-child psychotherapy. Psychiatry 17:267–275, 1954

Proskauer S: Focused time-limited psychotherapy with children. Journal of the American Academy of Child Psychiatry 8:154–169, 1971

Proskauer S: Some technical issues in time-limited psychotherapy with children. Journal of the American Academy of Child Psychiatry 8:154–169, 1979

Reibel S, Herz M: Limitations of brief hospital treatment. Am J Psychiatry 133(5):518–521, 1976

Turecki S: Elective brief psychotherapy with children. Am J Psychother 36(4):479–489, 1982

Volovik VM, Zachepitskii RA: Deinstitutionalization in Soviet psychiatry. International Journal of Mental Health 11(4):108–128, 1984

Woolston JL: Transactional risk model for short and intermediate term psychiatric inpatient treatment of children. J Am Acad Child Adolesc Psychiatry 28(1):38–41, 1989

✦ 18 ✦

Spectrum of Services for the Alcohol Abusing Patient

William R. Zwick, Ph.D.
Maurice Bermon, M.D.

The design of alcohol treatment services delivered by health maintenance organizations (HMOs) has differed widely across states and within communities (Levin et al. 1988). State-mandated benefits and available treatment options initially shaped these services. More recently, the design of managed alcohol treatment services has begun to shape services available in the fee-for-service community (Del Toro 1990; Shadle and Christianson 1989).

We believe four major assumptions should guide the design of a cost-effective managed care program for the treatment of alcohol abuse and dependence.

1. Early case identification is crucial in treating alcohol problems.
2. Successful treatment of alcohol problems is likely in many cases.
3. Reduced total health care costs can be achieved through the delivery of treatment services to alcohol abusing and dependent patients and to their family members.
4. Employers and employees want treatment services for those with alcohol problems.

Early case identification is crucial in the treatment of alcohol abuse and dependence. Alcohol abuse and dependence in the managed care setting, as in any other care setting, are best treated with early identification and aggressive intervention. Prognosis is improved if treatment is initiated prior to the onset of more serious later-stage complications (Babor et al. 1987a; Berg and Skutle 1984; Clark 1981; Hays and Spickard 1987; Kristenson et al. 1983). Client characteristics (e.g., age, marital status, social support, and psychiatric status) before the start of treatment are better predictors of outcome than are most aspects of the treatment delivered (Miller and Hester 1986). Capitalizing on positive client characteristics requires the earliest possible case identification.

Patient-treatment matching is an important concept in the design of substance abuse treatment programs. This approach has focused on refined assessment and assignment to subtly different treatment approaches after a member has been referred to a treatment setting. However, patient-treatment matching should be applied to the entire spectrum of primary health care services. For instance, failures in patient-treatment matching occur whenever a member is given Tagamet for alcohol-related gastritis or given antihypertensives for alcohol-related hypertension or treated for alcohol-related trauma but is not diagnosed as alcohol abusing/dependent and is not referred for treatment (Zwick 1986).

Primary health care provider attitudes in the identification and treatment of alcohol abuse and dependence are well documented (Bergen et al. 1980; Caswell and McPherson 1983; Chappel et al. 1984; Fisher et al. 1975; Griffin et al. 1983; Halon 1985; Kinney et al. 1984; Warburg et al. 1987). Most primary care providers are not trained in identification of alcohol abuse. Many primary care providers were trained in settings treating only patients with late-stage alcoholism. They seldom saw success; they were frustrated by patient noncompliance. They were not trained to recognize mild to moderate alcohol-related problems in patients being treated for other primary diagnoses. For example, if alcohol withdrawal symptoms were a problem for a patient during a hospital stay following elective surgery, the withdrawal symptoms were often treated with no referral for alcohol treatment. Because alcohol abuse leads to frequent use of medical services, providers have grown used to self-reports of six standard drinks per day as if that were normal. Among New York State adults, between 25% and 30% of the population drinks one drink or less *per year,* about 35% average three drinks *per week,* about 25% average one drink per day, and only 10%–15% average more than one drink per day (Barnes and Welte 1988).

Alcohol abuse or dependence is estimated to be present in 15%–

30% of cases in ambulatory care settings (Babor et al. 1986, 1987b; Clement 1986; Cyr and Wartman 1988; Kemerow et al. 1986; Persson and Magnusson 1987; Putnam 1982; Roberts and Brent 1982). Over years, a patient's reports of sleep disturbance, stress, trauma, depression, anxiety, hypertension, gastrointestinal tract complaints, and upper respiratory infections are usually not seen as a pattern of symptoms related to alcohol abuse but rather as a series of unrelated presentations to be treated individually. These presentations make up such a large part of the normal day-to-day work in all primary care settings that providers miss the forest of alcohol abuse in the endless trees of isolated complaints. Infrequent use of available, simple, inexpensive screening devices for alcohol abuse and dependence contributes to the problem. The combined impact of primary health care provider attitudes and missed diagnosis on delaying the onset of treatment should be seen as the major area in need of improvement in the delivery of cost-effective treatment for alcohol abuse and dependence (Kranzler 1987).

Emphasis on early identification of alcohol abusing and dependent members requires a commitment to train primary care and mental health providers in early identification. Emphasis on early identification of alcohol abusing and dependent members requires a concomitant emphasis on providing intervention strategies that are appropriate for early-stage alcohol abuse and dependence.

Successful treatment of alcohol abuse and dependence is likely in many cases. Numerous studies (Fink et al. 1985; Orvis et al. 1981) indicate positive outcome. The most likely course of events following the initiation of appropriate treatment for alcohol abuse and dependence is substantial periods of improved functioning, perhaps interrupted by relapses (Polich et al. 1981) that usually can be driven back into remission (Brownell et al. 1986). Through 1989, our own program has completed four separate 12-month follow-up studies of patients initiating detoxification treatment for substance abuse. Across the four studies, over the course of the follow-up period, the vast majority of patients—73%—required only the initial treatment episode. Approximately 20% of the patients required one additional treatment episode for redetoxification, approximately 5% of patients required two additional treatment episodes, and only 2% required more than two additional treatment episodes (Zwick 1992). The reality of this research is at odds with many clinicians' perceptions and biases concerning treatment outcome.

Reduced total health care costs can be achieved through the delivery of treatment services to alcohol abusing and dependent patients and to their family members. Cost-benefit analyses of alcohol treatment services consistently support the delivery of those services. There are a number of studies (Hayami and Freeborn 1981) that address this question; Luckey (1987) provides a review of this literature. One random assignment, prospective study demonstrates that patients identified sooner than traditionally show substantially less utilization of hospital and outpatient services (Kristenson et al. 1983). A second study (Holder and Blose 1986) emphasizes the reduction in utilization of medical services in patients who accept alcohol treatment. As of 1985, these reductions were substantial: on the order of about $110 per family per month (in 1985 dollars) over the 3 years following initiation of treatment.

The combination of these two studies provides powerful and compelling support for the notion that initiation of treatment for alcohol abusing and dependent members can reduce medical utilization, decrease patient morbidity, and save dollars. Advances in cost-effective delivery of treatment for alcohol abusing and dependent members improve the cost-benefit ratio further (Hayashida et al. 1989; Heather et al. 1986; Miller and Hester 1986; Rundell et al. 1981).

Employers and employees want treatment services for alcohol abuse and dependence. Over the past 15 years, there have been numerous studies of various types reporting that employers profit when employees have access to treatment for alcohol abuse and dependence (Orvis et al. 1981). Employee assistance programs (EAPs) are widespread and are strong proponents of treatment. Employers are moving toward drug screening programs in the workplace. These programs are targeted at illicit drug abuse but are certain to identify dually addicted individuals as well. Retention of trained employees is a significant financial concern; employers ask about substance abuse services when negotiating health care contracts. The availability of a credible treatment response for substance abuse in managed care systems is an important issue to many employers.

The stream of public figures who have gone into treatment over the past 10 years has greatly increased public awareness of at least some treatment modalities. The press has documented the popular, almost faddish concept of addiction (e.g., "Addicted to Addictions" 1990). Throughout the 1980s, state legislatures, reflecting a vocal and increasingly broad constituency, mandated services for alcohol abuse.

Managed care systems that avoid the delivery of high-quality alcohol treatment services are frequent targets in state legislatures (e.g., in Massachusetts between 1986 and 1990) and in the media (Roosa 1987). Notwithstanding the legitimate cries for reduced health care costs, the public clearly favors access to appropriate treatment for alcohol abuse. Managed care systems could be leaders in this area of health care delivery, because coordinated care can be expected to be more efficacious. By planning to deliver this care well, managed care systems can harness and lead public action in this area. As we will describe later in this chapter, high-quality alcohol treatment services stand up to cost-benefit analysis better than many other areas of medical care and show promise for continued improvement (Holder et al. 1991; Miller and Hester 1986; Sparadeo et al. 1982).

Impact on Costs

There are two cost issues to consider in developing alcohol abuse and dependence services consistent with our four assumptions. The first is the potential for great cost savings noted previously. Counting money not spent has never been a strength of most reporting systems. The savings are difficult to measure and assign to alcohol treatment services but are real nonetheless. The second cost issue is the cost of delivering alcohol abuse and dependence treatment services. Cost savings in this area have often been of the "reduced access," gatekeeper type. Throughout this chapter we will argue that a better approach is to increase access to early, less expensive alternatives to traditional late-stage treatment.

To control the cost of delivery of alcohol abuse and dependence services, managed care systems must address the historic pattern of utilization of inpatient care as the primary response to alcohol abuse and dependence (Miller and Hester 1986; Nace 1990). This is best done by developing alternative treatment programs that emphasize outpatient or partial hospitalization treatment (Holder et al. 1991). Our HMO achieved a 10% reduction in total costs per member per month, including inpatient and outpatient services, between 1984 and 1989. Utilization of an outpatient, early-intervention–focused program, including a day treatment setting, accomplished these savings while we *increased* the rate of cases entering treatment by approximately 50%. This 10% decrease in costs, paired with a 50% increase in the rate of cases treated, does not include the additional projected savings of avoided medical expenses. We believe this hidden saving (Holder 1987; Holder and Blose 1986) is larger than our savings from reduced delivery costs.

The coordination of care available in managed care settings, particularly staff model settings, allows us to achieve a tremendous advantage in costs while increasing the number of patients treated for alcohol abuse and dependence.

Staffing Alcohol Abuse and Dependence Services

The staff for alcohol treatment services sometimes fall under the purview of mental health services and sometimes stand alone as a separate department. The value of the integration of substance abuse and mental health services is discussed below.

Type of staff and staffing ratios. We believe that treating substance abuse requires an additional expertise beyond the delivery of general mental health services. Substance abusing patients present with the full spectrum of mental health problems seen in a traditional mental health practice plus the added complication of substance abuse (Osher and Kofoed 1989; Regier et al. 1990). The vast majority of traditionally trained mental health professionals are not equipped or inclined to address this fact. Substance abuse providers should be mental health professionals with additional training, experience, and interest in treating substance abuse. They should also be committed to the concept of early identification paired with aggressive outpatient treatment. Most of the frontline therapists should have master's-level degrees in mental health and be fully credentialed in substance abuse treatment as well. They should show a career commitment to substance abuse services and should have working experience in multiple substance abuse settings (e.g., inpatient, outpatient, partial hospitalization), if possible. Some of the staff should be master's-level nurses or psychiatrically certified nurses with advanced credentials in substance abuse. If possible, a doctoral-level clinician with a career commitment to substance abuse should oversee the delivery of substance abuse services. National credentialing processes exist for this field. Hiring preference should be given to credentialed individuals, and staff should be required to achieve full credentials within a reasonable time after being hired.

Well-trained, committed staff will insist on high-quality care and will be able to deliver it. Plan members and the treatment community will recognize the quality of the staff. As a result, they will more willingly accept the development and implementation of nontraditional outpatient focused care provided by obviously competent individuals.

Even assuming a high-quality staff of specialists, determining an appropriate level of staffing for delivery of alcohol-related services is still difficult. It is not uncommon to find staffing ratios of 1 per 30,000 members. Staffing ratios are also affected by the spectrum of services the HMO chooses to make available.

Specific staffing ratios should be based on an estimate of the likely incidence of alcohol abuse and dependence in the population to be treated. General membership demographics such as age and sex can be helpful in making this determination. Using one series of undocumented rules of thumb, we generated an estimation of our own staffing needs.

1. Assume that approximately 10% of membership over the age of 16 could be identified as alcohol abusing or dependent in a clinical interview.
2. Assume that in any given year, staff will target identifying 10% of that 10%.
3. Recognize that staff will have about three times as many cases presenting as this estimate yields. That is because they will have family members presenting for treatment before and in addition to the actual substance abuser.
4. Assume that a substance abuse staff member can manage approximately three new cases per week, plus crises.

The end result of this series of assumptions is that a staffing ratio of 1 to 9,000 total members is appropriate for our outpatient program.

In any case, it is important not to arrive at staffing levels by starting with one staff member, then overwhelming him or her, adding another, overwhelming that one, and adding another, and so on. Our experience suggests that this approach, time-honored though it may be, condemns staff to treating late-stage desperate cases, creates access problems, burns out staff, and overutilizes inpatient treatment options.

Limits of Service

This is a controversial area. Federally qualified HMOs cannot limit medically necessary detoxification care. Different states have mandated different levels of rehabilitation care for alcohol. The mandated care for drug abuse and dependence is often different from that for alcohol abuse and dependence. A common practice has been to have a combined limitation addressing yearly and lifetime services. In many cases, the limits have been tailored to meet regional assumptions of inpatient focused care and have neglected outpatient services.

Our HMO provides services in an area with mandated benefits of 30 outpatient sessions for the identified patient and 20 sessions for family members. Inpatient services are mandated as 30 days of rehabilitation per year as needed. A lifetime limit of 90 days of rehabilitation is also set. The same limits apply to cases of alcohol and drug abuse in our state. The state division of substance abuse has determined there is an excess of beds available for inpatient care for the insured population. There are a number of inpatient facilities competing in this environment through the use of radio and television advertising and other, more subtle campaigns.

In our HMO, these benefit limitations did not serve to define the nature of services provided. For members requiring inpatient admissions in the first halves of 1985, 1986, 1989, and 1990, the average number of inpatient plus day treatment days used by each case in the index admission plus any subsequent admissions in the following 12 months has decreased from 16.5 to 8.5 (Zwick 1992). This compares to a national average of 22 days for just the index admission (Holder and Blose 1991). Less than 2% of the members utilizing substance abuse services have used up their inpatient benefits in any given year since 1985. In a well-managed system of care, limitations on service are not an issue for the vast majority of cases. Readmissions for a small percentage of cases color many providers' perception of alcohol treatment outcome.

Managed care systems have a distinct potential advantage in both quality of care and cost savings compared to fee-for-service systems. Early identification procedures throughout primary care and mental health services, appropriately limited use of inpatient treatment, aggressive outpatient rehabilitative services, and coordinated follow-up with primary care and substance abuse specialists all can be expected to contribute to better treatment outcome and a lower cost of service delivery. Our HMO was able to provide inpatient, partial hospitalization, and outpatient services for cases of alcohol and drug abuse in 1989 for less than $1.25 per member per month.

Marketing of Alcohol Treatment Services

To ensure early case identification and appropriate treatment matching, alcohol treatment services must be marketed internally (to administrators and clinicians) and externally (to employees). Administratively, for the program to be creditable, administrators must have a way of knowing the plan is on track. Monitoring progress of the plan should include the following variables:

1. Readmission rates following initial treatment. This value should decrease annually toward a long-term goal.
2. Detoxification cases (inpatient plus outpatient) per 1,000 members. This value should increase annually toward a long-term goal.
3. Average inpatient days (detoxification plus rehabilitation) per case. This value should decrease annually toward a long-term goal.
4. Utilization of outpatient groups. This value should increase annually toward a long-term goal.
5. Total days of inpatient utilization. This value should decrease annually toward a long-term goal.
6. Total costs of direct alcohol treatment services as a percentage of plan income per member per month. This value should remain within acceptable annual budgetary limits while moving toward an agreed-upon long-term goal.

Primary care providers must become convinced that alcohol treatment services can contribute to the health of their patients. They must further be convinced that they play a crucial, central role in case identification (Babor et al. 1986; Goldman 1991; Helwick 1985; Kristenson et al. 1981; Nock 1980; Skinner et al. 1984; Smith et al. 1987). Project ADEPT (Lewis 1989) has developed a training program for primary care providers that addresses these issues (Dube et al. 1989).

Mental health providers must become convinced that alcohol treatment services can contribute to the health of their patients. Alcohol abuse and dependence should almost never be seen as only a symptom of another "deeper" disorder. Providers must recognize it as one of the three most common diagnoses they are likely to encounter in initial evaluations (i.e., depression, substance abuse, and anxiety disorders).

In-service training for primary care and for mental health providers should be presented with support from the highest clinical levels within their disciplines. Time and energy should be spent to ensure that these two groups of providers are aggressively identifying alcohol abuse and dependence in their case loads. For both groups of providers, direct experience of positive patient outcome is the most effective teaching tool. Barring that, staff should present regular reports to clinical staff addressing the improvements and outcomes for members treated for alcohol problems.

The corporate community, while very cost-sensitive, generally accepts the need for access to quality alcohol treatment services. HMOs have, at times, created the impression that they were more interested in restricting access to alcohol treatment services than in providing them. Managed care systems should make their corporate customers aware that they aggressively identify cases and provide high-quality care. The assumption that treatment is always synonymous with inpatient treatment must be challenged head-on. The managed care system should work as cooperatively as possible with EAPs; these programs have done a remarkable job of educating employers about the real cost and productivity benefits of substance abuse treatment. Fighting EAPs case by case will destroy the managed care system's credibility; working with them to develop cost-effective treatment responses will increase the managed care program's case identification rate and lower costs. Demonstrating an ability to respond rapidly to referrals is especially important when working with EAPs.

Integration of Substance Abuse in General Mental Health

A guiding principle of any successful alcohol treatment program is that alcohol abuse and dependence is a progressive disorder. The progression is reflected in the deterioration of various aspects of a person's life, including psychological, social, financial, occupational, and medical status. This disorder does not present a single manifestation but rather a continuum of symptoms. For a program to be successful, it must have the flexibility to intervene at any point along this continuum—the earlier the better. Alcohol treatment programs should be integrated with mental health and primary care to facilitate rapid, flexible, and early intervention.

People in the early stages of alcohol abuse and dependency rarely present with stated alcohol problems (Willoughby 1979). Rather, they present for treatment with early manifestations of alcohol abuse such as insomnia, anxiety, depression, impulsiveness, personality and mood changes, marital conflicts, job problems, school problems, and so on (Parker et al. 1987; Parsons et al. 1987; Ries 1989). These problems are those for which a person would often consult a mental health professional or his or her physician.

When an individual presents for an initial evaluation, it is essential that the evaluator be cognizant of the possible contribution of an underlying alcohol problem to the presenting complaint. In fact, it would not be an exaggeration to say that a guiding principle of every mental health evaluation should be that there is an alcohol problem (either with the individual or a close family member) until proven otherwise. Our experience over the last 15 years shows that about 35% of all patients who present to our Mental Health Department either have an alcohol problem themselves or have one in their family. For those presenting with a work-related problem, the percentage increases to more than 70%. There has been an increasing acceptance among mental health professionals of the value of substance abuse treatment (Kahle and White 1991).

There has to be a continuous process of education between mental health staff who do not specialize in alcohol abuse and those who do. That education can best flourish through close proximity and continuous interaction between the two staffs. It is important for the mental health department staff to have ready access to alcohol treatment options. An alcohol problem must be addressed immediately; treatment of other independent or related disorders will not progress if the alcohol problem is left untreated. Again, this is best accomplished by an integrated program.

In response to the general reluctance of mental health providers to see alcohol abuse and dependence as a primary problem, more traditional alcohol programs and self-help groups have tended to focus on alcohol as *the* primary problem. We believe that individuals who present with alcohol problems and with other disorders of an Axis I or Axis II nature do require monitoring and treatment of those disorders in conjunction with their alcohol problem. Although many, but certainly not all, affective episodes do resolve when alcohol abuse is treated, the interaction between the mental health and alcohol teams facilitates awareness on the alcohol team regarding other disorders and their treatment. Through this integration, individual members can be more comprehensively treated.

Differentiation of Substance Abuse From General Mental Health

The organizational structure of the delivery of alcohol-specific services within a mental health department can be problematic. There has been a history of conflict, mistrust, and disrespect between alcohol specialists and providers specializing in other areas of mental health. It is crucial that the alcohol program be administered by an individual respected by both sets of providers—one who must also clearly have alcohol treatment services as his or her primary responsibility. The director of alcohol treatment services within the mental health department must have credibility outside the department, in primary care, in administrative settings, and in the entire treatment community.

Staff who deliver alcohol treatment services should be supervised clinically by substance abuse specialists. The director of alcohol treatment services should report to the director of mental health or should be the director of mental health. Group and peer supervision should include both alcohol specialists and general mental health providers. Salaries and credentials of staff in alcohol treatment specialties should be comparable to those in general mental health.

Staff members should not treat outside their area of expertise. Those staff specializing in other areas of mental health care should not be assigned primary responsibility for alcohol cases unless they accept additional training and supervision. Similarly, mental health staff specializing in the care of alcohol-related problems should not be assigned general mental health cases without additional training or supervision. Sharing group leadership responsibilities is an excellent way to integrate the expertise of mental health staff specializing in alcohol treatment with those specializing in other areas.

Spectrum of Services for Alcohol Abusing and Dependent Members

The spectrum of services for cases of alcohol abuse and dependence should reflect a systematic organizational approach. The services should include two major areas of emphasis: primary care and specialty care for alcohol abuse and dependence.

Primary Care

The impact of primary care providers on early identification of alcohol abuse and dependence cannot be overstated. The role of primary care providers has been the focus of much recent work (Ewan and Whaite 1982; Magruder-Habib et al. 1991; Moore et al. 1989; Pokorny et al. 1978; Solomon et al. 1980). A recommended medical school substance abuse curriculum, developed at Brown University through Project ADEPT, focuses on primary care specialties including internal medicine, pediatrics, and obstetrics and gynecology (Dube et al. 1989). These authors suggest the primary care provider plays five critical roles in treating alcohol abuse and dependence in his or her patients: primary prevention, case identification, making and presenting the diagnosis, initiation of treatment, and follow-up. Primary care providers in the managed care setting should be trained thoroughly in each of these roles.

The *primary prevention* role is an ongoing task of member education and guidance. The goal is to help the patient avoid problems associated with alcohol use (Goldstein and Dube 1989). This primary prevention role is parallel to the provider's role in addressing cigarette smoking. Patients often ask or imply questions concerning the appropriate use of alcohol. They often need clarification about abuse, appropriate use, and abstinence. For instance, primary care providers' advice and direction can help patients avoid significant problems associated with alcohol use in temporary situations such as during pregnancy (Coles et al. 1991), in conjunction with taking prescribed medication, following a surgical procedure, or while in treatment for a psychiatric disorder (Frances and Franklin 1986; Grueninger et al. 1989). Other longer term conditions may be made significantly worse by a patient's use or abuse of alcohol. Primary care providers can alert patients to such risks and help patients avoid added problems in the face of such disorders as diabetes, hypertension, gastritis, and ulcers (Ashley and Rankin 1988).

The primary care provider can also educate a patient about the significant risks associated with using alcohol if one has a family history of substance abuse. The primary care providers' role in these common situations is to help the patient prevent abuse or avoidable consequences of use under moderate- to high-risk conditions. The question is not so much the avoidance of alcoholism as it is the promotion of health through informed decisions concerning alcohol use and abuse. Nevertheless, as with delaying or avoiding the onset of nicotine addiction, physician efforts in educating patients about the risks associated with alcohol use and abuse may prevent alcoholism (i.e., abuse and dependence), especially in an adolescent or young adult primary care setting (Dupont 1987).

The *case identification* role utilizes data from routine screenings and history, acute presentations, and extended assessments.

Because alcohol abusing and dependent members are such disproportionately heavy users of primary care services (Putnam 1982), the primary care setting provides an ideal opportunity for case identification. The long-term relationship between primary care providers and their patients can greatly facilitate identification. Case identification requires a knowledge of early medical signs and symptoms of alcohol abuse (i.e., sleep disturbance, palpitations, upper respiratory infections, trauma, gastrointestinal tract complaints, depression, anxiety, hypertension, self-reports of stress), recognition of acute presentations (i.e., withdrawal in hospital settings), and the ongoing use of standardized screening instruments (i.e., CAGE [Buchanan et al. 1991; Bush et al. 1987]; TRAUMA scale [Skinner et al. 1984]).

After primary care providers have gathered the necessary history and clinical data to *make the diagnosis,* how they *present the diagnosis* of alcohol abuse or dependence can affect the member's decision to accept treatment. Appropriate confrontational and nonconfrontational techniques for presenting the diagnosis have been discussed elsewhere (Cyr 1989).

Initiating treatment may be facilitated by the protocols and services available to providers in a managed care setting. Clear guidelines on how to access appropriate dispositions must be available. The primary care provider must be prepared to negotiate the treatment plan and contract with the patient to accept treatment (Cyr 1989). Whether treatment is accepted or not, primary care providers have *follow-up* responsibilities toward their patients. These responsibilities can increase the likelihood that appropriate treatment is being followed, or will begin at a later date. In substance abuse, as in most other medical conditions, patients are not always compliant after the first treatment intervention. Primary care providers' follow-up responsibilities include monitoring substance use, monitoring treatment adherence, treating medical and psychiatric complications or comorbidities, avoiding prescribing mood-altering medications, making rapid referral if relapse occurs, and if applicable, monitoring response to pharmacological treatments.

Specialty Care

The primary role of the alcohol treatment services program is to treat members in distress from their own alcohol abuse. A secondary role is to provide treatment to the families of alcohol abusing or dependent members and then to provide appropriate specialized services to alcohol abusing and dependent members and their families after a substantial period of abstinence has been achieved.

For patients in distress from their own alcohol use, the initial treatment of their families should be seen as a means to the end of providing treatment to the identified patient. Outpatient alcohol abuse services should be designed and coordinated to provide a high-quality alternative to inpatient treatment for the majority of members. Early intervention should be seen as a hallmark of providing quality services to alcohol abusing members.

Services are also provided to family members to address the consequences associated with living with an alcohol-troubled person, whether or not that person is in treatment. Such services for the young or teenage children of alcohol abusing members is an especially appropriate area for primary and secondary prevention.

Services for later stages of recovery might include such areas as marital therapy, group psychotherapy, family therapy, or pharmacological and psychological treatment for affective and thought disorders. When such services do not directly focus on substance-related issues, they should be delivered in a context of continual awareness of the patient's substance abuse history and risk for relapse.

Members should have *easy access* to detoxification evaluation services 7 days a week. On-call phone coverage should be available through mental health professionals with 24-hour substance abuse specialist backup. There should be minimal waiting time for an in-person detoxification evaluation (i.e., same day or next morning). The evaluations should be done by alcohol or substance abuse and dependence specialists. Whenever possible, the evaluations should be done in person, not over the phone, and at the managed care setting, not at an intensive inpatient treatment program admitting area. Members forced to wait for appropriate evaluations often eventually present in crisis and then require inpatient treatment.

Whether the evaluation is in person or by phone, when needed, there should be *rapid access* to appropriate outpatient or inpatient treatment. There especially should be minimal waiting for the beginning of detoxification treatment. All detoxifications should be begun on a same-day basis (or next morning from on-call). Access to individual, group, and family treatment modes should be available within 2 to 4 days. Noncrisis first appointments with alcohol specialists in general should have waiting times of no more than 1 to 3 days. Again, members forced to wait for access to appropriate outpatient treatment often eventually present in crisis and then require inpatient treatment.

Treatment participation should be closely *coordinated between treatment providers.* That is, primary care and medical providers involved in detoxification and individual therapists and group leaders should communicate sufficiently to ensure appropriate initial and ongoing support to the member. Further, consistent concepts and approaches to aiding the member in changing substance use behavior should be reinforced by all providers working with the patient and his or her family.

Treatments should be sequenced from early recovery topics to more advanced topics in a managed, orderly way. Clinical information, techniques, and support should be appropriate to the stage of change (Prochaska and DiClemente 1982, 1983) at which the patient can be assumed to be currently functioning. That is, treatment efforts should sequentially target the most likely clinical issues the member and his or her family are facing at the beginning and in the middle of treatment.

Self-help groups should be available on-site in the managed care setting. Alcoholics Anonymous (AA), Al-Anon, Alateen, Narcotics Anonymous (NA), Women For Sobriety (WFS), and others should be established on-site whenever possible. This greatly reduces member reluctance to begin self-help programs. These groups provide immeasurable support to recovering individuals; on-site groups improve the treatment community's understanding of the managed care program's commitment to alcohol treatment.

Clinical supervision by alcohol specialists should focus on critical choice points in the utilization of services. We often focus on five significant choice points, especially with newer HMO staff.

1. Does the patient require detoxification now? If yes, should the detoxification be done in an outpatient, day treatment, specialized inpatient, or medical acute care inpatient setting?
2. Does the patient require rehabilitation now? If yes, what setting is currently appropriate for that rehabilitation (i.e., outpatient, day treatment, etc.)?
3. Does the patient require treatment for a second psychiatric diagnosis now? If yes, should a referral be made for further evaluation or treatment now? What setting would be appropriate now for that evaluation or treatment?
4. Should significant others be involved in treatment now? If yes, should the involvement be in individual, couple, family, and/or group modalities?
5. Would the patient profit from Antabuse now? If yes, how should this option be presented to the patient?

Cases should be assigned in order of programmatic priorities. Some clinicians may favor working with particular subpopulations within the substance abuse treatment setting (such as adult children of alcoholics [ACOAs] or codependents). Although these subpopulations are important, rapid case assignment of the identified abuser must always take priority over other types of cases and services. This prioritization maintains the program's focus on alcohol abuse rather than collateral mental health issues. Services for identified patients are more likely to treat those at risk for hospitalization than are services for nonabusing codependents.

Outline of a Spectrum of Services

Given the priorities and program qualities presented previously, a spectrum of services (Zwick and Dube 1989) can be described as follows:

1. Education
2. Prevention
3. Early identification
4. On-call service
5. Treatment modes
   a) Detoxification

b) Rehabilitation/aftercare
c) Inpatient or intensive referral options
6. Follow-up after outpatient treatment

Major Treatment Disposition Options

In general, the concept of matching the *level of structured support* provided by the disposition to the *level of problem intensity* experienced by the member should guide disposition choices. (See Table 18–1 for a sample of specific guidelines.) Treatment dispositions should be considered sequentially, not as a packaged final decision. Evaluations first must address and resolve the question of the need for detoxification. If a detoxification is needed, then the question of an appropriate setting for detoxification is addressed. While the detoxification is in progress, an evaluation of rehabilitation needs is done and a rehabilitation disposition is made.

The major detoxification treatment disposition options can be ranked from low to high on structured support, as follows:

1. Outpatient detoxification (daily contact with physician and substance abuse therapist, medicated as needed daily, 3 to 5 days)
2. Intensive day treatment detoxification (6 to 8 hours daily contact, medicated as needed daily, 3 to 5 days)
3. Inpatient detoxification
   a) in a substance abuse specialty care setting
   b) in a psychiatric setting with a strong substance abuse treatment orientation
   c) in a medical hospital setting with a strong substance abuse treatment orientation

The major rehabilitation treatment disposition options can be ranked from low to high on structured support as follows:

1. Primary care diagnosis and primary care follow-up only;
2. Outpatient rehabilitation involving identified patient and family members;
3. Intensive day treatment rehabilitation;
4. Inpatient specialty care–based rehabilitation; or
5. Long-term residential placement (30+ days).

Table 18-1.   Treatment guidelines

Guidelines for selecting detoxification dispositions

A) *Refer to outpatient detoxification if all the following conditions are met:*
Medical complications:
1. the member has no history of seizures or delirium tremors,
2. the member does not have a current medical condition that is known to become difficult to manage during detoxification (i.e., insulin dependent diabetes mellitus, cardiac problems),
3. the member has not sustained a head injury that rendered him or her unconscious at any time during the past 2 weeks,
4. the member does not show signs of gastrointestinal tract bleeding, and
5. the member has no other complications or comorbidities requiring observation.

AND

Nature and level of substance dependence:
1. the member is alcohol dependent only (the member may have been using other substances but not in a manner associated with complicating alcohol detoxification), and
2. the member consumes less than 24 standard drinks on a drinking day.

AND

Social support:
1. the member will be able to stay with a person who is supportive of recovery and who can assist the member if further support is needed.

AND

Psychological functioning:
1. the member does not suffer from any psychological condition to such an extent that he or she cannot safely follow plans and directions when away from the outpatient setting.

AND

Treatment history:
1. the member has not been unsuccessfully detoxified in an outpatient setting in the past.

B) *Refer to a day treatment setting if outpatient criteria are not met but:*
Medical complications:
Same as outpatient.

AND

Nature and level of substance dependence:
Same as outpatient except
1. the member consumes up to 32 standard drinks on a typical drinking day.

AND

Social support:
Same as outpatient.

AND

Psychological functioning:
1. the member does not suffer from any psychological condition to such an extent that he or she cannot safely follow plans and directions when away from the day treatment setting.

Table 18–1. Treatment guidelines (continued)

AND

Treatment history:
1. the member has not been unsuccessfully detoxified in the day treatment setting in the past.

C) *Refer to an inpatient substance abuse specialty care setting:*
Whenever the member does not meet the criteria for outpatient or day treatment detoxification.

D) *Refer to an inpatient psychiatric specialty care setting:*
Whenever the member exhibits psychiatric symptoms of such a severity that the available inpatient substance abuse specialty care settings cannot be expected to provide an appropriate level of care. This may often be the case in acutely suicidal and psychotic patients.

E) *Refer to a general hospital setting:*
Whenever the member exhibits medical symptoms of such a severity that the available inpatient substance abuse specialty care settings cannot be expected to provide an appropriate level of care. This may often be the case in trauma and gastrointestinal tract bleeding cases.

Guidelines for referral to a level-structured rehabilitation

A) *Refer to a primary care provider if:*
Medical complications:
1. the member has no complications or comorbidities requiring continuous observation,
2. the member's concerns about health were a major factor in his or her decision to stop using alcohol.

AND

Nature and level of substance dependence:
1. the member was alcohol dependent only (the member may have been using other substances but not in a manner associated with addiction).

AND

Social support:
1. the member has strong social support for abstinence,
2. the member has a strong relationship with the primary care provider.

AND

Psychological functioning:
1. the member does not suffer from any psychological condition to such an extent that he or she cannot safely follow plans and directions when away from the outpatient setting.

AND

Treatment history:
1. the member has not been unsuccessfully detoxified in an outpatient primary care setting in the past.

AND

The primary care provider is trained in and committed to the delivery of substance abuse services.

B) *Refer to outpatient rehabilitation with a substance abuse therapist involving the identified patient and family members if:*

Table 18–1. Treatment guidelines (continued)

Medical complications:
1. the member has no complications or comorbidities requiring continuous observation.

AND

Nature and level of substance dependence:
1. the member was alcohol dependent and/or substance dependent.

AND

Social support
1. the member has at least some social support for abstinence, preferably the patient is living with the support person.

AND

Psychological functioning:
1. the member does not suffer from any psychological condition to such an extent that he or she cannot safely follow plans and directions when away from the outpatient setting.

AND

Treatment history:
1. the member has not been unsuccessfully treated in an outpatient rehabilitation setting in the past.

C) *Refer to intensive day treatment rehabilitation involving the identified patient and family members if:*
Medical complications:
1. the member has no complications or comorbidities requiring continuous observation but may profit from daily observation,

AND

Nature and level of substance dependence:
1. the member was alcohol dependent and/or substance dependent.

AND

Social support:
1. the member has at least some social support for abstinence even if the patient is not living with the supportive persons,
2. the member may have significant difficulties in forming social relations and could profit from the additional social support aspects of the day treatment setting.

AND

Psychological functioning:
1. the member does not suffer from any psychological condition to such an extent that he or she cannot safely follow plans and directions when away from the day treatment setting,
2. the member may show some significant psychiatric difficulties that could profit from daily monitoring and/or medication trials in the day treatment setting.

AND

Treatment history:
1. the member has not been unsuccessfully treated in a day treatment rehabilitation setting in the past.
2. the member may have been unsuccessfully treated in an outpatient-only rehabilitation setting in the past.

Table 18–1. Treatment guidelines (continued)

D) *Refer to inpatient based rehabilitation involving the identified patient and family members if the member does not meet the criteria for primary care outpatient or day treatment rehabilitation and if:*
Nature and level of substance dependence:
1. the member was alcohol dependent and/or substance dependent.
AND
Medical complications:
1. the member has complications or comorbidities requiring continuous observation. (Consider a 30-day or longer residential setting.)
OR
Social support:
1. the member has no social support for abstinence,
2. the member has a history of significant difficulties in forming social relations and could profit from the additional social support aspects of an inpatient setting. (Consider a 30-day or longer residential setting.)
OR
Psychological functioning:
1. the member suffers from a psychological condition to such an extent that he or she cannot safely follow plans and directions when away from the inpatient setting. The condition can be expected to resolve with treatment within the normal course of the inpatient stay.
2. the member may show some significant psychiatric difficulties that could profit from around the clock monitoring and/or medication trials. (Consider a 30-day or longer residential setting.)
AND
Treatment history:
1. the member has been unsuccessfully treated in a day treatment rehabilitation setting in the past. (Consider a 30-day or longer residential setting if the member has been unsuccessfully treated in an inpatient setting in the past.)

Following completion of the day treatment or inpatient-based rehabilitation, all members should be referred to the full sequence of the outpatient group-, couple-, family-, and individual-based rehabilitation program for a period of at least 6 months. Phone and/or letter follow-up contact should be established by a substance abuse treatment team member at the end of months 1, 2, 3, 6 and 12 following detoxification.

Assignment to each of these level-of-support options should be based on the clinical presentation of the member. Five variables should be considered for each case. These variables are medical complications, nature and level of substance dependence, social support, psychological functioning, and treatment history. The weight of these variables differs, depending on whether the decision concerns detoxification or rehabilitation.

In the spectrum of care we have described above, "aftercare" is a misnomer. Traditional views cast intensive inpatient care as "treatment" and what follows as "aftercare." This view negates the crucial role of each step in the recovery process and overemphasizes the role of intensive inpatient care. Treatment spans the full range of intensity. Treatment content and setting are individualized and matched to the needs of the member at any point in time. Given earlier identification and an appropriate range of treatment dispositions, many cases, perhaps the majority, will not require inpatient detoxification or rehabilitation.

The spectrum of specialty services described in this section implies the following:

1. The plan should be designed to span at least 6 months.
2. Coordination between primary and specialty care is crucial.
3 Self-help and substance abuse group participation should form the core of the treatment plan for the patient and his or her family.
4. Prescribing Antabuse should be considered, especially in cases where relapse has occurred.
5. Detoxified, abstinent members showing continued signs of psychiatric disorder beyond a point justified by their substance use history should be evaluated by a psychiatrist who is knowledgeable about substance abuse and should be judiciously provided with medication as needed.
6. Members who do not attend scheduled sessions should be followed up with phone calls and letters.

Members who have been identified as having alcohol-related problems should be aggressively pursued to aid in the initiation and continuation of their treatment. Members may decline treatment; if they do so, their primary care provider must note that decision but not accept it. Many members will come to address their alcohol abuse problems only over time. At each contact with a member, alcohol abuse must be reassessed and addressed. Any presenting complaint that can be tied to alcohol use should be explained to the member in detail, and the expected benefits of treatment for the member should be repeatedly pointed out and discussed.

The provider must treat an identified alcohol problem as what it is: a serious, potentially fatal, progressive disorder, easily treated early and excruciatingly difficult to treat late. The member should hear this view of the problems consistently in all contacts with the primary care setting. The member should be referred to begin or return to treatment at every opportunity. This may be frustrating for the provider. Acceptance of the member's refusal of treatment would give the member the message that his or her decision is correct. By failing to aggressively address an alcohol problem, the provider joins the member in denial of the problem and communicates a lack of hope for change.

The avoidance of relapse and the maintenance of abstinence from all mood-altering substances is a goal of alcohol abuse treatment. Most people treated for alcohol abuse will, at some point, use alcohol again at least once.

When relapse occurs, members should be supported in whatever ways are necessary to "drive the relapse into remission again." A relapse after an extended period of abstinence is not the same as a relapse during detoxification. If relapse occurs a considerable time after a particular level of care has been used, a return to that level of care may be sufficient. If relapse occurs during the delivery of a level of care, the level of care provided should be intensified or changed to a more structured setting. For example, a member abstinent for a year following outpatient detoxification and rehabilitation who has relapsed for 2 days may well be treated on an outpatient basis again. On the other hand, a member in the process of outpatient detoxification who relapses while on Librium prescribed for withdrawal probably should be referred to a more structured setting such as day treatment or inpatient-based detoxification.

Treatment plans should be reviewed in detail with a member after a relapse has occurred and areas of weakness or vulnerability addressed. Family members should be included in the plan review. Family issues of trust and continued support for the member should be addressed. A return to, or intensification of the use of, self-help programs should be recommended. Prescribing of Antabuse should be considered. The abstinence violation effect should be reviewed and negative self-statements challenged.

In some plans, members who refuse to follow recommended treatment plans and repeatedly present when they are in crisis and require intensive treatment responses are presented with a noncompliance treatment contract. This contract addresses the managed care plan's right to avoid financial liability for the care of a member refusing recommended treatment. Different plans will have different processes for implementing such a contract, and such contracts may not be permitted in some states. The contract should not be used lightly or be viewed as punitive. Members repeatedly refusing recommended treatment should be offered a new treatment plan. If they continue to be noncompliant, they then accept the financial responsibility of their medical care for any consequences of their alcohol abuse. If they comply with the treatment plan but relapse anyway, no plan-related financial consequence befalls the member, and the treatment plan is reviewed and strengthened and care is provided as usual. Compliance with the revised plan becomes the new contract.

This type of contracted treatment plan should only be used in extreme cases. It is designed for the financial protection for the HMO, not as a clinical limit-setting technique.

Managed and traditional fee-for-service care systems are both capable of providing high-quality, efficacious care for alcohol abuse and dependence. The cost of care is not strongly related to the quality of care or to treatment outcome (Bunn 1989; Miller and Hester 1986). In environments where there is general agreement about the components of quality care and where cost-effectiveness is a widespread concern, it would be expected that fee-for-service providers would be competitive on the basis of quality and cost. In such an environment, cost-effectiveness would be about the same for fee-for-service and managed care except for the theoretically positive effect of greater coordination of care in the managed care setting. When cost-effectiveness is not a central concern, fee-for-service providers would be expected to be about as efficacious as managed care systems but not as cost-effective; when quality of care is not a major concern, managed care systems would be expected to be less expensive than fee-for-service providers but no less efficacious.

Managed care systems are accused of achieving savings (and profits) by reducing quality of care. Fee-for-service providers are accused of increasing costs (and profits) without increasing quality. Throughout this chapter, we have argued that the best method to reduce costs (and increase profits) is through increased quality of care. Increased quality can be achieved through earlier identification and intensive outpatient treatment. Cost savings can be achieved the same way.

The greatest economic incentive for the delivery of high-quality care for treatment of alcohol abuse and dependence is achieved when one plan is at risk for both the direct services for alcohol abuse and for the costs of medical treatment for comorbidity. This configuration provides a massive incentive for early intervention and, therefore, better quality of care and better outcome.

"Carving out" direct services for the alcohol abuse portion from medical care of the comorbidity sets up exactly the wrong set of consequences for quality care. The provider at risk for costs of direct service may see powerful short-term advantages for restricting access to low-cost but ineffective treatment approaches to late-stage problems, because he or she is not at risk for the treatment of the comorbidity.

If a managed care plan must set up its services for alcohol abuse and dependence separately from the rest of its medical care, we suggest that the provider for alcohol treatment services be paid on a per case basis rather than per day or per admission. That is, once a case is identified for treatment, the provider is at risk for all subsequent alcohol abuse and dependence admissions of that individual. Although this approach does not address directly the issue of risk for comorbidity, the contracted provider now has an incentive to identify cases early so that more cost-effective treatments can be utilized. Efficacious treatment choices will be made at each stage of treatment intensity because of the ownership for the risk of repeated treatment. We are not aware of any system that has established this type of contractual arrangement.

Whenever possible when contracting for hospital care, a managed care plan should locate more than one provider of intensive services for alcohol abuse and dependence. Per diem rates are important but, over the long run, establishing a relationship with a setting open to variable lengths of stay is crucial to cost containment. Hospitals should be aware of the breadth of the outpatient services available through the plan. It is essential to educate the hospitals to the early identification nature of the provider's referral pool. Detoxification and rehabilitation should be authorized separately. Detoxification usually involves a set amount of time that can often be estimated at the point of initial assessment. If new information is discovered directly affecting the time needed for detoxification (i.e., a seizure episode or drug use unreported at the time of the detoxification assessment), more time may be authorized by the plan.

Criteria for admission to rehabilitation should be established in advance. At that time the plan clinician and the hospital should agree on an initial length of stay (LOS; usually 5 to 7 days). The LOS should be adjusted as needed for good clinical reasons, and any adjustments should be of sufficient size to resolve the problem. The clinician should avoid lengthening the LOS because of poor discharge planning on the part of the hospital.

The inpatient treatment team should be aware of the outpatient components available for discharge plans. An outpatient care representative could be available to go to the hospital to meet with members, answer outpatient planning questions, and confirm the postdischarge plans but not to negotiate the LOS.

It is important to work with the managers and clinical staff of the hospital to help them accept that an inpatient treatment stay is a part of a spectrum of care. Hospital staff and HMO patients should not be given the message that their shorter LOS is "inferior" care.

Settings that provide this type of flexibility in treatment planning must be located or developed. We would advise that members be freely transported up to more than 150 miles to receive such care. The coordination of care is much easier across large geographical distances than across large philosophical distances.

References

Addicted to addictions. U.S. News and World Report, February 5, 1990, p 62–63

Ashley MJ, Rankin JG: A public health approach to the prevention of alcohol-related health problems. Annual Review of Public Health 9:233–271, 1988

Babor TF, Ritson B, Hodgson RJ: Alcohol related problems in the primary health care setting: a review of early intervention strategies. Br J Addict 81:23–46, 1986

Babor TF, Korner P, Wilber C, et al: Screening and early intervention strategies for harmful drinkers: initial lessons from the amethyst project. Australian Drug and Alcohol Review 6:325–339, 1987a

Babor TF, Kranzler HR, Lauerman RJ: Social drinking as a health and psychosocial risk factor. Recent Dev Alcohol 5:373–402, 1987b

Barnes G, Welte J: Alcohol use and abuse among adults in New York State. Buffalo, NY, Research Institute on Alcoholism, New York State Division of Alcoholism and Alcohol Abuse, 1988

Berg G, Skutle A: Early intervention with problem drinkers. Paper presented at the Third International Conference on Treatment and Behaviors, North Berwick, Scotland, August 12–16, 1984

Bergen BJ, Price TR, Kinney J: Medical students' conflicting perceptions of alcohol patients. Journal of Medical Education 55:954–955, November 1980

Brownell KD, Marlatt GA, Lichtestein E, et al: Understanding and preventing relapse. Am Psychol 41(7):765–782, 1986

Buchanan DG, Buchanan RG, Centor RM, et al: Screening for alcohol abuse using CAGE scores and likelihood ratios. Ann Intern Med 115:774–777, 1991

Bunn G: Cost, quality not linked. Professional Counselor, July–August, 1989, p 10

Bush B, Shaw S, Cleary P, et al: Screening for alcohol abuse using the CAGE questionnaire. Am J Med 82:231–235, 1987

Caswell S, McPherson M: Attitudes of New Zealand general practitioners to alcohol-related problems. J Stud Alcohol 44(2):342–351, 1983

Chappel JN, Veach TL, Krug RS: The substance abuse attitude survey: an instrument for measuring attitudes. J Stud Alcohol 46(1):48–51, 1984

Clark WD: Alcoholism: blocks to diagnosis and treatment. Am J Med 71:274–285, 1981

Clement S: The identification of alcohol related problems by general practitioners. Br J Addict 81:257–264, 1986

Coles C, Brown RT, Smith IE, et al: Effects of prenatal alcohol exposure at school age, I: physical and cognitive development. Neurotoxicol Teratol 13(4):357–367, 1991

Cyr MG: Presenting the diagnosis and initiating treatment, in Project ADEPT Curriculum for Primary Care Physician Training, Vol I: Core Modules. Edited by Dube CE, Goldstein MG, Lewis DC, et al. Providence, RI, Brown University, 1989

Cyr MG, Wartman SA: The effectiveness of routine screening questions in the detection of alcoholism. JAMA 259(1):51–54, 1988

Del Toro IM: Design chemical dependency programs in HMOs. HMO Practice 4(1):19–23, 1990

Dube CE, Goldstein MG, Lewis DC, et al (eds): Project ADEPT Curriculum for Primary Care Physician Training, Vol I: Core Modules. Providence, RI, Brown University, 1989

Dupont RL: Prevention of adolescent chemical dependency. Pediatr Clin North Am 34(2):495–505, 1987

Ewan EC, Whaite A: Evaluation of training programs for health professionals in substance misuse. J Stud Alcohol 44(5):885–899, 1982

Fink EB, Longabaugh R, McCrady BM, et al: Effectiveness of alcoholism treatment in partial versus inpatient setting: twenty-four month outcomes. Addict Behav 10:235–248, 1985

Fisher JC, Keeley KA, Mason RL, et al: Physicians and alcoholics: factors affecting attitudes of family-practice residents toward alcoholics. J Stud Alcohol 36(5):626–633, 1975

Frances RJ, Franklin JE: Primary prevention of alcohol and substance abuse, in Primary Prevention in Psychiatry: State of the Art. Edited by Barter JT, Talbott SW. Washington, DC, American Psychiatric Press, 1986, pp 119–141

Goldman B: How to thwart a drug seeker. Emergency Medicine 23(6):40–61, 1991

Goldstein MG, Dube CE: Substance abuse prevention, in Project ADEPT Curriculum for Primary Care Physician Training, Vol I: Core Modules. Edited by Dube CE, Goldstein MG, Lewis DC, et al. Providence, RI, Brown University, 1989

Griffin JB, Hill IK, Jones JJ, et al: Evaluating alcoholism and drug abuse knowledge in medical education: a collaborative project. Journal of Medical Education 58:859–863, 1983

Grueninger UJ, Goldstein MG, Duffy FD: Patient education in hypertension: five essential steps. J Hypertens Suppl 7(3):S93–S98, 1989

Halon MJ: A review of the recent literature relating to the training of medical students in alcoholism. Journal of Medical Education 60:618–625, 1985

Hayami DE, Freeborn DK: Effect of coverage on use of an HMO alcoholism treatment program, outcome and medical care utilization. Am J Public Health 71(10):1133–1143, 1981

Hayashida M, Alterman AI, McLellan AT, et al: Comparative effectiveness and costs of inpatient and outpatient detoxification of patients with mild to moderate alcohol withdrawal syndrome. N Engl J Med 320:358–365, 1989

Hays JT, Spickard WA: Alcoholism: early diagnosis and intervention. J Gen Intern Med 2:420–427, 1987

Heather N, Whitton B, Robertson I: Evaluation of a selfhelp manual for media-recruited problem drinkers: six month follow up results. Br J Clin Psychol 25:19–34, 1986

Helwick SA: Substance abuse education in medical school: past, present, and future. Journal of Medical Education 60:707–711, 1985

Holder HD: Alcoholism treatment and potential health care cost savings. Med Care 25:52–71, 1987

Holder HD, Blose JO: Alcohol treatment and total health care utilization and costs. JAMA 125:1456–1460, 1986

Holder HD, Blose JO: Typical patterns and costs of alcoholism treatment across a variety of populations and providers. Alcohol Clin Exp Res 15:190–195, 1991

Holder HD, Longabaugh R, Miller WR, et al: The cost effectiveness of treatment for alcoholism: a first approximation. J Stud Alcohol 52(6):517–540, 1991

Kahle DB, White RM: Attitudes toward alcoholism among psychologists, marriage, family, child counselors. J Stud Alcohol 52(4):321–324, 1991

Kemerow DB, Pincus HA, MacDonald DI: Alcohol abuse, other drug abuse and mental disorders in medical practice. JAMA 225(15):2054–2057, 1986

Kinney J, Price TR, Bergen BJ: Impediments to alcohol education. J Stud Alcohol 45(5):453–459, 1984

Kranzler HR: A practitioner guide to the medical risks of social drinking. Resident and Staff Physician 33(2):80–85, 1987

Kristenson H, Trell E, Hood B: Serum-y-glutamyltransferase in screening and continuous control of heavy drinking in middle aged men. Am J Epidemiol 114(6):862–872, 1981

Kristenson H, Ohlin H, Hulten-Nosslin B, et al: Identification and intervention of heavy drinking in middle-aged men: results and follow-up of 24–60 months of long-term study with randomized controls. Alcoholism: Clinical and Experimental Research 7(2):203–209, 1983

Levin BL, Glasser JH, Jaffee CL Jr: National trends in coverage and utilization of mental health, alcohol, and substance abuse services within managed health care systems. Am J Public Health 78(9):1222–1223, 1988

Lewis DC: Putting training and alcohol and other drugs into the mainstream of medical education. Alcohol Health and Research World 13(1):8–13, 1989

Luckey JW: Justifying alcohol treatment on the basis of cost savings: the offset literature. Alcohol Health and Research World 12(1):9–15, 1987

Magruder-Habib K, Durand AM, Frey KA: Alcohol abuse and alcoholism in primary health care settings. J Fam Pract 32(4):406–413, 1991

Miller WR, Hester RK: Inpatient alcoholism treatment: who benefits? Am Psychol 41(7):794–805, 1986

Moore RD, Bone LR, Geller G: Prevalence, detection and treatment of alcoholism in hospitalized patients. JAMA 261(3):403–408, 1989

Nace EP: Inpatient treatment of alcoholism: a necessary part of the therapeutic armamentarium. The Psychiatric Hospital 21(1):9–12, 1990

Nock JJ: Instructing medical students on alcoholism: what to teach with limited time. Journal of Medical Education 55:858–863, 1980

Orvis BR, Armor DJ, Williams CE, et al: Effectiveness and cost of alcohol rehabilitation in the United States Air Force (R-2308-AF). Santa Monica, CA, RAND Corporation, December 1981

Osher FC, Kofoed LL: Treatment of patients with psychiatric and psychoactive substance abuse disorders. Hosp Community Psychiatry 40(10):1025–1030, 1989

Parker DA, Parker ES, Harford TC, et al: Alcohol use and depression symptoms among employed men and women. Brown University Digest of Addiction Theory and Application 6(4):48–51, 1987

Parsons OA, Butters N, Nathan PE, et al: Neuropsychology of Alcoholism: Implications for Diagnosis and Treatment. New York, Guilford, 1987

Persson J, Magnusson P: Prevalence of excessive or problem drinkers among patients attending somatic outpatient clinics: a study of alcohol related medical care. BMJ 295:467–471, 1987

Pokorny A, Putman P, Fryer J: Drug abuse and alcoholism teaching in US medical and osteopathic schools. Journal of Medical Education 53:816–824, 1978

Polich JM, Armor DJ, Braiker HB: The Course of Alcoholism: Four Years After Treatment. New York, Wiley, 1981

Prochaska JO, DiClemente CC: Transtheoretical therapy: toward a more integrative model of change. Psychotherapy: Theory, Research and Practice 19(3):276–288, 1982

Prochaska J, DiClemente C: Stages and processes of self-change of smoking: toward an integrative model of change. J Consult Clin Psychol 51:390–395, 1983

Putnam SL: Alcoholism, morbidity and care-seeking. Med Care 20(1):97–121, 1982

Regier DA, Farmer ME, Rae DS, et al: Comorbidity of mental disorders with alcohol and other drug abuse. JAMA 264(19):2511–2518, 1990

Ries R: Substance abuse intervention on inpatient psychiatry. Substance Abuse 10(1):28–32, 1989

Roberts KS, Brent EE: Physician utilization and illness patterns in families of alcoholics. J Stud Alcohol 43(1):119–120, 1982

Roosa N: One more hurdle. Massachusetts Health Care, November–December 1987, pp 22–25

Rundell OH, Jones RK, Gregory D: Practical benefit-cost analysis for alcoholism programs. Alcohol Clin Exp Res 5(4):477–508, 1981

Shadle M, Christianson JB: The impact of HMO development on mental health and chemical dependency services. Hosp Community Psychiatry 40(11):1145–1151, 1989

Skinner HA, Holt MB, Schuller R, et al: Identification of alcohol abuse using laboratory tests and a history of trauma. Ann Intern Med 101:847–851, 1984

Smith IE, Lancaster JS, Moss-Wells S, et al: Identifying high-risk pregnant drinkers: biological and behavioral correlates of continuous heavy drinking during pregnancy. J Stud Alcohol 48(4):304–309, 1987

Solomon J, Vanga N, Morgan JP, et al: Emergency room physicians' recognition of alcohol misuse. J Stud Alcohol 41(5):583–586, 1980

Sparadeo FR, Zwick WR, Ruggiero S, et al: Evaluation of a social setting detoxification program. J Stud Alcohol 43(11):1124–1136, 1982

Warburg MM, Cleary PD, Rohman M, et al: Residents' attitudes, knowledge, and behavior regarding diagnosis and treatment of alcoholism. Journal of Medical Education 62:497–503, 1987

Willoughby A: The alochol troubled person: known and unknown. Chicago, IL, Nelson Hall Publishers, 1979

Zwick WR: An advocate's view of substance abuse services in the managed care setting. Paper presented to the annual meeting of the Group Health Association of America, Minneapolis, MN, June 1986

Zwick WR: Time-effective treatment in a substance abuse day treatment program. Paper presented at Harvard Medical School, Harvard Community Health Plan Conference on Time-Effective Treatment in Mental Health, Boston, MA, March 1992

Zwick WR, Dube CE: Treatment, in Project ADEPT Curriculum for Primary Care Physician Training, Vol I: Core Modules. Edited by Dube CE, Goldstein MG, Lewis DC, et al. Providence, RI, Brown University, 1989

✦ 19 ✦

Treatment of Drug Abuse in the Managed Care Setting

Richard Caplan, M.S.W., L.I.C.S.W., M.P.H.

P roviding drug treatment for a prepaid population in a managed care setting has afforded a great opportunity for observing current trends in substance abuse care. With the increasing prevalence of drug use (especially freebase and crack cocaine) and the increasing demand for drug treatment from prepaid populations, managed care settings are confronted with tasks ranging from developing a comprehensive treatment philosophy to providing timely access to services. In this chapter, I will show how the philosophy of managed care and a clinically sound approach to drug treatment can be well integrated and outline the specific elements that make managed care settings different from the more traditional fee-for-service environment. I will then describe a treatment model developed for a staff model health maintenance organization (HMO) in which major clinical decisions are made using these elements in a clinical algorithm.

History

There has been little written about the history of drug abuse treatment in managed care settings. What is presented in this section is based on personal observation and conversations with other substance abuse program managers throughout the country. The development of drug treatment programs in prepaid plans seems to have more to do with the growth and progression of drug use in this country than with managed care per se.

Managed care settings that have been in existence for over 15 years developed substance abuse services primarily for alcohol abuse and alcoholism. Originally, the majority of hospital days and outpatient visits for substance abuse were for alcohol (New Jersey Business Group on Health 1986). The incidence of cocaine, opiate, marijuana, and other drug abuse was far lower than it is today. In fact, as recently as 5 years ago, the use of hospital resources for alcohol abuse and alcoholism at Harvard Community Health Plan (HCHP, a Boston-based staff model HMO) was significantly higher than the use of resources for drug abuse and addiction. The most recent estimates show that, since 1983, hospitalizations for drug treatment at HCHP have increased by 300%–400%, whereas alcohol hospitalizations have remained fairly constant (Harvard Community Health Plan 1987).

Although these data appeared to approximate national trends (Wise 1988), managers of substance abuse programs that had been designed to serve an alcoholic population were somewhat surprised at the demand for drug services. In the early 1980s, there was a fairly strong distinction between "alcohol" and "drug" treatment. Alcohol treatment was seen as 1) providing a medically safe environment for detoxification, and then 2) providing additional inpatient "rehabilitation" and/or additional outpatient counseling. Alcoholics Anonymous (AA) was considered a significant part of treatment regardless of which clinical route was chosen.

Drug-dependent patients presenting for treatment at that time were primarily members of minority groups who were from lower socioeconomic classes. They were seen as more likely to have serious character disorders and less likely to remain abstinent from their drug of choice. Drug addicts (especially intravenous heroin users) had very high relapse rates and were unlikely to comply with aftercare treatment (McAuliffe and Chien 1986).

Withdrawal from opiates was not considered a medically dangerous condition, so acute hospitalizations for patients addicted to opiates were avoided (Kauffman et al. 1984). Instead, most patients who were addicted to narcotics were referred to either outpatient methadone programs or long-term therapeutic communities (Simpson 1979). Those who were hospitalized were usually those who created so much anxiety in their caregivers that an administrative, rather than a clinical, decision to hospitalize would be made.

Also, at that time, patients who were addicted to cocaine used primarily intranasal and sometimes intravenous routes (many times in combination with heroin). Cocaine withdrawal was also not seen as needing medical attention, and acute hospitalizations for these patients were avoided. Patients who were addicted to cocaine were encouraged to remain in outpatient counseling in conjunction with Drug Abusers (now Narcotic Abusers) Anonymous (NA) (Colliver 1987).

Among HCHP members, the incidence of addiction to marijuana, PCP, LSD, or prescription drugs was so small that clinical decisions were made on a case-by-case basis with no clear protocol or algorithm for decision making. These drug-dependent or addicted members were only hospitalized when withdrawal presented a medical risk. When patients who abused drugs were offered outpatient groups or programs, they were expected to integrate into a largely white middle-class alcohol treatment population and were asked to simply substitute the name of their drug every time they heard the word "alcohol."

How Freebase Cocaine Changed the Treatment Structure

In the late 1970s, a new process of using cocaine called freebasing was introduced to the middle-class drug user. When a user "freebased" or smoked cocaine, additives were burned away so the resulting compound was much purer than street cocaine and the resulting high much more intense. The absorption of cocaine through the lungs was rapid, leading to a fairly immediate high and a rapid "crash," which led to further use (Paly et al. 1982).

The premade form of freebased cocaine, called "crack" or "rock," brought a much more potent, concentrated, yet inexpensive form of cocaine to a population of drug users who grew up in the 1960s and 1970s believing that cocaine was not a dangerous drug (Kleber 1988). For most recreational users who occasionally snorted street cocaine, that belief was accurate. By the time middle-class cocaine users got access to the drug, there was probably a much greater percentage of adulterates in it than actual cocaine.

The introduction of the process of freebasing to a middle-class population that viewed cocaine as harmless has been a great contributor to the current "epidemic" of cocaine addicts presenting for treatment (Adams et al. 1986; Grinspoon and Bakalar 1980). Thus, the introduction of crack brought in a much different population looking for drug treatment. Instead of patients who were poor or members of minority groups, middle- and upper-class white patients were presenting for treatment of their drug addiction. These are the people who are much more likely to be members of a prepaid, managed care plan. Most, if not all, of these care settings were caught totally unprepared for this new population of drug addicts.

The first approach of the HMOs was to integrate this new treatment population with already existing alcohol programs, with the expectation that the two populations would be fairly similar. Not only did this not work, but it also forced a tremendous reevaluation of existing programs. Soon after, the treatment programs and services were simply renamed "substance abuse" or "chemical dependency" programs. This approach basically views all mood-altering substances as having similar attributes and the addiction to them as having similar progression. Although in theory this may be true, a patient's recovery from these substances can look very different depending on the drug of choice.

Life-Style and Illicit Drug Use

For adults, the procurement and use of alcohol (including access to a safe, consistently pure supply) is no more a problem than walking to the corner liquor store. The same applies to nicotine. When one's drug of choice is illegal, it means time and energy must be spent to develop a network of reliable suppliers who can be trusted to provide the best drug for the best price. It also means contact with a criminal subculture. This subculture represents a departure from typical middle-class values. The middle-class user may experience a conflict between his or her usual life-style (with job, house in the suburbs, spouse, and children) and the seemingly more exciting subculture (complete with sexual and life-style experimentation).

Today, intravenous drug users have not only their addiction and conflicts of values to consider, but serious health risks as well. Most treatment programs now contain AIDS awareness groups, and the staffs of drug treatment programs are expected to take all safety precautions necessary when working with a high-risk population.

In addition, in recent years the threat of AIDS was bringing more people in for treatment. The prospect of becoming infected by sharing needles (or having intimate contact with someone already infected) scared some people who were addicted into coming in for treatment. For managed care settings, this meant that providing treatment now might prevent someone from contracting AIDS. Early case identification and timely intervention became even more important as the cost of drug dependency began climbing.

Psychiatric Considerations

The incoming population of people who freebased cocaine also brought a much higher incidence of psychiatric diagnosis (Gawin and Kleber 1986; Harvard Medical School Mental Health Letter 1989; Lowenstein et al. 1987). Treatment programs have had to be sensitive to this and to increase the sophistication of their clinical approach. Many traditional alcohol programs were staffed heavily with people who were recovering from alcoholism and who had some basic training in counseling (Kinney 1983). Programs now require psychiatric expertise as well as addictions experience in their staff and special clinical units or groups to deal with people diagnosed with psychiatric problems as well as chemical dependency.

Managed Care Considerations

There are several specific factors that make managed care systems different from the more traditional fee-for-service system. These include gatekeeping, affiliated (or preferred) providers, utilization management, claims review, and prepayment.

When a patient has a traditional indemnity policy, he or she has free choice of provider or hospital. The indemnity policy provides patients with immediate access to any desired clinical service. There is no permission, authorization, or "prescreening" needed. The indemnity policy also gives the hospital control over the length of stay. Hospital days beyond the state mandate for coverage (what insurance companies will usually cover) can be charged to the patient. Hospital programs generally build their length of stay around a state-mandated benefit. Most hospitals also offer outpatient care as a follow-up clinical service. These programs prefer to sell a "package" of treatment to each patient, based primarily on marketing concerns.

The insurance companies' costs rise as their admissions and hospital days stay consistently high. They have no control over how people spend their benefits. They also have no control over length of stay. They cannot "manage" how people enter the patient pool, how long they stay there, or what happens to them afterward. There is no mechanism for matching patients to the most appropriate care or for ensuring the quality and consistency of that care.

Treatment

Most current drug treatment programs contain the following phases:

1. Evaluation;
2. Stabilization (attending to the medical or psychiatric conditions, including withdrawal, that may develop during the initial period of abstinence);
3. Relapse prevention (psychoeducational and cognitive behavioral treatment and self-help programs); and
4. Maintenance (ongoing attention to a patient's life-style and life skills, development, and personal growth). This phase may include more traditional psychotherapy if indicated.

Although most drug treatment proceeds through these phases, there are clear differences between managed care and fee-for-service. Managed care settings require patients to appear for a screening evaluation. Based on that evaluation, patients will be directed to the most appropriate level of care. Managed care recognizes certain "choice points" throughout the treatment process (see Figure 19–1). Managed care settings often have clinical algorithms or protocols to help direct patients to the least restrictive care that is clinically appropriate.

Patients may believe managed care settings are more difficult to enter because of the emphasis on monitoring access to services (gatekeeper) and the screening evaluation. Patients sometimes see the evaluation phase as interfering with their ability to be treated and do not understand that they have begun the treatment process. They may also be unhappy with the affiliated or preferred providers that an HMO may offer and may disagree with the prescribed level of care.

To the hospital, HMOs can appear intrusive, demanding, or withholding. The utilization review or case management that HMOs use to help guide patients through hospital programs is sometimes seen as intrusive and requiring extra effort to reduce lengths of stay and refill

	PRETREATMENT		TREATMENT	
	Evaluation	Stabilization	Relapse Prevention	Maintenance
Access (Gatekeeping)	Authorized by ◆ primary provider ◆ screening service ◆ Mental Health Dept. or EAP* (◆ self-referral)	◆ Medical/psychiatric risk (self-refer) ◆ EAPs* ◆ Inpatient vs. outpatient—urgency?	Authorized by medical primary provider or substance abuse or mental health provider	Authorized by medical primary provider or substance abuse or mental health provider
Affiliated/ Preferred Providers	◆ screening service ◆ substance abuse providers ◆ mental health providers ◆ primary providers	◆ screening service ◆ substance abuse providers ◆ inpatient vs. outpatient	Substance abuse provider (or program)	Substance abuse provider (or program)
		REEVALUATION	REEVALUATION	
Utilization Management	Treatment matching ◆ quality of treatment ◆ level of care	Hospital liaison/ case review	Reevaluation for appropriate levels of care	◆ Benefit review ◆ Limits around rehospitalization
Claims Review	Timely membership check Authorization of treatment	Emergency membership check	Emergency membership check	Emergency membership check

*Some HMOs allow employee assistance programs (EAPs) direct access to evaluation and/or stabilization.

Figure 19-1. Phases of drug treatment across a managed care setting.

beds. For the HMO, there is more chance of high-quality, cost-effective care if decisions to treat are based on reasonable clinical criteria, and if a full spectrum of intensive services—not just hospitals—are available treatment options.

Effectiveness of Managed Drug Treatments

Figure 19–1 shows how a managed care system might handle the major phases of drug treatment. By viewing each phase of treatment across the elements of managed care, we can see how managed care is organized to provide efficient, high-quality, cost-effective treatment.

Evaluation

The purpose of the evaluation is to match the patient to the most appropriate level of care. Each level of care is based on specific medical, social, and psychiatric criteria. (A managed care screening should also include a timely membership and benefit check, as many addicted patients have recently lost jobs and coverage.) For drug-dependent patients, an evaluation would also include an appropriate medical screening (including blood and urine testing) to determine the extent of drug dependency and the need for hospitalization. Access to the evaluation should be quick and easy. The sooner a patient can be evaluated, the sooner the treatment plan can be put into place.

This is the area where employee assistance program (EAP) counselors have the greatest degree of trouble with HMOs. Quite often, an EAP counselor will call an HMO simply to authorize his or her treatment plan for the patient, and the HMO counselor cannot implement the plan until an evaluation is done at the HMO.

Some HMO models (i.e., independent practitioner association [IPA], group, network) do not staff their own substance abuse services. Instead, they contract with a screening service to evaluate all incoming requests for substance abuse treatment. Once an evaluation is completed, the patient will move on to the next step in treatment.

A special note must be made regarding response to court-ordered evaluation. Frequently, courts will order a specific modality and length of treatment, with regular reports to the court. Most HMOs offer patients only the care that is indicated by their evaluation and attempt to retain maximum confidentiality.

Stabilization (Detoxification)

Most managed care/HMO settings have a wide spectrum of services at their disposal. These include inpatient and rehabilitation, day treatment, evening treatment, and outpatient recovery groups. *The HMO clinician will try to choose the least restrictive treatment alternative that is clinically appropriate.* There is still much debate over who should be stabilized in an inpatient setting. For example, although the inherent risks for cocaine withdrawal have been documented (Lowenstein et al. 1987), there is still controversy involving the decision to hospitalize. Trials of outpatient cocaine treatment have been conducted using carbamazepine (Halikis et al. 1989), desipramine (Gawin et al. 1989b), flupenthixol decanoate (Gawin et al. 1989a), lithium carbonate (Gawin and Kleber 1984), and other medications, with varying degrees of success. The controversy regarding hospitalization extends to heroin addiction as well. Many studies are looking at clonidine as an antiwithdrawal agent (Gold et al. 1978; Kleber et al. 1987; Washton and Resnick 1980). Although clonidine hydrochloride (Catapres) has some positive effect on reducing the autonomic signs of withdrawal, it is less effective in relieving the subjective discomforts of withdrawal (Jasinski et al. 1985).

Relapse Prevention/Rehabilitation

Once a patient passes through "stabilization," there is a reevaluation process that determines the next step in treatment. Often patients look different or can offer better clinical information once stabilized. Based on that second look, decisions are made regarding where and how to rehabilitate. Managed care provides a wide spectrum of inpatient and outpatient choices including inpatient care, partial hospitalization, and intensive outpatient or regular outpatient care. Access to rehabilitation is only through the HMO clinician or case manager and takes place only at an affiliated program.

One of the major purposes of rehabilitation is to motivate the patient to remain in treatment. Of the few things we truly know regarding drug treatment outcome, time spent in treatment, as opposed to where the treatment takes place, seems to be the significant factor in a positive treatment outcome (i.e., abstinence, positive life changes, increased self-esteem, etc.; Simpson 1979). Programs designed to *keep* patients in treatment offer the best chance of success. HMOs may find that a generous outpatient benefit will provide better quality and ultimately save money.

Contracting for Services

When managed care facilities contract with outside resources for substance abuse services, there are several factors they take into account: quality of care, flexibility, cost-effectiveness, willingness to work within the philosophic framework of managed care, and willingness to work with managed care staff. Contracts may include goals of treatment, lengths of stay, and locus of decision making, as well as costs.

Most clinicians in managed care settings have a very clear idea of when they need to use hospital-based treatment. One way of managing the cost of health care is by moving people out of the more costly forms of treatment as quickly as possible without sacrificing quality of care. Additionally, managed care settings expect hospital programs to do what cannot be done on an outpatient basis: to remove the patient from a toxic environment and to provide a safe, chemical-free environment where a patient can be medically supervised. Freestanding (non-hospital) inpatient programs are also used to separate a patient from his or her environment so as to interrupt the pattern of drug use. These programs accept patients who are medically and psychiatrically stable, and they offer less expensive care than hospital-based units.

Utilization management (UM) is one way of monitoring quality and cost-effectiveness of care in a program. UM usually involves a mid-level clinician reviewing a patient's record and talking to the program staff. The UM clinician communicates treatment information back to the referring clinician so there will be no gap in services. At times UM (or a clinical liaison) can also screen a patient on-site for aftercare programs so that a smooth, clear referral can be arranged from one treatment site to another.

Maintenance

In this category, the focus is primarily on long-term recovery. This may include the ongoing involvement of a patient in a 12-step self-help program as well as in long-term recovery groups. This area may also include the ongoing psychological and emotional awareness of issues such as codependency or relationships with adult children. A complete long-term recovery program would include an ongoing relationship with a clinician, to whom patients (and significant others) could return periodically to review ongoing issues as they arose. Long-term recovery groups seem to provide the greatest ongoing success in drug treatment (Simpson 1979). Because of the nature of cocaine craving, short-term recovery is not the measure of a successful treatment outcome. In addition, many drug-addicted patients have concomitant psychiatric illness requiring ongoing care. Figure 19–2 presents a clinical algorithm for these treatment decisions, with examples of programs suitable for each phase of care.

Additional Considerations

Staffing

Providing high-quality, cost-effective services at the most appropriate level of care takes the time and effort of managers, administrators, and frontline clinicians. It is much harder and more complicated to treat someone or refer to an outpatient program than it is to hospitalize a patient. In managed care settings, there must be organizational support for clinicians working to avoid unnecessary hospitalizations. Work schedules, performance standards, and intradepartmental availability must all be designed to support the frontline clinician who is trying his or her hardest to fulfill the mandate of managed care.

The Case Manager

The role that most clearly differentiates managed care from fee-for-service is that of the case manager (Aquilera and Del Toro 1990). The case manager is responsible for evaluation and referral to the most appropriate level of care. He or she then follows patients from one level of care to the next, reviewing their progress and treatment plans while remaining available to consult with others in the treatment system.

Experience at the Harvard Community Health Plan suggests that patients who drop out of treatment return only at the next crisis, asking for another hospitalization. To retain patients in ongoing treatment, it is essential that one mental health or substance abuse

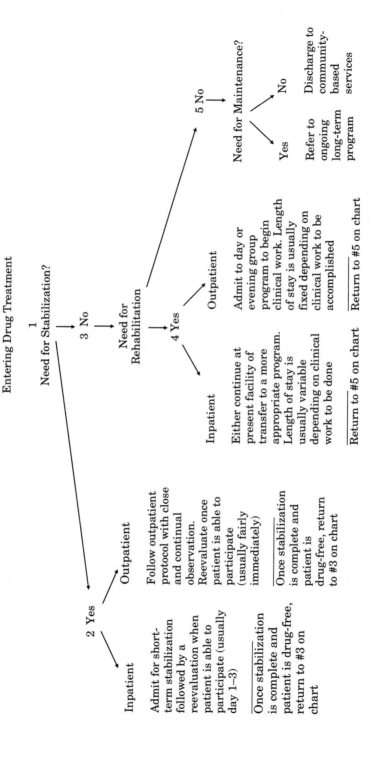

Figure 19–2. Decision points for drug treatment level of care.

clinician take primary responsibility for reengaging the patient after completion of each level of care.

Employer Groups

EAP counselors or work supervisors can be important allies in setting clear limits with substance abuse patients. Although HMOs can deliver the treatment, they have few means to make patients see the consequences of problem drinking or drug abuse. Working together, the employer/EAP and the HMO can make a powerful treatment team. Ideally, the EAP counselor and the HMO counselor can work together in forming a treatment-work contract, making clear to the patient the expectations and consequences of drinking or drug abuse behavior.

Chronic Relapsers

A percentage of all drug-abusing patients do not seem to comply with or respond to treatment. These are the patients who use up costly inpatient resources without having any sustained period of recovery or showing any discernible improvement in the quality of their lives.

For this population, several approaches are helpful:

1. *Performing a more complete evaluation to determine any missed diagnosis.* These might include posttraumatic stress disorder, gambling, eating, or sexual disorders; anxiety or affective disorders; or medical illness. There is a chance that a patient's return to chemical use may have to do with what has been left untreated.
2. *Increasing the intrusiveness into the patient's life.* This may involve engaging the patient's significant other, family, or work supervisor/EAP in treatment to help a patient connect his or her continuing chemical use with consequences to daily life.
3. *Having a patient assume more responsibility for his or her treatment.* This may involve asking the patient to do more and more of the work to get him- or herself into treatment with each additional request for detoxification.
4. *Treating chronic relapse as a clinical entity involving specific protocols or clinical programs.* Emphasis would be on arranging the treatment system to be more in line with the life-style of the pa-

tient who chronically relapses (e.g., providing a "drop-in" group at the same time each day). It would also be important to recognize the difference between relapse and noncompliance. Attention should be paid to the patient's environment and what life-style changes might be needed to allow the greatest chance for a long-term recovery.

5. *Structuring the benefit package to increase motivation to use care efficiently and discourage noncompliance.* This may include limiting coverage (if state regulations permit) with either a yearly or lifetime cap, or specifying criteria for noncompliance with consequences to future coverage.

Conclusion

Managed care does not have all the answers to the problem of drug addiction, nor should professionals in managed care systems make unrealistic promises regarding treatment outcome. Managed care can, however, offer a comprehensive spectrum of substance abuse treatments that can engage, support, and move a patient through a wide variety of treatment options based on the patient's clinical needs.

It is also important for managed care systems to support the timely collection of clinical data so that alternative treatment efficiency can be measured and compared to more traditional treatments.

As hospital-based programs become more expensive and care is increasingly reviewed, more traditional insurers (and providers) are now incorporating elements of managed care into their own systems. Managed care currently offers an excellent opportunity to provide and review the technology we have available to treat addictions. As we continue to record and review outcome data, we will have additional opportunities to modify our treatments to produce the best outcomes for our patients.

References

Adams EH, Gfroerer JC, Rouse BA, et al: Trends in prevalence and consequences of cocaine use. Adv Alcohol Subst Abuse 6:49–71, 1986

Aquilera C, Del Toro I: Using case management to enhance provider effectiveness. Paper presented at the annual meeting of the Group Health Association of America, New Orleans, LA, January 1990

Colliver J: A decade of dawn: cocaine-related cases 1976–1985. Washington, DC, National Institute on Drug Abuse, Division of Epidemiology and Statistical Publication, U.S. Government Printing Office, 1987

Gawin FH, Kleber HD: Cocaine abuse treatment: open pilot trial with desipramine and lithium carbonate. Arch Gen Psychiatry 41:903–909, 1984

Gawin FH, Kleber HD: Abstinence symptomatology and psychiatric diagnosis in cocaine abusers. Arch Gen Psychiatry 43:107–113, 1986

Gawin F, Allan D, Humblestone B: Outpatient treatment of "crack" cocaine smoking with flupenthixol decanoate. Arch Gen Psychiatry 46:322–325, 1989a

Gawin F, Kleber H, Byck R, et al: Desipramine facilitation of initial cocaine abstinence. Arch Gen Psychiatry 46:117–121, 1989b

Gold MS, Redmond DE Jr, Kleber HD: Clonidine in opiate withdrawal. Lancet 1:929–930, 1978

Grinspoon L, Bakalar JB: Drug dependence: non-narcotic agents, in Comprehensive Textbook of Psychiatry, 3rd Edition. Edited by Kaplan HI, Freedman AM, Sadock BJ. Baltimore, MD, Williams & Wilkins, 1980

Halikis J, Kemp K, Kuhn K, et al: Preliminary indication of differential treatment responsiveness to carbamazepine for cocaine addiction, based on differential personality psychopathology. Biol Psychiatry 25:10A–13A, 1989

Harvard Community Health Plan: Hospital Information System, Yearly Hospital Reports, 1981–1986. Brookline, MA, Harvard Community Health Plan, 1987

Harvard Medical School Mental Health Letter 6:5, November 1989

Jasinski DR, Johnson RE, Kocher TR, et al: Clonidine in morphine withdrawal. Arch Gen Psychiatry 42:1063–1066, 1985

Kauffman JF, Schaffer H, Burglass ME: A strategy for the biological assessment of addiction, in The Addictive Behaviors. Edited by Schaffer H. New York, Haworth Press, 1984, pp 7–18

Kleber HD: Cocaine abuse: historical, epidemiological and psychological perspectives. J Clin Psychiatry 40(suppl 2):3–6, 1988

Kleber HD, Topazian M, Gaspari J, et al: Clonidine and naltrexone in the outpatient treatment of heroin withdrawal. Am J Drug Alcohol Abuse 13:1–17, 1987

Kinney J: Relapse among alcoholics who are alcoholism counselors. J Stud Alcohol 44(4):744–748, 1983

Lowenstein DH, Massa SM, Rowbotham MC, et al: Acute neurologic and psychiatric complications associated with cocaine abuse. Am J Med 83:841–846, 1987

McAuliffe W, Chien J: Recovery training and self-help: a relapse prevention program for treated opiate addicts. J Subst Abuse Treat 3:9–20, 1986

New Jersey Business Group on Health: Mandated health care benefits, in The Cost of Insurance Coverage of Alcoholic, Drug Abuse and Mental Health Treatment. Trenton, NJ, New Jersey Business Group on Health, April 1, 1986, pp 212–234

Paly D, Jatlow P, Van Clyke C, et al: Plasma cocaine concentration during cocaine paste smoking. Life Sci 30:731–738, 1982

Simpson D: The relation of time spent in drug abuse treatment to post treatment outcome. Am J Psychiatry 136(11):1449–1453, 1979

Washton A, Resnick R: Clonidine vs methadone for opiate detoxification: double blind outpatient trials, in Problems of Drug Dependence: National Institute on Drug Abuse Research Monograph #34 (DHHS Publ No ADM-81-1058). Edited by Harris LS. Washington, DC, U.S. Government Printing Office, 1980

Wise R: Assuring quality in chemical dependence treatment program. Paper presented at the annual meeting of the Group Health Association of America, Seattle, WA, October 1988

✦ 20 ✦

Employee Assistance Programs

Dale A. Masi, D.S.W., L.C.S.W.
Richard Caplan, M.S.W., L.I.C.S.W., M.P.H.

Employee Assistance Programs (EAPs) were introduced in the 1940s at Kemper Insurance, Eastman Kodak, and the DuPont Corporation. These programs were initiated not by the companies themselves, but through the efforts of employees who were recovering from alcoholism. These employees went to upper-level management stating that if their supervisors had confronted their job performance problems earlier and had been less understanding about their "problem," they could have broken the denial of their illness earlier, thereby saving the companies thousands of dollars in lost productivity as well as improving the employees' health and happiness. These employees asked to be able to start programs to help their fellow workers whom they knew had similar problems. The rationale for having the program in the workplace was based on the recovered workers' claim that the threat of losing their jobs was leverage to motivate alcoholic patients who had jobs into accepting treatment (Masi 1982).

These early programs were called Occupational Alcoholism (OA) programs and dealt strictly with the alcoholic employee. In that model, supervisors were trained to look for symptoms of alcoholism and to confront the employee with those symptoms. The employee was then expected to see an alcoholism counselor (a recovering alcoholic) within the company for treatment of this addiction or run the risk of losing his or her job.

Such programs continued, but they were not developed to a great extent until the passage of the Hughes Act (Public Law 91-616 1970).

Senator Harold Hughes, a recovering alcoholic, testified in the U.S. Senate on behalf of separate legislation for alcoholism. The Hughes Act mandated the establishment of the National Institute on Alcoholism and Alcohol Abuse (NIAAA) as separate from the National Institute of Mental Health (NIMH). This Act also mandated the establishment of an Occupational Branch for the NIAAA that granted funds to each state to hire two Occupational Program Consultants (OPCs). These consultants developed programs in the private and public sectors (Masi 1982).

The Hughes Act also mandated the development of programs for the prevention, treatment, and rehabilitation of federal employees with alcohol and drug problems. (One of us [D. A. Masi] was privileged to direct the model Employee Counseling Services [ECS] for the federal government in the office of the Secretary of the U.S. Department of Health and Human Services from 1979 to 1984.)

Another major development occurred in 1971, when a group of individuals in the field came together in Los Angeles to develop an organization called the Association of Labor-Management Administrators and Consultants on Alcoholism (ALMACA). It was developed as a nonprofit international organization of practitioners involved in occupational alcoholism programming and employee assistance programming. This organization continues to serve as the professional body for the OA/EAP practitioner (Masi 1984); in 1989, it changed its name to Employee Assistance Program Association (EAPA).

Other legislative action serving to promote awareness of the need for OA/EAPs was the Rehabilitation Act of 1973 (Office of Personnel Management 1979). Section 504 guarantees the rights of handicapped people. The implications for the workplace are that employers must offer reasonable accommodation to employees with handicapping conditions. The U.S. Attorney General has defined alcoholism and drug addiction as handicapping conditions (National Institute on Alcohol Abuse and Alcoholism 1976).

Meanwhile, changes began to occur in the area of occupational programs as practitioners began to report that programs that included other types of employee problems, as well as alcoholism, were more effective and tended to avoid the stigma associated with OA programs. Also, it was becoming harder to justify turning away employees who needed assistance in other areas besides alcoholism. The evolution of this new, broader model was the birth of the Employee Assistance Program (EAP).

The EAP's scope included other problem areas such as marriage, emotional, and financial problems. It also had a focus on a supervisory referral to the program based on observation of poor job performance rather than on a diagnosis of alcoholism. Because it usually utilized untrained staff members who were recovering from alcoholism, the OA model often referred employees out for treatment of problems other than alcoholism. Today, however, this practice is changing with the influx of mental health professionals into the EAP field. Most EAP programs currently are operated by outside contractors and offer members 6 to 8 counseling sessions by mental health professionals.

EAPs as "Managed Systems"

In recent years, "quality of work life" has become a term used to describe values some believe have long been pushed aside by industrial societies. These values relate to the quality of human experience in the world of work. Structures for new benefits have developed to ensure and promote this quality of life. At the same time, there is considerable concern about the ways and means of increasing industrial productivity in the face of international competition and the increased shortage of skilled, educated workers.

Currently these dual concerns are converging and focusing attention on the relationship between quality of work life and productivity. EAPs have been developed in acknowledgment of that relationship. The employee assistance movement addresses the interconnections between work problems and personal/family life conflicts and the resulting effects of stress and strain on workplace productivity.

The OA/EAP saved the company money, because employees whose alcoholism went untreated used up leave and health benefits and had more frequent accidents. This was a unique benefit of the EAPs, which made them distinct from traditional counseling services. In recent years, EAPs have operated from a systems perspective and have evolved to assess and modify more broadly "troubled" behaviors. Although problems are now addressed more holistically, the basic emphasis remains on improving work performance and lowering the costs associated with workers' problems.

Program components and procedures vary, depending on whether the program is developed by the company staff in the medical or human resources department or by outside contractors. EAP models have developed to meet the growing needs of a wide variety of companies. The major program types are the in-house model, the out-of-house model, the consortium model, and the affiliate model.

✦ *In-house model.* In this model the entire assistance staff is employed by the company. The company directly supervises the program's personnel, sets policies, and designs all procedures. It could be housed physically in the company or located in offices away from the company.

✦ *Out-of-house model.* In this model the company contracts with a vendor to provide an employee assistance staff and services. This model usually provides 8 counseling sessions to an employee. The company sets and agrees to specific policies and procedures for the EAP contract that the vendor must follow. The vendor might provide services in its offices, the company's offices, or a combination of both. One pattern that has emerged with this model is that there are fewer referrals to community providers for treatment and counseling.

✦ *Consortium model.* In this model several companies pool their resources to develop a collaborative program at one location to maximize individual resources. Generally, this model works best for companies with fewer than 2,000 employees. Services are shared and provided in one central office, although separate supervisor training programs can be offered.

✦ *Affiliate model.* In this model a contracted EAP vendor subcontracts with a local professional when there is neither sufficient clientele nor employees to warrant hiring full-time staff. The vendor can then reach employees in a company location in which the vendor might not have an office. Usually this model is used in conjunction with one that involves paid staff (Masi and Friedland 1988).

Today most EAPs are staffed with social workers or individuals with master's-level education and training. Psychologists with doctorates, for the most part, make up the affiliate/subcontractor group. Future directions show this continuing, with more emphasis on hiring licensed clinicians. Internal programs are often staffed by employees who are recovering from alcoholism, some of whom have gone back to school and obtained graduate degrees. However, the self-identified alcoholic individual in the EAP field is less visible as the mental health professionals in EAPs increase in number.

Ingredients of Effective EAPs

EAPs should include the following ingredients to be effective:

1. A policy statement that includes the purpose of the program;
2. Organizational and legal mandates;
3. The roles and responsibilities of various personnel, especially managers, in the organization and procedures;
4. Staffing with mental health professionals who have at least 2 years' training and experience in treatment of alcoholism and addiction;
5. Confidential record-keeping in accordance with federal alcohol and drug regulations issued in 1987 by the U.S. Department of Health and Human Services;
6. Union support;
7. Supervisory training in problem identification and proper referral techniques;
8. Employee outreach and education; and
9. Sensitivity to special populations in the work force.

Criteria used to measure the success of outcomes vary considerably, and few rigid scientific studies support many of the claims of EAPs. There is considerable concern in the employee assistance field that as staffing patterns change to include more licensed professionals and fewer recovering employees, less attention is being paid to treatment of addictions. A relationship appears to exist between contracted programs (employing fewer recovering staff) and a lower number of alcohol and drug cases treated by the EAP.

EAPs have traditionally been confined to providing information and assessing performance problems of employees and referring them to appropriate community resources for treatment. Many EAPs are now able to offer their own short-term treatment/counseling sessions, because they have added professional staff who can provide the same services as referral agencies. EAPs reduce a company's health benefit utilization by providing counseling services in a contained environment. The provision of such counseling services made it a natural development for EAPs to move into providing managed mental health care.

EAPs and HMOs

Most American corporations offer health maintenance organizations (HMOs) as part of their benefit plan. HMOs and EAPs are similar in that they are both funded through a prepaid per capita system rather than a fee-for-service system. They both attempt to manage care so as to contain costs and use limited resources to provide care to a population. To do this, they usually use a specified panel of providers, and specified referral sources, which act as gatekeepers to mental health and substance abuse services. Both types of organizations train and supervise their staffs and have standards for clinician performance and quality of care.

However, there are several important differences between EAPs and HMOs:

✦ HMOs offer medical as well as mental health and substance abuse services. This means that HMOs can offer more comprehensive treatment of serious mental illnesses and provide coordination between medical, psychiatric, and addictions care (to provide alcohol detoxification, for instance). EAPs offer a variety of social and vocational services (child care, elder care) that are less focused exclusively on health.

✦ HMOs are insurance companies as well as service providers. This means that the HMO is financially at risk for *all* health services needed by its members. The EAP is responsible only to provide those services specified in its contract or scope of operations. This means that if an HMO clinician decides that a patient needs hospital care, day treatment, or continued counseling, the HMO must cover the costs within its benefit package, even if it does not directly provide these services.

✦ HMOs provide mental health or substance abuse care to patients referred by themselves or their primary physicians. This care is totally separate from the work environment. Clients of EAPs are often referred by their supervisors, and care is provided in the context of the work environment. This means there are different guidelines for confidentiality in the two systems, and different ways in which work and work performance are included and used in counseling.

✦ HMO service is provided in a medical or clinic setting. EAP service is provided on-site in the workplace, or as close to it as possible. It is most often under the auspices of the personnel department, rather than a medical department.

✦ HMOs are usually available to families of subscribing members. Many EAPs are not available to family members.

✦ HMOs and EAPs have different historic traditions. Although both arose from the efforts of organized labor, HMOs were traditionally medical institutions, employing professional clinical staff. EAPs were begun by recovering employees who were not professionally trained.

These differences may lead to clashes in the two systems when it becomes necessary for them to work together. Because HMOs are increasingly prevalent as a dominant form of employee health insurance, an EAP is often faced with a referral to an HMO for hospital services or continued counseling.

When working with an HMO member, the EAP counselors must approach the work much differently than with a privately insured employee. With a privately insured employee, the EAP counselor is the sole decision maker regarding disposition of the patient's case. If the counselor decides to admit the patient to a hospital, he or she also decides which hospital to admit to (traditionally, a fixed length-of-stay 28-day program). The aftercare is also provided, post-hospitalization, by the EAP counselor.

When working with an HMO member, the EAP counselor usually has to call the primary care provider for a mental health referral so he or she can speak to a substance abuse counselor regarding the case. The HMO counselor would then ask to do his or her own evaluation. This is often seen as a delay tactic by the EAP counselor. Even if the HMO counselor did not need to do a face-to-face evaluation and did an immediate phone screening, the two clinicians might disagree on disposition of the patient's case (i.e., need for hospitalization). The EAP counselor might see this as a denial of substance abuse services and would react accordingly, whereas the HMO counselor might believe that reaction to be inappropriate and intrusive.

Even when there is agreement to hospitalize a patient, there can be disagreement over which treatment facility to use and for how long. Once the patient is in treatment, neither clinician would believe there was a collaborative effort.

There are several reasons why this HMO/EAP interface is difficult to maintain.

1. *Clash in gatekeeping role.* Because both the EAP and the HMO clinicians believe their job is to make the appropriate clinical match between a patient's/employee's needs and available resources, there are two people doing the same job. The EAP clinician sees no need for the HMO clinician's evaluation, because he or she has already completed that piece of work. Meanwhile, the HMO clinician wonders why the EAP clinician is asking for a particular treatment, because the evaluation has not yet been done.

2. *Clash in preferred providers.* EAP counselors often wish to refer patients to the inpatient substance abuse programs with which they are most familiar. Because EAPs do not have to cover the costs of such programs, they sometimes prefer traditional 28-day programs. Although EAP counselors do not have contracts with these facilities, this resource network represents *their* preferred providers. The HMOs usually use short-term inpatient detoxification programs, or outpatient detoxification, as well as rehabilitation programs with shorter lengths of stay. These represent their preferred providers. They usually have contracts with each and work closely with in-house utilization review programs. Often preferred providers of an EAP and an HMO are mutually exclusive.

3. *Lack of communication.* Because EAPs and HMOs are different systems, with differing costs, traditions, and objectives, it is often difficult for clinicians in these systems to collaborate in treatment planning. There is limited literature on efforts by EAPs and HMOs to grapple with these problems and work together (Fallon and Lenney 1987; Lee 1988).

The Harvard Community Health Plan, a Boston-based staff model HMO, recently conducted a 6-month pilot project with an EAP for a large municipal employer. During these 6 months, the 5 senior EAP counselors could admit patients directly to the HMO's contracted short-term, in-hospital detoxification unit without prior approval by the HMO. The EAP counselors would be able to phone the unit, 24 hours a day, 7 days a week, and if the unit staff thought it was appropriate, the member would be immediately accepted for admission. The HMO also brought in a clinical liaison to work with the hospital staff and meet every one of the members admitted through this system. Once stabilized, the patient would meet with the liaison to determine any additional treatment. Admission criteria were written up and agreed on by the HMO and the EAP.

Through follow-up phone conversations, the EAP counselors reported being greatly relieved at the ease they had in admitting the HMO members for in-hospital treatment. They were now allowed to act as gatekeeper for urgent substance abuse cases and referred appropriate patients. During the 6 months, the program generated 13 admissions, which represents about 5% of the year's detoxification admissions. It is difficult to determine how many of these patients would have been admitted if prior approval had been required, but it is clear that the admissions represented some additional cost to the HMO.

However, at 3- and 6-month review meetings, the atmosphere between EAP and HMO was totally changed. There was a sense of collaboration that never before existed. For the first time, the HMO and the EAP counselors thought they had worked together to accomplish a difficult goal.

Problems between the EAP and the HMO still remain, but because the project was so successful, the HMO developed a 24-hour telecommunications system that connects *all* their employer groups to an immediate phone screening service.

EAPs and Health Promotion

Some EAPs market health promotion activities. This must be considered carefully, because there is a real difference between health promotion and counseling assistance for employees with problems. Though they are not contradictory systems, the expertise each needs is not the same. An example is the U.S. Department of Health and Human Services, which placed health promotion and education in the Office of Public Health and its EAP in the Office of Personnel. Table 20–1 may simplify the differences between the two (Behrens 1983).

Utilization of EAPs

It is estimated that 18% of the members of any work force are affected by personal problems that can affect job performance. Of the entire work force, 12% have alcohol- and drug-related problems, and 6% have emotional problems.

The numbers of employees seen in the EAP are generally expressed in terms of a penetration rate that is a measure of the extent to which a program is reaching its target employee population. It is

Table 20–1. Distinctions between Health Promotion Programs and Employee Assistance Programs	
Health Promotion Programs	Employee Assistance Programs
Strictly voluntary.	Uses coercion and threat of job loss as stimuli for seeking assistance.
Deals with healthy employees.	Deals with employees with personal problems.
Aimed at all employees and often deals with employees in groups.	Focuses on individual employees.
Concentrates on all types of health education, along with other life-style topics.	Involved with diagnosis and treatment of alcohol- and drug-addicted employees.

derived by dividing the number of employees seen by the total employee population. A typical penetration rate for the first year of an EAP is between 4% and 6%, which is expected to stay approximately the same from year to year, as long as it is a new 4% to 6% of the employee population that is being reached. Statistically, the demographic proportions existing in the company population at large should be reflected in the demographics of the EAP clientele. The philosophy of the EAP is to try to reach all groups in the company's work force. In fact, employee outreach and education is aggressively performed by EAP staff.

Executives are often underrepresented in these statistics. Minorities and women may also be over- or underrepresented in program statistics. If an EAP is not representative of the employee population at large, charges of singling out employee groups may be made, which greatly undermines a program.

Future Trends and Issues

Certain major trends, both in the organization of employee assistance services and in the larger social and economic picture, have implications for the future of EAPs.

There are four factors that will have a direct impact on EAPs as they continue to prosper:

1. The role of EAPs in managed mental health;
2. The focus on drug abuse in the workplace;

3. The increasing number of persons with or affected by AIDS; and
4. The need for quality management by objective third parties.

At one end of the managed mental health continuum, EAPs are becoming the HMOs of mental health services. Increasingly, companies request that an EAP provide up to eight counseling sessions for an employee. As a result, the EAP is able to facilitate problem resolution without referring the client. Thus the client avoids use of health care benefits while receiving *bona fide* professional assistance.

However, if the EAP emphasizes short-term general mental health services, it may dilute its mandate of reaching the addicted employee.

Both public- and private-sector employers are seeking to combat drug abuse in the workplace. Drug testing is currently receiving the most attention. The American Management Association in its research report *Drug Abuse: The Workplace Issues* (1987) stated, "There has been a rapid increase in the number of companies testing [for drugs], and the trend will continue. . . . EAPs will be increasingly called upon for assistance as companies attempt to develop policies on drug testing and related issues" (p. 10).

EAPs may also contribute to an emphasis on rehabilitation in combating drug abuse (Masi 1987). This is evidenced in the Federal Executive Order of September 15, 1986, "The Drug Free Federal Workplace," which states, "Agencies shall initiate action to discipline any employee who is found to use illegal drugs, provided that such action is not required for an employee who . . . obtains counseling or rehabilitation through an employee assistance program" (p. 176).

Increasingly, employers are having to address the issue of AIDS in the workplace. The EAP could take the lead in assisting companies to address this highly sensitive issue by providing a number of services. For example, short-term EAP counseling can be made available to employees who are HIV positive. EAP intervention in the workplace would include ongoing education on AIDS, supportive counseling to co-workers and supervisors of persons with AIDS or who are HIV positive, and facilitating implementation of the company's policy on AIDS. Education on AIDS will be the key means of intervention, and the EAP should not wait to begin this effort only after an employee who is HIV positive or who has AIDS is identified within a company. Education efforts may include counseling family, friends, and co-workers in how to better understand the employee's needs and how to cope with the problems presented by the disease on a day-to-day basis. Another large group of employees whom the EAP could assist would be those who have family members or significant others with AIDS or who are HIV positive (Masi and Montgomery 1987).

As programs develop over time, a critical need will be for evaluation by objective third parties. Knowing that at this time there is no regulatory body for EAPs, company attorneys are asking that there be some built-in protection for the companies they represent. Third-party clinical evaluation will be necessary to protect both client and company. Companies are being asked to justify the cost of programs. Thus, the trend toward evaluating from a cost-effective dimension will also grow.

References

American Management Association: Drug Abuse: The Workplace Issues. New York, AMACOM, 1987

Behrens R: The distinction between health promotion programs and employee assistance programs. Lecture to DHHS EAP Administrators in Employee Counseling Service Units Directors at a workshop, Washington, DC, February 14, 1983

The Drug Free Federal Workplace. Washington, DC, Federal Executive Order, September 15, 1986

Fallon AB, Lenney JR: EAPs and HMOs: the genesis of a new partnership. EAP Digest 7(4):29–32, 1987

Lee FC: EAPs and managed care: a blurring of the line. EAP Digest 8(5):20, 1988

Masi DA: Human Services in Industry. Lexington, MA, Lexington Books, 1982, pp 74–75

Masi DA: Designing Employee Assistance Programs. New York, AMACOM, 1984, p 14

Masi DA: The Drug-Free Workplace. Washington, DC, Bureau of National Affairs, 1987

Masi DA, Friedland SJ: EAP actions and options. Personnel Journal, June 1988, pp 63–64

Masi DA, Montgomery P: Future directions for EAPs. ALMACAN 17(3):20–21, 1987

National Institute on Alcohol Abuse and Alcoholism: Rights of alcoholics under federal law: advisory memorandum from the Ad Hoc Forum on Occupational Alcoholism convened by the Occupational Branch of NIAAA. Washington, DC, National Institutes of Health, Fall 1976, p 3

Office of Personnel Management: Handbook of selected placement of persons with physical and mental handicaps in federal and civil service employment (Document 125-11-3). Washington, DC, U.S. Government Printing Office, March 1979

Public Law 91-616 (42 U.S.C. 4582): Comprehensive Alcohol Abuse and Alcoholism Prevention, Treatment and Rehabilitation Act of 1970, 3 August 1970

✦ 21 ✦

The Future of Mental Health Care

Daniel Y. Patterson, M.D.
Steven S. Sharfstein, M.D.

The future of mental health care is closely tied to its past, the current organization and financing of medical care in this country, and the potential for new clinical and research breakthroughs.

A Historical Note

Barely six decades ago there were no fiscal "third parties" that were responsible for underwriting the cost of medical care. Physicians were free to charge what they wanted in an open marketplace, define illness according to their own training and judgment, and institute "technologic advances" as they deemed appropriate. Practice was more closely a two-party system between doctor and patient. Treatment was neither regulated nor prescribed on the basis of outcome studies, and the era was unabashedly procompetitive, without federal or state regulation or consumer protection—to the patient *caveat emptor*.

Before 1850, people who were mentally ill were lumped together with those who were criminals or who were indigent. Responsibility for care fell to local jurisdictions and was inconsistent at best. Dorothea Dix and her allies began the process of separating out the mentally ill population from jails and poorhouses and, after an early defeat in trying to get the federal government involved, turned to state government as the locus of care and responsibility. By the early 1900s, psychiatric treatment of seriously ill patients was primarily in the state hospital, with few options in the private sector.

Since the 1930s, control of health care policy and financing has been dominated by the so-called "unholy trinity" of government, insurers, and hospitals. Medicine has become more effective, and the medical and legal professions have begun to tighten up practice, with payment becoming more and more contingent on quality standards. Until very recently, the basic theme in medicine might be articulated as "medical care is good, and more of it is better."

Indeed, in the 1950s and 1960s, enormous federal resources were poured into resource development, which expanded the numbers of physicians and health care professionals, hospital beds, and high-cost technology. The passage of Medicare and Medicaid in 1965 led to the federal government becoming the primary payor of medical care. With the tax incentives embodied in health benefits as a tax-free wage supplement, employers expanded private health insurance as well. The method of payment was retrospective, usual and customary, and mostly fee-for-service. This led to unprecedented cost inflation during the 1970s and 1980s (Figure 21–1) and to current efforts at cost containment in the 1990s (Figure 21–2).

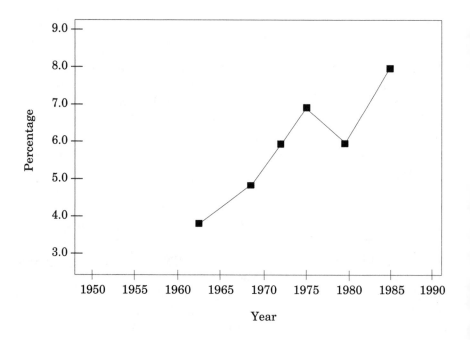

Figure 21–1. Cost of health care in the United States as a portion of gross national product (GNP).
Source. U.S. Department of Commerce 1990.

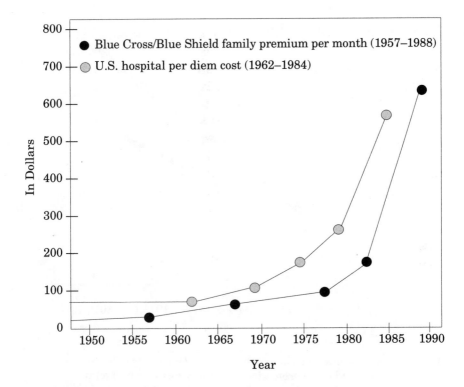

Figure 21–2. Comparison of hospital per diem cost and Blue Cross/Blue Shield family premium per month.
Source. American Hospital Association, Equitable Life Assurance Company, and Blue Cross/Blue Shield of Washington, DC.

During the same time period (the 1950s and 1960s), mental health care continued to remain primarily the responsibility of state government, with growth in third-party private health insurance, Medicare, and Medicaid, leading to an increasing number of private beds in short-term general hospital psychiatric units and private psychiatric hospitals throughout the country. On February 5, 1963, President Kennedy, in the only presidential address to Congress solely devoted to mental health, proposed the first major involvement of the federal government in mental health services through the establishment of the National Community Mental Health Centers Program (Kennedy 1963). This program, plus the National Institute of Mental Health support for the training of mental health professionals, led to an expansion and diversification of the overall mental health portfolio (Figure 21–3). Private hospital companies began to develop and market

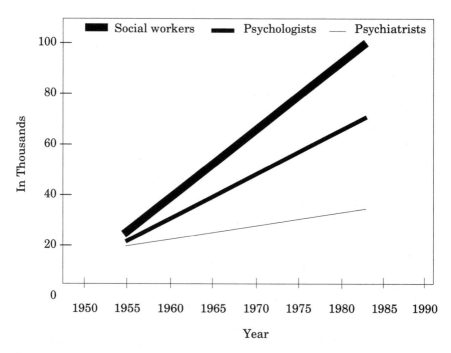

Figure 21–3. Mental health manpower development. The dramatic increase of mental health professionals is the direct result of NIMH manpower development support.
Source: American Psychiatric Association 1987, p. 55. Used with permission.

private psychiatric facilities and to hospitalize patients aggressively (Figure 21–4). Cost inflation became the major fact of life for mental health services through the 1980s as well.

We had the privilege of being part of health policy discussions and decisions made in the 1970s regarding the Health Maintenance Organization (HMO) Program (D. Patterson) and the Community Mental Health Centers Program (S. S. Sharfstein). These decisions laid the groundwork for future policy issues that will affect the practice of psychiatry and the opportunities for treatment of people who are mentally ill. The struggle of the 1970s was a classic one between the proponents of liberal solutions as embodied in the Great Society programs (which included the Community Mental Health Centers Program) and conservative solutions that favored procompetitive and industrial solutions to health care cost and distribution problems. The HMO Program was an example of the procompetitive strategies. The

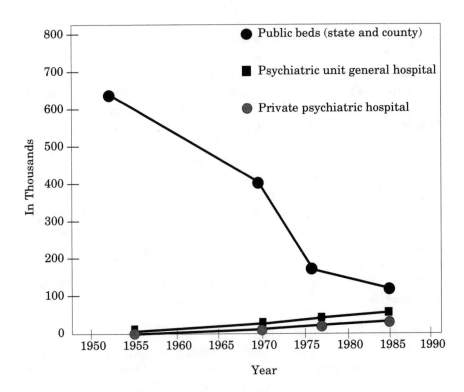

Figure 21–4. Psychiatric hospital beds. With the introduction of the use of neuroleptics for the treatment of schizophrenia in the 1950s came the closure of state hospital beds. In spite of this impressive trend in deinstitutionalization, there has been a clear growth in private psychiatric hospital beds over the past 20 years.
Source. National Institute of Mental Health 1989.

HMO was to be a wedge driven into the long-standing "benign" health monopolistic triad of physician, hospital, and third-party payor. The conservative capitalist Richard Nixon won out over the socialist liberals of the Kennedy/Johnson era. Then President Nixon issued a clarion call to the captains of industry to become prudent buyers of health care for their employees—not just payors, but principals, not mere brokers. Businesses that had stayed at arm's length in the health care transaction became more aggressively involved through self-insuring for employee health benefits and then through aggressively utilizing managed care approaches.

It should be noted that the business sector was not only disappointed in Blue Cross/Blue Shield and indemnity carriers, but also in the first generation of managed care HMO approaches. To businesses, some less responsible HMOs seemed to compete, causing traditional insurers to be adversely selected by the sickest patient (who could ill afford to break the continuity of benefits and care) and leaving the well patient to move to the HMO. A marketing research consulting firm based in San Rafael, California, claims that by using their market segmentation methodology, an HMO or preferred provider organization (PPO) can attract at least 5% more enrollees from low-user categories and decrease the number of high-user categories by the same amount. "A hypothetical PPO (and presumably HMO) with 100,000 covered lives can save 2.8 million dollars annually" (Kight 1988, p. 34). This type of market segmentation may prompt more governmental regulations to prevent mischievous selection by managed care companies.

Today big business is looking for new, alternative, *genuine* managed care. At present, the following is taking place:

1. Employers are poised to become the major player in health care.
2. HMOs are perceived as inadequate and in some ways defective (e.g., gatekeeping prevents access, yearlong lock-in is onerous, market segmentation appears pernicious [see above]).
3. Health care, and especially mental health and substance abuse care costs, are rising at a rate between two and three times the general inflation rate (Foster Higgins & Co. 1988).
4. Federal and state support for public mental health care is declining.

One Scenario for the Future

By the year 2000, employers will continue their trend to self-insure and will no longer offer traditional indemnity benefits that allow free and unmanaged choice of provider. They will move toward integrated "point of service choice" health care delivery systems. For those employers who do not self-insure, the products of the large health insurers will evolve into managed care products. Mental health and substance abuse care currently garners up to one-fourth of employer-sponsored health care dollars and is the fastest rising health care cost (Foster Higgins & Co. 1988). Employers, therefore, may move to "carve out" programs for mental health and substance abuse. Managed care companies providing mental health services will offer a "point of service choice" for covered employees. Cost sharing will be minimal for the "in-system" care, but will be based on employer equity should the patient choose to opt out of the system. Employer equity means that employers will pay essentially the same overall amount for in-system or out-of-system care. Patients, however, will pay considerably more if they make the out-of-system choice, and these higher copay costs are likely to be significant deterrents to out-of-system care for most employees.

This is different from the current second opinion and concurrent utilization review organizations we see today. Employers have become increasingly disenchanted with these approaches because of the adversarial nature of the approach and the tendency by providers to "game" such systems.

It is also likely that by the year 2000 we will have a modified form of national health insurance that will provide a minimum level of benefits for all Americans, paid for by either employers or government or a mixture of the two. In essence, Congress is likely to mandate by law that employers provide a "minimum wage" in health care benefits for all employees. The "minimum wage" in annual mental health benefits is likely to be in the range of 10 to 45 hospital days and 20 outpatient visits (or visits with substantial copayments). This legislation may aggravate the growing rift between employer-sponsored managed care and the public mental health sector, because the patients who exceed their insurance benefit will shift to the public system at a time when the public system increasingly feels the impact of reduced support. The combination of state hospital patients deinstitutionalized into a community, pressures on community mental health centers to be self-sufficient, and fewer state resources could lead to an exacerbating of what is the new "shame of the states," the mentally ill homeless person.

It is ironic that *The Shame of the States*, written by Albert Deutsch in 1948, eloquently described the gross mistreatment of the mentally ill population within asylums. A current "shame of the states" could describe the mistreatment of people who are mentally ill outside the psychiatric hospital. Past is prologue; it is time for another Dorothea Dix to help America separate the mentally ill population from the indigent or criminal population and provide them with humane care within sanctuaries. But will we recreate the large, custodial facilities that existed 100 years ago? Business coalitions on health care, mental health professionals, managed care companies providing mental health services, and mental health agencies of government will form blue-ribbon commissions to assess the problems described above and formulate recommendations and proposals.

Who is responsible for people who are seriously mentally ill, and who will fund needed treatment and support? We believe that the result of these deliberations and decisions could lead to an even sharper definition of public versus private responsibility. In essence, the private insurance sector as funded by employers will be responsible for acute mental illness treatment, leaving state and federal government to support and fund treatment for people who are chronically ill, disabled, or elderly. States may provide a fixed capitation payment to community mental health centers and other local programs (care service agencies) to take care of the mental health needs and other concerns of all citizens who are enrolled in such an agency (Dorwart and Schlesinger 1988). Direct funding of state psychiatric hospitals would be eliminated, and these care service agencies would be free to contract with state hospitals or private alternatives for chronic care. This "mental health HMO" could lead to a creative, public/private partnership if adequate funds were made available.

Private companies that provide mental health care management services will look to the use of more cost-effective approaches in the delivery of care by developing and using freestanding, integrated, non-hospital "spectrum" facilities that would include 24-hour emergency service, day treatment, detoxification, intensive substance abuse rehabilitation during the evenings, crisis intervention, home visits, crisis beds, and residential treatment approaches. However, these hospital alternatives will not totally replace traditional inpatient care, but prospective patients will use these spectrum resources whenever appropriate before being hospitalized.

The mental health professionals will have more clearly delineated roles. Psychiatrists will be medically oriented, caring for the sickest patients. Nonphysician clinicians will serve as the mental health "family practitioners" and will undertake short-term treatment approaches with adolescents, adults, couples, and families. Long-term psychotherapy and psychoanalysis will continue, but patients will increasingly have to pay out-of-pocket, because private and public financing is likely to be quite scarce.

In summary, the future suggests more managed care in the offing. This includes a clearer definition of private versus public responsibility for mental health care, a clearer assignment of duties consistent with training and compensation among the medical and nonmedical mental health professions, more direct involvement by employers in health care, and, one hopes, professional training programs capable of preparing clinicians for the 21st century.

References

American Psychiatric Association: Economic Fact Book for Psychiatry, 2nd Edition. Washington, DC, Office of Economic Affairs, American Psychiatric Association, 1987

Deutsch A: The Shame of the States, 1st Edition. New York, Harcourt, Brace, 1948

Dorwart R, Schlesinger M: Privatization of psychiatric services. Am J Psychiatry 145(5):543–553, 1988

Foster Higgins & Co.: Yearly Health Care Benefits Survey: Health Care Costs. Princeton, NJ, Survey & Research Services, 1988

Kennedy JF: Message from the President of the United States relative to mental illness and mental retardation to the 88th Congress, First Session, House of Representatives, Document No. 58. February 5, 1963

Kight D: Larger HMOs consider targeted marketing to shift enrollee mix. Contract Healthcare 13(6):34, 1988

Section III:

Special Topics

Introduction

Managed care systems can be ideal settings for the development of innovative treatment techniques and programs. Clinicians and managers, faced with case pressures and service demands, are eager to embrace new ideas that may be cost-effective. With appropriate clinical review and outcome assessment, some of these programs may prove to have lasting benefit to patients and be a real addition to the spectrum of available services.

In the private sector, many innovative programs fail for lack of third-party reimbursement. Managed systems can decide internally to "cover" any program that they develop.

In addition, a managed system has access to a large patient group (and often a centralized medical record) providing a population base for specialized programs. The availability of special programs relieves the burden on busy clinicians and provides the patient with easy access to subspecialists and to the support of patients with similar conditions.

Development of special programs may have a positive marketing effect for a health maintenance organization (HMO) or other managed system. Programs for patients with severe mental illness must be marketed cautiously, however, as they may pose adverse risk for an organization.

Following are two examples of such programs developed within managed settings. Both are outpatient programs designed for patients with mild to moderate illness and set up to handle large groups of patients. Both provide an approach that may be useful in other settings as well.

✦ 22 ✦

Adult Development and Brief Computer-Assisted Therapy in Mental Health and Managed Care

Roger L. Gould, M.D.

I n a managed care setting, many different mental health services are provided to a broad array of age and diagnostic categories. In this chapter, I will be addressing only the large subset of services provided as brief therapy to adult outpatients.

The history of brief therapy has been reviewed elsewhere (Ursano and Hales 1986) and need not be repeated here. In those settings where brief therapy is accepted and used to determine the delivery of services, therapists approach the treatment with their own idiosyncratic model and method based on their training and comfort with various theories, as well as their personal experiences as patients or trainees. In a department that aspires to be more than a collection of therapists sharing space and administrative support, this total diversity presents two almost insurmountable problems. The first is training of new professional staff; the second is quality control.

While awaiting a consensus-driven agreement as to the model of brief therapy that should be applied in an HMO setting, I will present a candidate model, a method that reflects this model, and a standardized technique (computer-assisted therapy) that delivers the method in a highly replicable way. This model and method are based on principles of adult development. The method and technique have been tested in a computer-assisted therapy program, the Therapeutic Learning Program (TLP), with more than 7,000 patients in various clinical settings, including HMOs and psychiatric hospitals.

Although the use of computers in therapy is a radical departure from traditional methods, the model underlying the method is not at all radical. It is essentially a distillate of clinical common sense based on easily observed and agreed-upon clinical phenomenon. In fact, the method that will be described has often been commented upon by both junior and senior therapists: "Of course, that's what I do already, albeit not in such a systematic fashion."

I believe that the method presented here is already in widespread use throughout the country (even though often called something else) and that the model of adult development is already the commonly understood and accepted context of most brief therapies (even when there is a preoccupation with the deep unconscious and distant past history).

Adult Development Model

There are many implications for brief treatment to be derived from the understanding of adult development, but two are of outstanding importance.

The first was described by Cummings and then by Bennett as intermittent focal therapy (Bennett 1984). Their position is that because adults continue to develop and run into various roadblocks along the way, brief therapy should be intermittently delivered during the course of a lifetime when patients are stuck in their attempt to change. Then the goal is to bring the patients back into the stream of experience where they can continue their development on their own. In this view, brief therapy is not just a bandage or a watered-down version of long-term therapy, it is a form of treatment solidly grounded and attuned to the phenomenon of the life cycle.

The second important implication for treatment comes directly from the life cycle descriptive studies. Every adult is constantly making life course decisions as he or she is faced with the new adaptational demands that come with age, an always-changing situation, new expected and unexpected events, and significant changes in significant others. In short, the therapist is reminded that patients live in reality, and that a current life situation drives their need for therapy. Their past history does not directly cause them to seek treatment.

The life cycle studies describe the typical age-related adaptational demands patients encounter. When these demands are not responded to effectively, there is a tension between the patient and his or her construed reality. However, there is no recommendation for therapeutic approach implicit in this understanding.

To create an adult developmental paradigm that does have therapeutic implications, therapists must integrate the understandings of childhood and adolescent development as reflected in the epigenetic framework of Erikson (1959). Erikson reminds us that, although we may lose or sacrifice various potentials and functional capacities during our early development, we have many opportunities to repair and continue development throughout the adult phase of the life cycle. Development, developmental blocks, and repair of previous developmental blocks occur at all ages.

Therefore, when a patient presents him- or herself for therapy, he or she is always experiencing direct pain because of some developmental block. The patient is unable to meet a current adaptational demand, because in order to meet that demand, he or she would have to utilize some unfamiliar pattern of behavior (e.g., expressing feelings, standing up to unfairness, taking risks, etc.). These patterns of behavior are off-limits because of earlier adaptational learning that has been institutionalized (blocked development). The presenting clinical picture is composed of the current reality demand, the blocked development in the form of being unable to experiment with a wider range of appropriate behaviors that might address that demand, and the symptoms that are secondary to this tension system.

It is out of this paradigm of adult development that a short-term treatment method can be derived that does justice to the deeper issues (the developmental block) while staying in touch with presenting phenomena that constitute the conscious preoccupation of the patient. The life cycle problem and the developmental problem are coterminous with the patient's experience of being "stuck" (i.e., the problem that brings the patient to treatment).

Clinical Methodology

Once this model is understood and accepted, the focus and goals of the method become self-evident: to find and to resolve the current developmental block from the past that is interfering with a higher level adaptation in the present.

Finding the developmental block within the complex life narrative of the patient is surprisingly easy compared to the more difficult task of resolving the block. To find the developmental block, the clinician has to work with the patient to uncover a special kind of volitional conflict. When a patient says "I would like to be more loving (or patient, or confrontational, etc.) but I can't get myself to take the risk or do the work," then the patient recognizes a palpable and real conflict within him- or herself and the therapist has the developmental block in focus.

The question "But what stops you from experimenting with these new behaviors?" leads therapist and patient into the more complicated domain of the beliefs, emotional responses, and catastrophe predictions that keep the patient frozen in past history.

Each of the fears and excuses that come out of that questioning process must be pursued until the patient recognizes that the fear sensation is not a valid indicator of real-life danger and that there is no good contemporary reason not to experiment with the new behavior. The length of this process varies with the difficulty of the block and the discipline of the therapist.

Once the patient has experimented with the new behavior and received and integrated the feedback from reality that, in fact, he or she can safely and proudly incorporate the new behavior into the concept of self, then a piece of psychological work has been accomplished. This discrete piece of work that starts with a volitional conflict and ends with the resolution of a particular developmental block can be considered as a "unit of work" in the adult developmental saga.

This unit of work can be studied, named, monitored, and quantified. The implications for outcome, process, and comparative studies are obvious.

The phenomenon of psychological work is more familiar to the clinician than the concept of a "unit" of psychological work. When a clinician struggles with a patient to achieve clarity, he or she is expending therapeutic effort. When the patient achieves clarity, a bit of psychological work has been accomplished. Similarly, work is accomplished when a defense is replaced with more mature behavior and insight is transformed from intellectual acceptance to a real shift away from unrealistic expectations.

The concept of a developmental unit of psychological work subsumes the many different pieces of psychological work that are accomplished during repair of a specific developmental block.

All brief therapies are predicated on the need to focus. What is focused upon is a useful basis for comparing the models behind the method. The focus in this model is the inability of the patient to act in a way that he or she deems highly desirable. In other short-term methods, the focus is upon transference resistance or upon some core neurotic pattern.

Although focusing upon a simple action conflict seems simplistic and superficial compared to the foci recommended by other dynamic short-term therapies, that appearance is misleading. The "depth" comes from the fact that the volitional conflict represents the developmental conflict that is ripe for repair. The developmental conflict from the past that interferes with necessary function in the present is the natural center of attention for the patient as well as the therapist. The depth of importance comes not only from the origins in the past, but also from its pertinence in the present.

The method of brief treatment based on accomplishing a unit of adult developmental work is easy to master, already familiar, and excludes almost no part of the patient population ordinarily seen in managed care settings. The conflict line is easy to find, requires no special training, and can be accomplished in a friendly conversational manner by an active therapist.

The resolution of a developmental block is a process that can be minutely described as a linear series of interventions that are spelled out in the computer-assisted therapy technique that will be described in the next section. Because these steps are spelled out in detail (with branching logic to cover most variations) and a comprehensive training manual is available, it is easy to train clinicians on content and process simultaneously.

The Method Translated Into Computer-Assisted Therapy—The TLP

The TLP (Therapeutic Learning Program) is a computer-assisted brief therapy program that helps patients define a specific problem, propose an active solution, and resolve their conflicts about taking the action.

The program represents the condensation of years of therapeutic experience designed into a very explicit model and then translated into a computer program. The course consists of 10 interactive computer sessions. Each session is a sequential unit and cannot be taken out of order. The patient works with a therapist at the end of each session to accomplish a specific work assignment. This is done either one-to-one or in a group.

At each step of the way the computer helps translate thought processes into external visual print that patients can hold on to, talk from, think about, and carry with them during the time between sessions. By presenting menus for each step of the process, the computer helps individual patients gain an appropriate vocabulary, make discriminations, and transform slippery feelings and thought processes into examinable pieces of information. A patient thus has a controlled and private relationship directly with the program and learns to think about problem resolution in a slow and stepwise way. From the patient's point of view, the program focuses on three important questions:

1. What hurts and what can you do about it that you are not already doing?
2. Would taking this action be a wise and safe thing to do?
3. What deeper fears stop you from taking the intended action?

In Sessions 1 and 2 of the TLP program, the patient is helped to find a volitional conflict that is at the center of his or her being "stuck." In Sessions 3 through 9, the patient is helped to resolve the underlying developmental conflict in a series of generic steps that are customized to his or her thinking patterns. Although this approach appears mechanical on paper because it is so structured, the patient's passage through these steps is highly emotional. Not all sessions are equally meaningful to the patient, but the cumulative effect almost always adds up to an emotional learning experience with strong impact.

Table 22–1 gives a glimpse of the program and allows the reader to "see" the relationship between the model and the method that has already been described.

Although the TLP is a different way of investing therapeutic effort than conventional treatment, the goal of treatment is the same. The goal of brief therapy, in particular, is to help patients resolve the immediate conflicts they are having within themselves about how to act and respond to a current life situation.

The therapeutic talk often is about interpersonal relationships. Although that is the topic, it is not the centerpiece of the therapeutic effort. The centerpiece is an intrapersonal dialogue about a conflict situation. Even in long-term treatment where transference is inter-

Table 22–1.   Therapeutic Learning Program (TLP) session goals

Session 1: Identifying stress-related problems, conflicts, and symptoms
a. to identify sources of stress and ineffective responses
b. to sort out stressful issues from developmental stress problems
c. to prioritize one clearly stated stress problem that calls for some action

Session 2: Clarifying goals and focusing on action
a. to identify the developmental goal that addresses the adaptational demand
b. to clarify and define the action or behavior change that is necessary
c. to build an action intention that represents the recovery of the underdeveloped function

Session 3: Thinking through the consequences of taking action
a. to distinguish realistic dangers from exaggerated dangers
b. to isolate and expose the fears as predictions confused with memories
c. to reach a conscious cost-benefit positive decision about the intended action

Session 4: Uncovering hidden motives and fears of failure and success
a. to clarify that certain strongly felt fears are not objective dangers
b. to weaken the hold of irrational fears
c. to learn to identify thinking errors as a useful concept
d. to distinguish between healthy and unhealthy motives
e. to demonstrate that fears of failure and success rarely point to real dangers

Session 5: Exploring anger and guilt as obstacles to action
a. to clarify that certain strong anxiety feelings are not indicative of external dangers
b. to demonstrate that angry feelings are controllable by rational considerations
c. to demonstrate that the feeling of guilt is information that can be processed to clarify values
d. to continue to confirm that the intended action is safe and doable

Session 6: Confronting issues of self-esteem
a. to identify and acknowledge self-esteem sensitivities
b. to begin to accept the universality and mystery of these sensitivities
c. to entertain the thought that this powerful inner voice represents a historical fiction
d. to understand that the self-esteem sensitivity is the biggest block to resolving the developmental conflict

Table 22–1. Therapeutic Learning Program (TLP) session goals (continued)

Session 7: Examining old and detrimental patterns of behavior
a. to identify the deepest vulnerability that is being challenged by the action intention
b. to see how the self-doubt triggers the ineffective protective behavior
c. to examine and demonstrate how the self-doubt system feeds itself
d. to begin to challenge the automatic response

Session 8: Understanding the history of self-doubts
a. to expose the illusion of permanent damage
b. to see that responses to early events were limited and naturally protective
c. to see that these early protective behaviors were automatic responses to feeling inadequate
d. to view the self-doubt as an initial response to events by the immature mind

Session 9: Analyzing a current incident involving the self-doubt
a. to demonstrate and diminish self-fulfilling prophecies
b. to identify the erroneous thinking that currently feeds the powerful self-doubt
c. to understand that feeding the doubt by misinterpretation is a choice, not a necessity
d. to recognize that to continue to do this is to avoid growth

Session 10: Evaluating the changes experienced during the course
a. to see that fears are to be overcome and not submitted to
b. to see the action intention as part of ongoing recovery of function
c. to understand that recovery of function and individuation are necessary
d. to consolidate new views of reality

preted, the interpersonal conflict focus is used to help the person get back to the primary intrapersonal conflict focus. In the final analysis, only the patient can act, and all the therapist can do is facilitate the recognition and resolution of conflict. The more clearly the conflict is stated and the more the stated conflict accurately represents the central issue to be resolved, the more likely the resolution will take place with accompanying desired results.

In conventional therapy, the focusing and refocusing of the process is the responsibility and the work of the therapist. He or she has to sort through the confusions of the patient and work through the stories and dramas of the patient's life in order to frame the conflict line in the intrapersonal form in which it can be resolved.

The TLP uses the computer, the printout, and the underlying model to frame the conflict as follows.

First, the TLP software helps the patient explore the *domain* of the problem and sort out, amongst the many possible candidates, the central issues that have to be addressed. This is accomplished by presenting the patient with a comprehensive list of possibilities. The patient is guided to make distinctions, establish priorities, and recognize the difference between external stressors and intrapersonal conflicts. Once the domain of the problem is specified in detail, the conflict itself has to be spelled out in understandable, concrete, and easily acknowledged terms. When the patient is helped to state a conflict about action, he or she has to make a decision about what he or she wants to do. It is an *intrapersonal* conflict: "me versus me" or "one part of me versus another part of me." The locus of the problem and the locus of potential control are aligned in the intrapersonal conflict framework.

The patient is the one who, with the help of the computer, defines and redefines the conflict line until he or she discovers the most accurate version. With that discovery, he or she owns the conflict; whatever results will be obtained from resolving the conflict are to his or her benefit. The patient is not satisfying the therapist or the therapist's version of the conflict.

One of the reasons people stray from working on the intrapersonal conflict is because, once it is clearly stated and framed, it sometimes seems at first inspection to be unresolvable. The process steps necessary for resolution are not seen as the orderly process defined in the TLP, but collapse into one huge, apparently insurmountable and ineffable obstacle. The work of the model and the TLP computer program is to break the resolution of the conflict into small digestible decision steps that have a cumulative learning effect and cause transformation of perspective. As patients resolve the earlier and easier steps, they begin to develop confidence that they are not helplessly stuck—that there is a knowable process that they can master at their own rate of learning. Each success builds confidence as the next and more difficult obstacle is challenged.

The result of these processes is that patients continue to move through the steps of resolving a conflict with little or no resistance to learning and sharing with therapists (and often with other group members). The spookiness of irrational and powerful thought processes is diminished in favor of an objective learning process that can be mastered. Patients are rewarded for sticking to the intrapersonal conflict line by insights and a growing sense of being able to control their lives in areas in which they felt stuck, helpless, and symptomatic.

As patients work with the computer "auxiliary therapist," the relationship to the flesh-and-blood therapist is modified. In interpersonal, noncomputer, one-to-one therapy, the therapist is seen more as a "guru" and wise parental figure who has much information to dispense but can only dispense it in small quantities at each session. The experience of being childlike in a therapy situation is common, because the therapist is seen as having the experience and wisdom needed to guide a successful life. In the TLP therapy, this transference phenomenon does not appear to any significant degree. The therapist is cast and accepted as facilitator and teacher in a class setting. The responsibility for the patient's success in life clearly rests with the patient. The therapist is not confused with an overlaid parental image where the responsibility lies with the parent/ therapist.

In summary, the TLP program helps keep the patient on the intrapersonal conflict track by giving him or her the opportunity to systematically and slowly discover the conflict and then recognize that there is an orderly process that can lead to resolution of the conflict. With this empowerment, the distraction of an intense dependent relationship with the therapist is minimized, allowing the energy of the developmental imperative to be focused primarily in development progress.

Advantages of a Standardized Computer-Assisted Therapy

Training, Quality Control, and Research

Because the model, method, and delivery are all of one cloth, research on questions of effectiveness and efficiency of treatment is easier to design and likely to result in clearer outcomes than usual in this field. The psychological work is spelled out in detail and is contained within the framework of psychological work accomplished by the patient. As a result, measurement of process progress can be accomplished and compared with outcome measure in a systematic way. Because the therapist's work is described in detail and related explicitly to each step of the process, this variable can finally be isolated in a relatively simple manner.

A commonly held model and method makes the training of staff easier. Having a computer program and therapist manual as teaching aids increases the reliability and replicability of training, and quality control can more naturally become an extension of the training mission. The computer program serves as its own quality control device because, at the end of the 10 sessions, the patients summarize their learning and evaluate the program and the process of their learning.

Diverse Viewpoints Can Be Explored

The model being presented here is coherent, yet it is composed of many easily recognized elements from other popularly endorsed and familiar models. It is basically an adaptational dynamic model but is heavily laden with cognitive and interpersonal elements, as well as a touch of behaviorism with the emphasis on action. Deeper psychological structures and past/present confusion, as well as reality testing, are all important parts of the model. Because all of these important phenomena are included in the model, therapists that represent different viewpoints have a common language with which to discuss their differences.

This model of adult development is not divisive. It is prepared and presented in the spirit of integration.

Delivery Workhorse Without Sacrifice of Quality

The TLP can be considered as a workhorse program in managed care settings where resources are limited and demand for services is high. This can be done without sacrifice of quality or patient satisfaction.

Outcome studies in the first 2,000 patients using the TLP in CIGNA Healthplan indicate a very high patient satisfaction with the program immediately following the program and at intervals of 6 months and 3 years. In fact, patients report that they have learned a new generalized approach to stress and attribute their lower stress level to this approach. Therapists trained in the TLP method universally endorse the program, find it useful for a wide variety of presenting problems and clinical diagnoses, and claim it makes their work burden easier (R. Klein, personal communication, July 1988; D. S. Schag, T. Larsen, L. Read, personal communication, April 1985; J. L. Talley, personal communication, November 1987).

The model of adult development and the unit-of-work concept help the therapists committed to brief treatment explain the rationale of their work to critics who claim brief treatment is just a new way of shortchanging patients from what is "always" necessary (i.e., long-term treatment).

One of the outstanding problems of mental health care in a managed care setting is the large panel of patients assigned to each therapist. When the therapist has to keep too many people "in mind," it is easy to be overloaded and resort to coping mechanisms that diminish the quality of care despite the best intentions. The TLP lends itself to intensive group work and large psychoeducational class formats. Both of these mechanisms help relieve the load while providing intensive and quality care to the panel patient. The TLP keeps the focus and records the detailed interaction, leaving the therapist free to do what he or she does best.

References

Bennett MJ: Brief psychotherapy and adult development. Psychotherapy 21(2): 18–20, 1984

Erikson EH: Identity and the Life Cycle (Psychological Issues, Vol 1, No 1). New York, International Universities Press, 1959

Ursano RJ, Hales RE: A review of brief individual psychotherapies. Am J Psychiatry 143(12):1507–1517, 1986

✦ 23 ✦

Management of Chronic Benign Pain in a Prepaid Practice

Steven R. Tulkin, Ph.D.
Gerald W. Frank, M.D.
Allan Bernstein, M.D.
Bridie Aubel, R.N.
Marie Lehn, R.N.

The cost of treating chronic pain is enormous, both in terms of number of patients affected and of health care dollars spent to treat them. Estimates from the National Institutes of Health put the cost of chronic pain at over $40 billion a year (Aronoff et al. 1983). More specifically, it has been estimated that 25 million Americans suffer from recurring headaches (with a loss of 180 million workdays annually), and an additional 15 million suffer from lower back pain (with a loss of 93 million workdays annually).

Another way in which chronic pain impacts the health care system is its effect on provider morale. Most health care providers will admit that chronic pain patients are among the most difficult to treat. A large part of the problem is that both patient and provider are working toward the goal of *treating* the pain (i.e., reducing or eliminating the nociceptive symptoms). Even those patients and providers who accept that the pain is chronic are unable to bring about the life-style changes necessary to "learn to live with the pain."

Over the past 15 years, since the publication of Fordyce's (1976) book, many pain clinics have been developed. They range from a one-person acupuncture office, to private practices involving neurologists, anesthesiologists, physical therapists, and psychologists, to comprehensive multidisciplinary centers that provide inpatient or day treatment services over a 30-day period. The purpose of this chapter is to describe the methods for management of chronic benign pain that we have developed over the past 10 years at the Kaiser Permanente Medical Center in Hayward, California. Several reports appear in the literature describing multidisciplinary pain clinics (Ghia 1988; Turk and Holzman 1986), but very little has been published about chronic pain programs in HMOs (see Kempler 1991).

The program to be described in this chapter was started in 1980 as a joint effort of the Departments of Medicine, Psychiatry, Neurology, and Orthopedics. A description of the start-up of the program is contained in a paper by Tulkin and Frank (1982).* One of the main incentives in developing the program was to offer a viable treatment option to primary care providers as well as specialists who had been frustrated by continuous complaints from chronic pain patients. By supporting this program, the Psychiatry Department contributed a unique resource to the other departments in the Medical Center. Other interdisciplinary programs in the Behavioral Medicine Service are described in other papers (Tulkin and Frank 1985; Tulkin et al. 1989).

Modalities and Management

There are two major components required in the treatment of chronic pain: modalities and management. In the modalities phase, patients need to have symptoms evaluated by an appropriate specialist and every attempt made to diagnose the pain. Specialists that may be involved in this process include neurologists, physiatrists, anesthesiologists, physical therapists, psychologists, rheumatologists, and neurosurgeons. Diagnostic procedures are needed in order to 1) determine that no malignancy is present, 2) determine that no surgical procedure is indicated, and 3) establish a diagnosis. After a diagnosis is made, it may be appropriate to attempt treatment through a specific modality. Treatment could include nerve blocks, biofeedback, transcutaneous electrical nerve stimulator (TENS) units, physical therapy evaluations and treatments, and various drug protocols (e.g., tricyclic

---

* This program, originally developed by Dorothea Lack, Ph.D., is currently staffed with a psychologist at 20 hours per week, an internist at 10 hours per week, a neurologist and a physiatrist, each at 2 hours per week, and two registered nurses, each at 32 hours per week.

antidepressant and nonsteroidal anti-inflammatory drug for fibrositis). The reason that we are emphasizing these modalities is that unless the patient is satisfied that "everything has been done" to evaluate and treat the pain, chances of success in a pain management program are very low. (For an excellent description of the office management of diagnosis and modality treatments for chronic pain, see Covington 1989a, 1989b.)

There are two types of specialist evaluation and treatment that we will discuss in detail: headaches and back pain. Because these are the most common pain complaints and frequently can be treated successfully with modalities, it is important to describe the specific evaluations and interventions commonly used.

Headache and Facial Pain Clinic

Because headache is one of the two most common causes of chronic pain, headache sufferers constitute a large population of potential chronic pain patients. In all cases, a "hands-on" exam is extremely reassuring to the patient and is also medically appropriate. Many patients arrive at a headache clinic never having had a physical exam directed at this specific problem. At the conclusion of the initial visit, a diagnosis can usually be made based on the history and physical exam alone. If there is any question about the diagnosis, further testing may be needed.

Treatable causes of headache and face pain are then appropriately treated. A certain number of patients with such diagnoses as chronic cervical headaches, tension headaches, mixed headaches, posttraumatic headache, atypical facial neuralgia, trigeminal neuralgia, and myofascial pain syndromes are best referred to a pain management program. Analgesic-induced headaches, which may be from either prescription or nonprescription drugs, are also best treated in a comprehensive pain management program. When this is the case, the findings are discussed with the patient (and the spouse, if there is one), and the rationale for referral to the Pain Management Program is explained.

Low Back Care Clinic

The Low Back Care Clinic, located in the Department of Medicine, Kaiser Oakland, is available for patients who do not respond to the "usual conservative treatment protocol." The most common referral problem is persistent low back pain and/or sciatica not responding to a 2- to 3-month trial of conservative treatment.

The patient is counseled in regard to his or her diagnosis, prognosis, and limitations. Treatment in the Low Back Care Clinic includes an emphasis on proper body mechanics, posture, and an ongoing exercise program. If appropriate, steroid injections as well as selective nerve root blocks may be offered. Other interventions might include a TENS unit and antidepressants. When necessary, the patient is evaluated for surgery.

Patients who are referred to the Pain Management Program typically have minimal physical findings, have not responded to the above interventions, and have been severely incapacitated from work and social activities. Most have not complied with prescribed exercise suggestions and clearly need the structure of an intensive, behaviorally oriented program.

Screening for the Pain Management Program

If pain persists and interferes with daily functioning after all diagnosis and intervention is completed, it is appropriate for the provider to consider referring the patient to a pain management program. When a patient is referred to us, the following procedures are followed:

1. A letter is sent to the referring physician indicating the criteria for acceptance (e.g., all diagnostic work and all attempts to reduce the pain are complete; the patient accepts that the pain is chronic and the only intervention left is to learn to live with it; and the patient is willing to be withdrawn slowly from all analgesic and sedative-hypnotic medications, including nonsteroidal anti-inflammatory drugs). We also discuss the importance of physician involvement with the behavioral contract established in the Pain Management Program: being very positive about improvements in mood and daily functioning, refusing to listen to complaints about the same symptoms for which the patient was referred to the program (obviously any new symptoms, including pain symptoms, are evaluated carefully), and—most important—not prescribing *any* medication for the chronic condition.

2. A letter is also sent to the patient outlining the goals of the pro-

gram: "Although we cannot do anything to reduce your pain, we can help you to increase your activities, improve your mood, and help you get off pain medications." The patient is also told that he or she must be able to commit to being at the program for 4 hours per day, 4 days per week, for 1 month. During that time the patient is not allowed to work and can expect to have home assignments to complete each day that will take an additional 2 hours. Finally, the patient is told that he or she must have a family member (the spouse, if the patient is married) or a friend accompany him or her to the initial evaluation as well as to one 90-minute Family Group Meeting each week for 5 weeks.

3. A chart review is done. The purpose of the chart review is to ensure that the medical workup has been adequate and that, if possible, a diagnosis has been established. We also want to differentiate chronic pain from chemical dependency as a primary diagnosis. Finally, we need to determine that the patient is capable, physically and emotionally, of participating in the program. (Additional details regarding the screening criteria are available from the authors.)

Intake Evaluation

Present are two physicians, one of our nurses, and the psychologist. The patient is told that we have spoken with the referring physicians so we know medical details of the pain, but we would like to hear directly from the patient about how the pain has affected his or her daily functioning, mood, and relationships. During the interview we want to accomplish the following:

1. Give the patient the experience of our having listened attentively to his or her pain complaints, attempts at treatment, and anger at practitioners. We assure the patient that we believe the pain is real (giving a diagnosis if necessary); make sure that the patient is satisfied that everything medical has been done; and make sure that the patient accepts that we will not be trying to relieve pain in the program.

2. Explain the requirements of the program, especially the necessity of strict adherence to the rules. The patient is told that he or she must attend every day regardless of how he or she feels—in fact, if the patient does not feel well, it is still important to attend in order

to be evaluated by the physician who is available to see patients
daily. The patient is also told that he or she must obey all of the
behavioral requirements even though it may seem very controlling.
We tell the patients and family members that we will be teaching
the patient to manage his or her pain so that it will not be possible
to tell if the patient is having a good day or a bad day, and we will
be teaching family members to ignore all communications about
pain.

3. Take a detailed inventory of all medications (prescribed and over-
   the-counter) that the patient is taking. We also ask about alcohol
   and nicotine consumption. We describe the process of medication
   withdrawal and offer assurances that going off medicines has not
   been difficult physically for our patients.

Physical Examination

A primarily musculoskeletal evaluation is done before the patient enters the program. The examination involves measurement of range of
motion of all the major joints of the body as well as an evaluation of
muscle strength.

Physical examination is also another screening sieve. Occasionally
diagnoses have been made that were previously missed, including
illnesses such as underlying malignancy and multiple sclerosis. Once
we have determined that the patient is medically stable and physically strong enough to participate in the program, arrangements can
be made for a start date.

Program Components

Medication withdrawal. The overwhelming majority of patients
beginning the Pain Management Program are taking some analgesic
and/or sedative hypnotic medication. Our approach to medication
withdrawal (or more accurately, medication fading) is similar with
each patient. At the order of the internist, the pharmacy makes up a
series of "pain cocktail" bottles for each individual patient. The pain
cocktail contains the same medications as that person was taking at
the start of the program. This varies all the way from nonsteroidal
anti-inflammatory agents to morphine sulphate. Patients take 2 tea-
spoons of this liquid every 4 hours around the clock, and in bottle num-

ber one they receive approximately the same amounts of the same medications they were taking at entry. Every 3 days the patient picks up a new bottle. The directions are the same, but the concentration of active ingredients is decreased by small amounts. By using this system, we can keep medication levels fairly constant in the patient's bloodstream and achieve small decrements every 3 days with little or no withdrawal symptoms. Using between 7 and 10 bottles for each patient, we are able to get almost all patients to taper off their medications during the first month of the program.

When the patients begin taking the pain cocktail, they turn over to us whatever medicines they have in their possession, including old prescriptions for analgesics or sedative hypnotics that they are no longer taking. These are saved in a locked safe and given to the patient at graduation to flush down the toilet.

Daily availability of physicians.   One of the most important aspects of the program is the availability, on a daily basis, of one of the team physicians. At the beginning of the program, patients need the "security" of knowing that they can see a physician to discuss any new symptoms they have or to ask about specific aspects of the program. In addition to diagnosis and treatment of conditions such as urinary tract infections or minor upper and lower respiratory infections, considerable attention needs to be paid to fine-tuning the treatment of hypertension or diabetes mellitus because of changes resulting from increased activity.

Patients complain that "the pain is getting worse," or "the exercises make the pain worse." They are told that it is expected that the pain will be worse as new muscles are used and more energy is expended. They are told to continue their exercises and eventually told to stop complaining about the same symptoms. Sometimes the patient and the physician will discuss discontinuing the use of walkers, canes, or braces. This is done gradually over a period of weeks.

A third topic discussed with the physician involves complaints about other staff members (e.g., "the nurses are treating me like a kid in school"). This "divide and conquer" technique is common to chronic pain programs and is treated initially by telling patients that we understand it is difficult for adults to accept instructions and corrections for simple behaviors such as what to talk about, but it is a critical part of the program that will eventually be beneficial.

Finally, there are times when patients discuss emotional issues with the physician, because the topic "is too threatening to bring up in the group." With rare exceptions, patients are encouraged to talk in the group and told that similar issues have been discussed previously.

Meditation. Each day starts off with a brief 10-minute meditation designed to bring about a relaxed state of mind. Breathing and guided imagery are the major components (Bensen 1975). By teaching patients the value of a short meditation, we emphasize that they can bring about a relaxed state in a short period of time in many settings in their daily lives.

Exercises. The exercise program consists of a series of stretching and strengthening movements that involve all of the major muscles and joints of the body. Baseline data are collected for the first 3 days of the program, and a schedule is then developed for each patient. The increase in repetitions in each group is plotted on graphs to give the patient a visual record of the increased activity and an opportunity to take pride in this accomplishment. In addition, the staff nurses provide considerable positive reinforcements as the patients improve their form on the exercises and eliminate pain behavior.

Activities of daily living. In the initial days of the program, patients are given a list of activities of daily living, including personal grooming and hygiene, home maintenance (cooking, cleaning, gardening, etc.), recreation, and vocational activities. They are asked to note which activities they are "currently doing," which they "cannot do," and which they "would like to do." In addition they are asked to write any goals they have for their daily activities. This information is incorporated into demonstrations and practice of body mechanics and discussions about the need for realistic pacing of activities and for understanding that there are likely to be limitations that the patients need to accept.

Walking. The patients are required to walk outdoors every day. The distance is charted and increased gradually. The goal of walking 1 mile is reached by the end of the first month for most patients.

Pain diary. Because the patients are not allowed to talk about their pain, they need some means to "validate" their experience. This is accomplished by keeping a "pain diary" for the first month of the program. On an hourly basis throughout their waking hours, patients assess their pain and rate it on a scale of 1 to 10. At the same time they note any medication taken and the activity during the preceding hour. We emphasize that the diary allows them to have a specific time to think about the pain, which can free them during other times to *not* think about it. In addition, the diary is an important tool for discovering which activities or times of day may be associated with increased pain. Behaviors can then be altered if necessary.

Behavior modification.   One of the most important aspects of the program is behavior modification. Both verbal and physical pain behaviors are targeted. Patients are not allowed to talk about pain, disabilities, or medical histories or to use any medical terminology. In addition, we have found it necessary to disallow all negative discussion (traffic, weather, insensitivity of staff, etc.). Similarly, patients are not allowed to moan, groan, or sigh.

We differentiate between complaints and problems. Problems have solutions; we encourage problem solving in the daily group session.

Discussion at the lunch table is an especially good forum for developing positive social interaction. All patients are required to eat lunch together with the two nurses. Discussion of positive topics (hobbies, trips, parties, etc.) is encouraged, and all negative conversation is stopped.

Physical pain behaviors (e.g., rubbing a part of the body, resting one's head in one's hands, and leaning against a wall or piece of furniture) are also modified. Our response is to remind patients that the behavior is not acceptable and then to tell them that if it continues, they will not be allowed to remain in the program.

During program hours patients are expected to take responsibility for themselves. They are each required to take out and replace their own exercise mats, move their own chairs, open doors for themselves, and pick up anything that they drop.

No props are allowed, including pillows, collars, heat or ice packs, or special shoes. Patients may use a wheelchair to come to the door of the program room, but they must be able to walk (with cane or walker if necessary) in order to participate. Gradually, the use of wheelchairs, walkers, and canes is reduced as muscles are strengthened by exercises. The first step is to bring the cane or walker to the room but not use it, then to leave it in the nurses' station and use it only for the walk outside, and finally to not bring it at all.

Relaxation training. Audiotapes are used for a daily relaxation training period of 30 to 45 minutes. The patients are exposed to a variety of methods of relaxation such as progressive muscle relaxation, autogenics, visualization, and guided imagery. They are encouraged to purchase the type of tape that is most beneficial to them and to use it at home or at work. The nursing staff works with the patients on the mechanics of achieving maximum response to the tapes and directs the patients to discuss any emotional responses in the daily support group meeting that immediately follows the relaxation training period.

The emphasis on relaxation is important. We discuss the role of stress in exacerbating chronic pain and encourage patients to take time on a daily basis to detach from the pressures in their lives and "nurture themselves." In the Daily Group Meeting, assertiveness is discussed as a necessary component of setting limits on activities that take care of others while making time for activities that take care of oneself.

Daily Group Meeting. The group meeting is held for 30 minutes at the end of each day. The group is cognitive-behavioral in orientation (Turk et al. 1983), with the general goal of helping patients to accept those aspects of their lives that they cannot change, to learn the skills to change the aspects of their lives that they *can* change, and to develop the "wisdom to know the difference." Patients are told when they first enter the group (the day they start the program) that no complaints are allowed, but they are invited to bring up problems for which solutions might be possible. Some of the themes that are discussed most often are the following:

1. *Accepting their condition and their limitations.* It is clear from the program descriptions given to the patients, both in writing and in person, that their entry into the program is based on their having accepted that their condition is chronic and their pain cannot be "cured." We have found, however, that patients still hope that the activities of the program will reduce their pain. In fact, some patients do find that the severity of their pain is reduced, but that no one's pain is cured. When this becomes clear to the patients (usually around the third week of the program), many experience a sense of hopelessness and depression. This response is treated in the group by differentiating pain from suffering, pain being the

physical sensations and suffering the effect on their lives. The most powerful method of counteracting the feeling of hopelessness is to have program graduates describe how their lives have changed since graduating.

Positive planning is also used as a means of reducing negative life consequences of the physical pain. Patients are encouraged to pace themselves. We emphasize that they need to monitor their physical and emotional condition (which they learn to do with the pain diary) and to recognize when they are approaching their limit. At that point they are advised to curtail activity so that they do not risk exhausting themselves and increasing their pain.

Another way to differentiate pain and suffering is to emphasize that patients and family members can have fun despite pain. Patients are *required* to plan a weekend activity that will be fun, and they are taught to use that activity for guided imagery to divert their attention from pain and/or feelings of hopelessness during the rest of the week.

Occasionally it has also been helpful to utilize the grieving process as a model for dealing with the permanence of the pain. The stages of denial, anger, bargaining, depression, and acceptance (Kubler-Ross 1969) are described and the appropriate methods of dealing with the depression are discussed. Patients are encouraged to grieve the activities they can no longer do (e.g., tennis, track, certain careers) and advised that after they have grieved appropriately, it will be easier to move on to the next chapter in their lives.

2. *Guilt about not being able to do as much for others or not living up to their own expectations.* Patients are told that people often grow up with the hope that by performing with high standards they will be able to obtain approval from other important people (e.g., parents), but it is critical as adults to counteract this internal pressure and work on accepting ourselves as we are. Internal dialogues are discussed and practiced. Sometimes it becomes clear that a patient could benefit from individual therapy in the future, but during the first month of the program the focus is kept on the "here and now" and rarely is an attempt made to deal with deeper emotional issues.

A specific problem that is often used as an example of the need to take care of themselves is that patients are frequently reluctant to take time at home to do the exercises and relaxation because they don't want to be unavailable to family members and friends.

These patients are encouraged to put up "do not disturb" signs, to take the phone off the hook, or to say to family and friends, "This is my time and I need to do these things to take care of myself." Family members are told that patients who complete the program are not lazy, because they are exercising twice a day and completing other program requirements. Rather, when they "set their limits," they are taking responsibility for themselves in a way that will enable them to sustain their activity level on an ongoing basis.

3. *Pain behavior as power in relationships.* Sometimes patients become aware of how different their relationships will be if interactions do not revolve around pain. They become aware that they may have used their pain to avoid activities or intimacy and that *not* using the pain as an excuse will require more honest communications. Patients often express fear that more honest communication will increase marital conflict, and we tell them that this is sometimes true, but not always. Most patients have reported that their marriages have improved without additional therapy because they have learned to have more fun and to communicate better.

4. *Dealing with negative behaviors of other people.* Patients ask how to deal with family and friends who continue to ask them how they are feeling, what new doctors they have seen, and so on, or who accuse them of not having "real pain." We advise the patients to describe the Pain Management Program briefly and tell their friends and family that they no longer want to be asked about their pain problem because talking about it is counterproductive. This is also emphasized in the Family Group Meeting. The support people attending that meeting are encouraged to talk to other family and friends about the fact that the patient's pain is real but talking about it undermines their progress in learning to live with it.

Family Group Meeting. Patients attend five meetings of this weekly 90-minute group with the significant other who came with them to the initial interview. The purpose of the group is to provide education for the significant others and to encourage generalization of the program's behavioral principles into the patients' social environments.

Each meeting starts with a description of the basic philosophy of the program. By the time the patient graduates, each significant other has heard this talk five times, yet they tell us that each time they seem to hear something new. It is emphasized that this is a program for people with real physical pain that doctors and therapists have been unable to eliminate. It is also noted that this meeting is held because chronic pain is difficult not only for the patient, but also for those who love someone with a chronic pain problem. Family members and friends need to understand that there is nothing they can do to make the pain go away, and that communication about the pain only intensifies its effect. Significant others have an important role to play in reinforcing positive behaviors. When they see improvements in mood, activity, appearance, and so on, it is important to offer compliments. Patients will be more assertive about setting their own limits, and it is important for their loved ones to understand this change. It is not because patients have become lazy; rather, it is because they have learned that pacing is a process that they can use to maximize their energy.

Patients are asked in the Daily Group Meeting if there are specific points they would like brought up in the Family Group Meeting. These points are presented as part of the general discussion with no indication that it originated from a specific patient. Some of the points patients ask to have repeated include the importance of not being interrupted when doing exercises and relaxation, the importance of the spouse stopping his or her own complaining, and the importance of fun and reducing "workaholic" life-styles.

1. *Videotape of patients' progress.* Patients are videotaped on the first day of the program and once a week thereafter. On the videotape patients are shown walking, turning their heads to both sides, sitting, crossing their legs, standing, and holding both arms straight up. For each patient, the group watches the first tape and the most recent tape. Considerable positive reinforcement is given for the changes that are quite obvious even after 1 week in the program. Significant others are asked for comments about the patient's progress at home, and staff members address any specific questions or issues that may be brought up.

2. *Graduation.* Following the videotapes, a graduation ceremony is held for patients completing the program that week. Graduating patients receive a diploma and a cassette tape of the exercises, including the voices of the nurses and a group of patients. A photograph is taken of the patient and staff members for the program scrapbook. Each patient is also photographed getting a kiss or a hug from their significant other, who is reminded of the *ongoing*

importance of ignoring the patient's chronic pain while responding enthusiastically to positive behaviors.

An important part of the graduation is flushing the medicines down the toilet. A short talk is given about the limitations of most medicines in the treatment of chronic pain. Patients and family members are reminded that chronic use leads only to addiction and side effects such as further energy loss and depression. The patient then accompanies the physician to the rest room and dumps the pills in the toilet while a picture is taken. A round of applause usually greets the patient when he or she returns to the meeting room, followed by comments by patient and family about how relieved they are to no longer have to worry about the pills. A brief discussion is held about the risks of relapse (Marlatt and Gordon 1985), and patients are reminded that there *will* be bad days but that they should remember that medications are not the answer.

Graduating patients may also turn in various props such as special pillows or blankets as well as braces, crutches, canes, and other appliances. These are kept on display on a table in the clinic under a sign that reads: "We don't need these anymore."

Finally, opportunities are available for individual patients or significant others to ask questions or make comments, and some group discussion usually takes place.

Dictated summary. Following the graduation the internist dictates a summary report to the referring physician, noting the progress the patient has made in areas of strength, flexibility, and endurance. It is noted that the patient is now completely off of analgesic and sedative hypnotic medications, and the referring provider is cautioned against prescribing these types of medications for the chronic problem. It is noted, however, that all new symptoms should be evaluated fully, and the patient should be treated no differently than anyone else in prescribing medications for other problems. Referring providers are also informed that the program offers follow-up care (as described below) and that patients may return for a "tune-up" if for some reason their functioning is again compromised by chronic pain.

Follow-up visits. Patients are given appointments for follow-up visits once a week for the first month, once a month for the next 3 months, once at 6 months, and once at 1 year. They are also told that they can call us if they need to come more frequently, or if they "fall off the wagon" and find that their functioning has again become impaired. In such cases, we invite the patient to return for a full week (four visits of 4 hours in length), followed by weekly follow-up visits for 1 month.

Program evaluation. The effectiveness of the Pain Management Program is currently being evaluated, both in terms of the program's effectiveness in reducing functional impairment (measured by activity levels, ratings of quality of life, prescription use, etc.) as well as the impact on utilization of health care resources. A preliminary analysis of some of the data on medical utilization (Tulkin et al. 1990) indicates that 44 patients completing the program decreased the number of outpatient medical visits from 29.9 in the 2 years before entering the program to 18.1 in the 2 years after graduation. A comparison group of 42 patients who were referred to the program but declined to participate showed no change in their utilization over that 4-year period (27.7 visits in the 2-year period prior to referral compared to 26.3 visits in the 2 years after referral). A repeated measures analysis of variance showed that this difference was significant (interaction of condition × repeated measure yielded $F = 6.218$, $P < .02$). These data argue convincingly that a pain management program is cost-effective in a prepaid health care plan.

References

Aronoff GM, Evans WO, Enders PL: A review of follow-up studies of multidisciplinary pain units. Pain 16:1–11, 1983

Bensen H: The Relaxation Response. New York, William Morrow, 1975

Covington EC: Management of the patient with chronic benign pain: diagnosis. Modern Medicine 57:75–81, 1989a

Covington EC: Management of the patient with chronic benign pain: treatment. Modern Medicine 57:82–100, 1989b

Fordyce WE: Behavioral Methods For Chronic Pain and Illness. St. Louis, MO, CV Mosby, 1976

Ghia JN (ed): The Multidisciplinary Pain Center. Hingham, MA, Kluwer Academic Publishers, 1988

Kempler HL: The treatment of chronic pain, in Psychotherapy in Managed Health Care. Edited by Austad CS, Berman WH. Washington, DC, American Psychological Association, 1991, pp 220–233

Kubler-Ross E: On Death and Dying. New York, Macmillan, 1969

Marlatt GB, Gordon JA: Relapse Prevention: Maintenance Strategies in the Treatment of Addictive Behaviors. New York, Guilford, 1985

Tulkin SR, Frank GW: Introducing behavioral medicine into the HMO: systems and clinical issues. Paper presented at the annual meeting of the American Psychological Association, Washington, DC, August 1982

Tulkin SR, Frank GW: The changing role of psychologists in health maintenance organizations. Am Psychol 40:1125–1130, 1985

Tulkin SR, Buchman NA, Frank GW: Interdisciplinary treatment of chemical dependency. International Psychologist 29(5):39–48, 1989

Tulkin SR, Frank GW, Bernstein A, et al: Changes in medical utilization after treatment in a pain management clinic. Paper presented at the Sixth World Congress on Pain, Adelaide, Australia, August 1990

Turk DC, Holzman AD: Chronic pain: interfaces among physical, psychological and social parameters, in Chronic Pain: A Handbook of Psychological Treatment Approaches. Edited by Holzman AD, Turk DC. Elmsford, NY, Pergamon, 1986, pp 1–5

Turk DC, Meichenbaum D, Genset M: Pain and Behavioral Medicine: A Cognitive Behavioral Perspective. New York, Guilford, 1983

✦ 24 ✦

Managed Care of the Acutely Ill Psychiatric Patient: Development of a New Delivery System

Robert A. Wise, M.D.

ffective management of the care and cost of the treatment of
acutely psychiatrically ill patients remains a poorly solved but
pressing problem. This group of patients, requiring intensive and
expensive treatment, represents a small percentage of the patients
who present themselves for psychiatric service, but a group that consumes a disproportionate percentage of expended resources. As all
managed care systems have a fixed budget from which all services are
expected to be financed, there is the very real possibility that these
few patients have the potential of using up such a high proportion of
resources that inadequate resources will be available to the majority
of patients who require more routine types of services.

When a small group consumes a disproportionate amount of a total
budget, the how and why of the consumption needs to be carefully assessed and managed. At the same time, this expensive population contains the most unstable and the sickest patients, and thus the patients
most likely to have catastrophic outcomes from errors in clinical judgment. Great care and an extra dose of caution must be administered to
any system that attempts to reduce costs primarily through the typical utilization review mechanisms of aggressively cutting down on
number of admissions and reducing hospital length of stay. Clinical
failures that at times can be catastrophic (such as a successful suicide)
caused by underutilization of the hospital will result in demoralization

of the staff, significant legal exposure, and severe criticism of the entire managed care system.

To respond to these concerns by increasing patients' lengths of stay has serious financial and clinical ramifications. In these days of shrinking benefits, the hospital time available to an acutely ill patient is a scarce and precious resource. This is especially true for a patient who has a resistant or recurrent form of a serious illness and who likely will require several hospitalizations over the benefit year. The exhaustion of the benefit prior to a substantial remission of the illness can mean disaster. For example, a common situation may be seen in the case of a bipolar patient undergoing destabilization of the illness because of severe life stressors such as a serious illness in a family member or a divorce. The injudicious use of the inpatient benefit in the early part of the benefit year might very well mean that this patient will be without coverage toward the end of that year. This will result in the patient being sent to a public facility or receiving no treatment.

Another common problem is deciding when to switch from an antidepressant medication to electroconvulsive therapy (ECT) in the depressed and suicidal patient. The doctor may use most of the benefit while administering an antidepressant and patiently waiting through the latency period for the expected delayed response. By the time it is clear that the patient will not respond to the drug regimen, there is insufficient time to institute a series of ECT or even a different medication. If the patient must be transferred to a state-funded facility, the appropriate treatment modality, ECT, is frequently unavailable to them (in Illinois, this is a treatment that is available in few state-funded facilities). These scenarios suggest some of the pressing reasons to develop methods that are capable of managing this shrinking precious resource, the inpatient benefit, that is acceptable to patients, providers, and insurers.

Before suggesting a new method of managing this resource, I will review some commonly used methods. Typical techniques of managing this benefit can be divided up according to whether the financial and clinical responsibilities are split between insurer and provider, respectively, or both responsibilities are placed with the provider.

The typical technique used to manage cost when the insurer is financially responsible is various forms of concurrent/retrospective hospital review. Essentially, in these methods a utilization reviewer determines appropriateness of care by communicating with the clinician and/or reviewing the chart. Through the information gathered, a decision by the insuring body is made concerning an appropriate length of hospitalization. This separation of clinical and financial decision making puts insurer and provider in adversarial positions. To polarize these positions: the insurer is primarily concerned about the insurance company's financial health, and the provider is primarily concerned about his or her patient's remuneration or the patient's clinical needs without a thought to the cost-effectiveness of the care.

A series of other systems have evolved that place both clinical and financial responsibility in the hands of the provider. The typical form that this type of system takes is payment for services based on a capitated or fee-per-case arrangement. As the provider is at direct financial risk, there is a vested interest in providing high-quality care at the lowest cost.

As providers and insurers seek innovative ways to lower cost, they begin to demand that the available mental health care system deliver care more efficiently. The present system, which developed in an environment that valued quality without a serious regard to cost-effectiveness, can be expected to show its inherent limitations as it is stressed to act in a cost-effective manner.

Let's take a quick tour of the typically available system. This system of care consists of two tiers. The first tier is a treatment dominated by the hospital. The patient is treated in a therapeutic milieu by a treatment team usually available 24 hours a day. Typically, the doctor is the head of the treatment team. The doctor, who sees the patient three to six times per week, is intensively supported by the hospital's resources and personnel. The second tier is the outpatient setting where a therapist is totally or predominantly responsible for the patient's care. In this setting, the patient is typically seen anywhere from 45 to 90 minutes a week to as little as 15 minutes or less per month.

These two settings have different clear capabilities. The hospital is uniquely capable of treating very sick patients who require multiple interventions at unpredictable intervals. The outpatient setting, as it is run by a single practitioner with few auxiliary resources, does best treating patients with limited and predictable needs. The patient requiring repeated adjustment in medications, or one who is feeling unsure of self-control, or who needs multiple therapeutic interventions on a daily basis, would overwhelm the resources of a typically busy outpatient practitioner. These patients must be hospitalized. On the other hand the patient who requires no or minimal unplanned therapeutic contact between sessions will be satisfactorily treated in an outpatient setting.

These two types of patients have been picked from the extremes of patient needs. Most patients, at some time in their illness, require care beyond the outpatient setting but are not unstable enough to require around-the-clock care. Acute psychiatric symptomatology usually recedes gradually. As most severely ill patients pass through multiple stages to their premorbid baseline, different levels of care are required. Thus, at some point in the recovery process the outpatient setting would be insufficient to offer adequate care, whereas the inpatient setting offers more than what is required.

To clarify this point, take as an example a psychotically depressed woman who is admitted to a hospital because of the high risk of suicide. At the time of her admission, the 24-hour-a-day observation of the hospital is a necessity. Within 10 days, significant amounts of the initial presenting symptomatology (e.g., severe insomnia, constant crying, severe anxiety) have abated, but the patient still is significantly depressed with some feelings of helplessness and hopelessness. Though the risk of suicide is small, a regression is still very possible. The patient is subjectively improved and prefers the more familiar and less restrictive environment of her own home. She requests a discharge with outpatient follow-up. Although a 24-hour-a-day supervised setting is no longer needed, a traditional once- or twice-weekly outpatient treatment is wholly inadequate. The patient's request for discharge must be denied. The hospital is overly restrictive and expensive, but the traditional outpatient setting is inadequate and thus dangerous.

Herein lies the inherent problem with our traditional delivery system that must treat limitless varieties of clinical needs but has only two settings in which to offer care. Even if at the time of admission the needs of the patient are well matched to the setting, it is likely that at some time in the treatment there will be a significant mismatch of services purchased to services required.

The goal of balancing resources expended to resources needed is just not possible to achieve in our present limited two-tier system. What is needed is a system that has improved flexibility to alter the amount of resources expended in response to changing patient needs. In the past I have analogized this problem to the inefficiencies that would be produced by having only a high and a low gear in a car that should be equipped with a five-speed transmission. This hypothetical car will optimally perform in two situations: start-ups or uninterrupted highway driving. Its ability to handle in-between demands would be exceedingly limited, inefficient, and, frankly, dangerous. It is time for our two-gear delivery system to receive some additional options (Wise 1987).

This discussion of the limits of our present system leads into a description of a new system—one that can improve the efficiency by more closely matching resources expended to patient needs. What is needed is a system that can safely transfer a patient from a hospital that has extensive resources but is inflexible in the amount it can expend, to a setting that can supply resources in a variable fashion. To help set the stage, it is worth a moment to look at factors affecting the timing of a hospital discharge.

How is a decision concerning the timing of a hospital discharge made? It is not solely, nor even predominantly, the patient's clinical condition that determines length of stay in the hospital, but rather the *capabilities of the receiving treatment setting* to safely and effectively deliver needed care that is the major factor in determining the timing of a discharge. It is important to appreciate that viewing the time of discharge in this fashion is very different than determining discharge by when the patient no longer needs the specialized services of the hospital.

This nuance in determining timing of hospital discharge can explain much of the disagreement that occurs between utilization review personnel and providers of service. Currently the hospital not only acts as the sole environment that is able to give lifesaving care, but also as the setting that is capable of rendering intensive treatment on multiple days per week and for multiple hours per day. As hospitals discharge most patients to resource-limited outpatient settings, the typical practice is to treat the patient to the point that the available resources of the receiving system are adequate to meet the patient's needs. To do otherwise would potentially jeopardize the patient's health. Therefore, the timing of the discharge will frequently occur long after the life-threatening issues that necessitated hospitalization have been resolved.

How does one go about designing a delivery system that realizes that impossible dream of reducing costs, maintaining or improving quality, and being acceptable to insurers, providers, and consumers? The first step in this creation is to delineate the unique functions that the current acute care hospital fulfills that other treatment settings cannot. Once these functions are identified, an attempt will be made to recreate them in a less costly, less restrictive ambulatory setting. To put it another way, what are the crucial features of a hospital setting that must be partially or wholly duplicated in an outpatient setting to allow acutely ill patients to rapidly leave the hospital? These features are the ability to provide the following:

1. Constant observation and ongoing evaluation (important for resolving complicated diagnostic problems and essential for safety);
2. Immediate psychotherapeutic, pharmacological, and/or physical interventions;
3. Concentration and coordination of diverse resources to complete complicated diagnosis workups; and
4. Compliance with treatment.

What are the characteristics of the hospital that give it these unique abilities? Most, if not all, of these capabilities are derived from two characteristics: 1) the locked door, and 2) 24-hour-a-day multidisciplinary staffing.

The locked door ensures that the patient is always available in a controlled environment. This is the most significant advantage an inpatient unit has over any other setting. First, long uninterrupted periods of time are available to assess and reassess the patient before therapeutic intervention or after an intervention. Second, "showing up" for the next appointment, a never-ending issue in outpatient work, is now guaranteed. It makes no difference if the next therapeutic intervention is at 3 A.M., as the patient waits for another dose of medication, or at 3 P.M., as the patient prepares for the beginning of a community meeting; his or her presence is ensured. Third, the closing of the unit door succeeds not only in "locking" in the patient, but also can "lock out" stressors. The unit can provide a partial respite from work, a malignant relationship, or intolerable pressures from home responsibilities. The closed unit creates an insular environment in which the patient can recuperate in a relatively relaxed manner, preparing for return to outside life.

The other unique aspect is 24-hour-a-day staffing. This allows a depth and breadth of clinical observation unavailable in any other setting. Staff is always available to handle both planned (e.g., medication) and unplanned (e.g., need for seclusion or restraint) interventions. Lastly, this environment allows a multidisciplinary evaluation to be coordinated so that information can be readily exchanged, analyzed, and used in the patient's care.

Although no ambulatory setting can be constructed that *exactly* duplicates the capabilities of a hospital unit, altering the physical structure and adding some new resources can substantially extend existing capabilities, thus allowing increasing numbers of acutely ill patients to be treated in a new "outpatient" setting. The limits to which these treatment capabilities can be extended will be significantly determined by how well the inpatient functions can be transplanted to a new setting. The following modified goals of the previously stated essential features of a hospital will be achieved in the "new" ambulatory setting:

1. Rapid access to evaluation, reevaluation, and treatment;
2. Adequate time and resources required to correctly place the patient in the appropriate intensity of treatment;
3. Ensuring patient compliance with treatment (especially in regard to attending scheduled appointments and taking prescribed medications); and
4. Rapid access to a hospital when an outpatient setting is not appropriate.

There are many effective strategies to achieve these goals. As an example of one way to construct this setting and develop a program, I will describe some of the parts of the program developed at the Michael Reese HMO.

Rapid access to evaluation, reevaluation, and treatment. Evaluations are available 24 hours a day, 7 days a week, either by one of the program staff during the regular work week, or by the psychiatrist on call after hours with backup from an emergency room. Any important information obtained during off-hours is relayed to an answering machine by the psychiatrist on call. This machine is reviewed every morning by program staff, and appropriate changes in treatments are initiated.

Adequate evaluation time. Frequently the hospital is used because the clinician thinks that an insufficient amount of time is immediately available to assess the patient and then to mobilize the necessary resources to safely treat in an outpatient setting. The clinician cannot take the risk that a patient will remain safe without this effort and prefers to use the hospital for an extended evaluation in a controlled situation. In our setting, we have the resources to allow evaluations of several hours' duration. This period of time allows the staff to obtain additional history by contacting knowledgeable persons, to ensure that a supportive social system exists, and to initiate pharmacological interventions and then assess the patient's response. To make it easier to conduct these evaluations, we have made sure that there is sufficient staff time to conduct the interviews and evaluations, and a comfortable environment that includes two rooms with beds, a full kitchen, leisure activities, and a nursing station with a wide variety of parenteral and oral medications.

Rapid access to the hospital. As we are treating a seriously ill population, it is our expectation that, on occasion, patients deteriorate to the point that hospitalization is required. Our outpatient program has close ties to a hospital unit. This unit, which is about one-third of a mile away, is dedicated to the treatment of our patients. Administrative systems have been developed and implemented so that patients can move with ease from one program to the other.

Ensuring patient compliance. The program would be unable to maintain credibility if acutely ill patients were discharged from the hospital and lost to follow-up. Our solution has been to subcontract with a local taxicab company and offer rides, when needed, to and from the program. If a patient misses an appointment, we have the capability to send a taxi to the patient's home and bring him or her to the program.

I have highlighted some special program characteristics that allow treatment of acutely ill patients outside of a hospital. These become support structures that allow the patient to receive intensive treatment in a safe and acceptable environment. The actual treatment rendered is an integration of traditional care and special programming. The special programming targets the areas that are viewed as most significant in helping the patient return to his or her premorbid level of functioning and helping to avoid relapse. To clarify this area of "special programming," I will outline two examples.

The first area is responsible and accurate self-administration of medication. An unstable patient will not be given control of medication. However, as soon as possible, he or she will be encouraged to initiate control of the medication. Most patients are issued medication-dispensing boxes that allow a week of medication to be presorted. Patients, under staff supervision, sort their own pills at the start of each week. If a patient is considered an overdose risk, the filled box is left at the program or given to a family member. As soon as is clinically appropriate, the patient will take control of the medication. The boxes are brought to the program where they are regularly checked by staff so that early medication noncompliance can be observed.

The other area is the intensive effort made by staff to assist patient and family in early detection of relapse. Patients and families are educated about factors (e.g., high-stress job, alcohol use) that have precipitated exacerbation of symptoms in the past and are taught to recognize early signs and symptoms of another episode (e.g., sleep disturbance, isolation from family).

The special emphasis programming is integrated into ongoing treatment modalities that include activity and therapy groups, individual therapy, and family and multifamily therapies.

As a final note, it is worthwhile to consider what managed care settings are best suited and will be preferentially used to explore alternative-to-hospitalization programs. The creation and support of these systems requires three situations: access to a consistent patient base, ready availability to insurance dollars, and a flexible administration that will allow the use of these resources in innovative ways. An example of how these three requirements work together in my present system is the ready access of transportation for patients to and from the Spectrum Program. As I have already described, to be able to ensure the attendance of acutely ill patients to an alternative-to-hospitalization program is a basic requirement of a competent program of this type. At times this means using taxicabs to bring patients into our systems from as far as 35 miles away. We have spent as much as $100 a day in cab fares to ensure a patient's attendance. This cost is in lieu of a daily hospital cost of more than $400 a day. Few delivery systems have this level of control of resources. One is most likely to find this in a managed care system, particularly in a staff model system where the unique combination of large patient populations and control over insurance dollars exists. As these types of programs show their ability to maneuver in these new markets, other payors will become more willing to reimburse this valuable but nontraditional method of care.

As alternative-to-hospitalization programs are created, the final structure of the facility and program will vary widely depending on the population served, the resources available, and the ingenuity of the program architect. Successful systems will not only contain costs but will allow patients to receive sufficient treatment in an environment that is carefully geared toward their constantly changing needs.

Reference

Wise RA: Management challenges in mental health service delivery. Paper presented at the conference of the Group Health Association of America, Minneapolis, MN, September 18, 1987

✦ 25 ✦

The Harvard Community Health Plan: An Evolving Model of Managed Mental Health Care

Richard J. Fitzpatrick, Ph.D.

The Harvard Community Health Plan (HCHP) was founded in 1969 as a nonprofit corporation having a close affiliation with the Harvard Medical School. It is a staff and group model health maintenance organization (HMO) serving about 520,000 members in the New England (primarily Boston) area. The original staff model (310,000 members) currently has 14 sites, each with its own mental health department, multidisciplinary staff, and on-site chief who is either a psychiatrist or psychologist. A merger with a group model HMO in 1987 added 140,000 members, and a staff model HMO in 1990 added another 70,000 members in geographically more diverse areas.

The original mental health benefit at HCHP provided services for acute conditions only; mental health staff were viewed as consultants to primary care clinicians. Patients with chronic problems (approximately 15%) were not covered and were referred outside the Plan. The early 1970s saw the development of brief group therapies for people with adult developmental problems. By the mid-1970s, programs were developed with primary care to treat alcohol abuse. In 1976, the Massachusetts legislature mandated minimum mental health benefits and, as a result, chronic patients could no longer be excluded from treatment. Continuing care programs were established to care for this steadily growing population. With this change the mental health program shifted from the role of consultant to that of primary provider, and resources began to shift to the treatment of members with mental illness and those who were at risk for hospitalization.

Over the years HCHP has taken enormous pride in its ability to recruit an exceptional mental health staff that has been supported by a culture of innovation, creativity, and scholarship. A large proportion of clinical staff retain teaching appointments at area medical schools, and significant numbers of clinical studies, many supported by HCHP, are published yearly.

The Problem

In only a few years HCHP had more than quadrupled in size. Organizational and programmatic support lagged behind as a diverse clinical population of patients demanding services dramatically increased. With this growth the dynamics affecting the delivery of quality services became exceptionally complex. Externally, employers, employee assistance programs (EAPs), educated consumers, and various state agencies vigorously advocated for competitive premiums, member satisfaction with services, and demonstrated quality of care. Internally, rapid growth resulted in a dilution of the core clinical culture. Many new clinicians were hired with significant productivity expectations, but without well-honed skills in brief modalities or practice management. The result was an enormous increase in systems stress.

Since 1987, HCHP has sponsored a comprehensive review of the Mental Health Department and benefit. The enormous scope and depth of this 5-year project is the result of the consistent support of HCHP's Corporate Medical Director, John Ludden, M.D. His clinical perspective as a practicing psychiatrist at HCHP, combined with his active guidance as a senior manager with a national perspective on mental health issues, has created and nurtured this project. Nearly $2 million in resources have been spent to research and understand the complexities. We have been in the process of implementing a restructured program and benefit that will attempt to articulate a rational model of managed mental health group practice in the prepaid setting. The following is a summary of the key findings that have laid the groundwork for the development of this redesigned model.

The Clinicians

The HCHP staff model employs nearly 300 mental health clinicians divided roughly equally among psychiatrists, psychologists, social workers, and nurses. During 1987 and 1988, extensive formal interviewing and surveying of this group revealed considerable diversity about the purpose of the mental health program. Without a corporate mental health mission statement or a guiding treatment philosophy, clinicians experienced much confusion about which patients should be seen and what services should be offered.

Marketplace pressures to satisfy plan members ran into conflict with available resources. Pressures to deliver quick access to care resulted in a front-loaded system in which treatment decisions were driven by limited availability of return appointments rather than clinical indications for necessity of care.

Clinicians also found difficulties with the advertised mental health benefit (which was marketed to employer groups). Members were receiving an *average* of 6 visits in the form of brief or intermittent treatment, but they often felt "entitled" to the 20 sessions as a covered portion of long-term treatment.

Time management was also a source of stress. Clinicians thought that there was not enough time for consultation with peers, coordination of care with outside agencies, adequate documentation of care, training and skill enhancement, or clinical supervision with mentors. They believed that they needed to work overtime to see all the assigned new patients, chronic patients, and returning old patients. Moreover, the implementation of productivity expectations for bookable and delivered clinical hours fueled growing feelings of resentment, guilt, and anxiety. At a time when clinicians were feeling less support in managing their practices, they were also feeling increasingly overcontrolled and micromanaged.

Clinicians cited need for improvements in systems and services to support clinical care. These included liaison between hospital and ambulatory settings, coverage for patients in crisis both during the day and after hours, and a full range of hospital, day treatment, and intensive outpatient services for people with substance abuse problems as well as for children, adolescents, and adults with acute psychiatric illness. The burden of care fell back on the clinicians in the outpatient setting, who had few resources to manage the patients' presenting needs.

Although surveys of patients revealed dissatisfaction with the benefit and access to care, they consistently showed that the clinical talent and caring attitude of the clinicians was the number one asset of the mental health program.

The Members

Formal surveys and focus groups of HCHP members have shown fairly consistently over the years that about 85% of members have been satisfied with services in the departments of Internal Medicine, Pediatrics, and Obstetrics and Gynecology. Comparatively, overall satisfaction with care and benefits in the Mental Health Department has averaged much less (67%). Members have been the least satisfied (43%) with the amount and accuracy of the information they received regarding mental health services before beginning treatment. Patients balked at the confusion between their sense of the "right" to care that has been prepaid and the perceived arbitrariness of a clinician's description of the term "medically necessary."

Patients were also confused by the referral procedures to Mental Health. A member would have to first speak with his or her primary provider in Internal Medicine, or select one to see if he or she was without one, in order to get a paper referral to Mental Health. Then a phone screening by a mental health clinician might be required before assignment, followed by another call to schedule a first appointment. Members perceived these actions as deliberate barriers to care.

Member ratings of access—telephone access, appointment access, on-call services, visit frequency, and length—were also low, averaging 63%. Interestingly, although only 15% of patients who are seen in the Mental Health Department participate in groups at HCHP and many of these patients are in concomitant individual therapy, it was widely perceived that "all you can get at HCHP is group therapy."

Despite these problems, nearly 75% of patients were pleased with their therapists, whom they considered both competent and caring. Empathic support from their clinician was rated by members as the single most important aspect of satisfaction. The real core of members' unhappiness with mental health services was with the issue of *choice:* they could not choose to self-refer to Mental Health, or have a choice of provider, or have free choice among treatment type or modality, or even have the choice to extend treatment if desired. Everything had to be negotiated with a system that seemed cumbersome and inflexible.

The Community

HCHP's tremendous growth over the past 10 years has forced the local professional community to shift its perception of HCHP from a curious social experiment to that of a major alternative to indemnity insurance in the area. Being a closed panel HMO for most of its history, HCHP has generally focused inward, and outside contracts were held to a minimum. As a large and rapidly growing but still isolated player, HCHP had been viewed by the community with considerable suspicion.

Local employer groups have been exerting pressure for HCHP to hold the line on increasing premiums. A few believe that increasing mental health benefits may reduce overall medical expenses; others think that larger copays, deductibles, and benefit limits are necessary. They insist that HCHP improve its flexibility in price and service options and also demonstrate in measurable terms its relative and comparative quality of care. Expectations increasingly focus on outcome studies of clinical efficacy and ratings of member satisfaction with services.

Local EAPs have had, until recently, a largely adversarial relationship with HCHP. Their lobbying efforts with key state politicians pressured HCHP to open the doors for immediate access on demand for inpatient detoxification and rehabilitation for substance abuse. Although drug and alcohol abuse is a very significant problem, ironically, utilization did not dramatically increase without the gatekeeper function. Creating guidelines that support collegial intersystem interchange has become a priority.

Local community mental health centers (CMHCs) have also been generally unhappy with HCHP, and other area HMOs, because patients who have exhausted their benefit often come to the CMHC without continuing insurance coverage. They also feel the crunch of losing "market share" as their patients select HCHP coverage in large numbers. The state psychiatric hospitals also balk at assuming the long-term care of severely ill HCHP members who have exhausted their 60-day inpatient benefits. The boundary between private and public responsibility for chronic care is vague, and with the Massachusetts budget crisis, the need for joint planning looms as a top priority.

Other private psychiatric hospitals, particularly child and adolescent hospitals, have perceived HCHP's efforts to integrate care across the continuum as intrusive. Finally, there is the community of clinicians in private practice who see HCHP as providing too little care to too many. These "outside" clinicians cannot bill HCHP for insurance coverage, because all services are provided in-house. Although HCHP has the reputation of providing excellent care to the sickest patients,

the cohort of patients who seek longer term, insight-oriented psychotherapy are forced without continuing insurance coverage into fee-for-
service (FFS) practices.

The Management

HCHP management noted with increasing alarm the distress signals
coming from clinicians, members, and the wider community. Simply
spending more of the premium dollar on mental health did not seem to
help. From 1986 to 1990, cost increases for the Mental Health Department averaged 14%. Cost increases for the rest of the delivery system
rose just 8%.

During this same period the mental health staffing ratios increased from 1 clinical full-time equivalent (FTE) per 2,500 members
in FY84 to 1:2,900 in FY88. Moreover, the number of visits per FTE
clinician per year increased by approximately 150, from 1,200 to
1,350. Two hundred and twenty clinicians (123 FTEs) delivered
121,646 sessions with patients in 1989 in the health centers (staff
model). By 1991, this had risen to 151,627 visits. The mental health
outpatient visit rate over the 8-year period 1984–1991 was essentially
stable at 475 visits per 1,000 members (see Figure 25–1). However,
the percentage of membership receiving mental health services in-

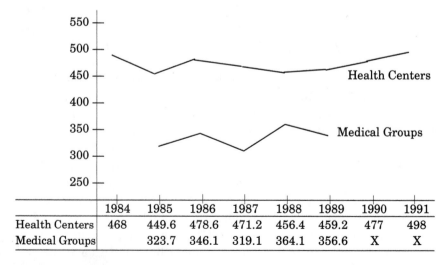

	1984	1985	1986	1987	1988	1989	1990	1991
Health Centers	468	449.6	478.6	471.2	456.4	459.2	477	498
Medical Groups		323.7	346.1	319.1	364.1	356.6	X	X

Figure 25–1. Mental health visit rate per 1,000 members for Harvard
Community Health Plan.

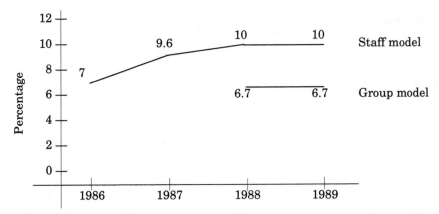

Figure 25–2. Mental health patients as percentage of Harvard Community Health Plan members.

creased from 7% to 10% (see Figure 25–2). Thus, the average number of total visits each patient received dropped from 6.8 to 4.6 (see Figure 25–3). In short, a greater proportion of the HCHP membership was asking for and receiving services in mental health, but were receiving less total treatment time.

Total costs during FY90 of $33 million were approximately evenly split between inpatient hospital and ambulatory mental health sites. Total per-member per-month (PMPM) costs for mental health rose from $4.77 in FY87 to $6.12 in FY89 (see Table 25–1). In just 5 years, total mental health costs had risen from $18 million to $33 million.

Although the overall costs for ambulatory care remained relatively stable and consistent with medical inflation, inpatient costs rose dra-

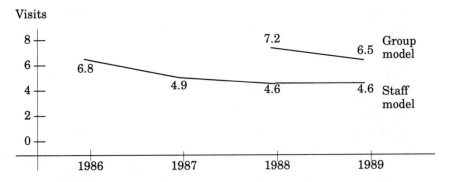

Figure 25–3. Average visits per patient per year to Harvard Community Health Plan's ambulatory mental health facilities.

Table 25–1. Harvard Community Health Plan (HCHP)'s mental health
costs as percentage of premium revenue

	FY87	FY88	Annualized FY89
HCHP total premium revenue PMPM	$82.98	$88.84	$100.67
HCHP mental health costs PMPM			
Ambulatory	2.27	2.49	2.82
Inpatient	2.50	2.82	3.30
Total mental health cost	$ 4.77	$ 5.31	$ 6.12
Costs as % of premium revenue	5.8	6.0	6.1

Note. PMPM = per member per month.

matically. From FY84 to FY88, substance abuse days per 1,000 members increased from 3.5 to 31.8. Psychiatry days per 1,000 members during the same period rose from 26.8 to 48.6 (see Table 25–2).

Interestingly, the average length of stay per admission during this period was relatively constant: approximately 13 days. It was the significant increase in numbers of admissions that accounted for the rise in hospital days. Was this caused by adverse selection by sick patients into HCHP because of the cutbacks in services in the public sector? Was it some unknown variable contributing to patient recidivism? Was it a function of a lack of appropriate services and inadequately

Table 25–2. Inpatient mental health days per 1,000 members per year for Harvard Community Health Plan

	Health care days
FY84	
Substance abuse	3.5
Psychiatry	26.8
Total	30.3
FY88	
Substance abuse	31.8
Psychiatry	48.6
Total	80.4
FY90	
Substance abuse	27.1
Psychiatry	59.0
Total	86.1
FY91	
Substance abuse	19.87
Psychiatry	51.70
Total	71.57

developed alternatives to hospitalization? Was it related to outpatient clinician burnout, or inadequate skill development in crisis management, or fears of malpractice? At that time we simply had very little idea of the underlying causes. What we did know was that the compound annual growth rate for inpatient care at HCHP was a startling 32.4%. Nationally, mental health costs were increasing 10% over the increase in total medical expenditures. Nonetheless, HCHP management was faced with the task of addressing problems with satisfaction while simultaneously containing costs that were escalating out of control.

The Process of Change

John Ludden, M.D., has described the HCHP Mental Health Redesign Project as a "major endeavor to develop and evaluate models that would improve psychiatric and substance abuse service delivery and benefit design in the managed care setting" (Harvard Community Health Plan 1988, p. 1). Since 1987, our efforts have included intensive surveying, formal interviewing, and focus groups of administrative staff at all levels; of clinicians practicing in and outside of HCHP; of new, old, and disenrolled members; and of local and national leaders in the health care and legislative sectors. We have conducted a national HMO survey of trends in mental health service delivery, and we have commissioned a consumer survey by the Lewis-Harris Corporation. We have completed extensive cost and utilization analyses, and we have reexamined our concept of work expectations and productivity.

The results of this work were a series of conclusions about what was and was not working in the mental health program, a set of guiding principles for change, a mission statement that articulated a philosophy of care, and treatment modalities to support this philosophy. Our efforts at this point were to develop a *rational process* that would lead to a redesign of benefits, programs, and systems. The next step was to move the project from the data collection and theoretical phase to an action phase in which a new benefit and supporting programs could be implemented.

We learned that employer groups and consumers generally rejected the idea of increasing the premium to support program enhancement in mental health. Therefore, our efforts have been devoted toward the reallocation of existing resources and the creation of new ones. For example:

✦ Operationally defining "medically necessary" services would establish boundaries such that increased treatment is made available to the neediest patients.
✦ Savings from program and systems improvements that result in decrease of inpatient utilization could now be diverted and used to improve ambulatory services.
✦ Discretionary treatment (not medically necessary) could be made available and supported by cost sharing for members who want and value this service.

Our primary objective, which is admittedly ambitious, has been to tackle the meaning of the term "medically necessary." If this can be accomplished, the mental health benefit no longer needs to be solely defined and constrained by arbitrary criteria such as number of visits, copays, or deductibles.

To do this, we would have to develop a methodology for understanding a patient's presenting and evolving needs, and a means for linking these indices to treatment guidelines that are organized according to type of treatment and duration, frequency, and intensity of that treatment. Therefore, we would need to learn more about which treatments are most appropriate for which kinds of patients to ensure quality of care. We would have to be able to identify and demonstrate standards of care and define appropriate outcomes. We would also need to develop a formal mechanism for case review by clinicians to support efforts to appropriately match patients to treatments and to follow progress toward desired goals. Finally, we would need to learn on a large scale much more about who our patient population comprises so that we could proactively organize the programs and services to meet these diverse needs. Each of these goals represents major initiatives that have been undertaken to address the problems that have been identified.

At the beginning of this phase, six initial work groups were established, each with a specific charge and composed of HCHP mental health clinicians. These groups reported to an Advisory Committee whose role was to integrate the process. In turn, the Advisory Committee would present formal progress reports at key points to a Review Team comprised of mostly senior medical managers. Finally, implementation of the new benefit was subject to approval by the HCHP Policy Group, the Chief Executive Officer, the Medical Director, the Physicians Council, and the Board of Directors. The entire process was conceived and had the approval of top management from the beginning of the project.

The newly designed benefit for mental health includes an evaluation for anyone requesting mental health or substance abuse treatment. The type and duration of treatment following the evaluation is determined by the clinician. Visits in that treatment plan carry the following copayments: one to eight, basic copay level (usually $5). As of January 1991, visits 9 through 20 cost $35 for individual therapy and $15 for group sessions. Thereafter, sessions are billed at FFS marketplace rates. Benefits automatically renew each calendar year. Specific services for treatment of the medical aspects of mental illness and substance abuse (medication evaluation and management, hospital prescreening or diversion, case management, etc.) would be provided on an ongoing basis *without escalating copay or benefit limits* to those patients who qualify for the services according to the newly designed formal assessment process.

Concomitant with the benefit redesign, the process of implementing multiple new programs and systems has been in full swing. Examples of new improvements that fill in the continuum of care include a series of flexible day and evening treatment programs for adults, people with substance abuse problems, and adolescents; a centralized 24-hour crisis service with holding beds to supplement local programs and assist in hospital treatment planning; an intensive outpatient service to support those in need of daily appointments as a form of hospital diversion; a morning outpatient alcohol detoxification program following a formally designed screening process; an expanded group program including specialized services for AIDS patients, incest survivors, and patients with eating disorders, chronic medical illnesses, chronic pain, or character disorders; a formalized intake protocol that supports improved decision making for access of self-referring members; a utilization management/peer consultation network for both hospital and ambulatory settings; an automated appointment scheduling system; implementation of voice mail for clinicians throughout the system; and an updated medical record documentation process.

During 1990–1991, multiple work groups of HCHP clinicians met to design, validate, pilot, and implement a new *Patient Assessment Tool* (PAT). These scales assess:

✦ Substance abuse (current and historical)
✦ Duration of abstinence
✦ Ranking of severity of diagnosis
✦ Lethality (dangerousness to self or other)
✦ Scaled limitation of functioning (revised from the Global Assessment of Functioning from DSM-III-R [American Psychiatric Association 1987])
✦ Change in scaled limitation of functioning (rates change in status in recent past)
✦ Severity of psychosocial stressors (environmental, interpersonal, social, physical)
✦ Impairment of support systems (personal, interpersonal, social/institutional)

This assessment tool produces eight scores that are treated independently and facilitate a prescriptive approach to treatment planning. The tool provides consistent language and uniform standards to assess level of need. Thus, it serves as a decision-making vehicle for placement into appropriate treatment. These scales help to determine initial access to treatment, type of service, session frequency, and both length and duration of therapy. Linked with the treatment guidelines, the assessment tool also prescribes markers during the treatment process that will serve as flags for reevaluation and peer review.

A series of clinical algorithms are in continuous development and review and serve as a guide for clinicians in the diagnostic and treatment planning process. For example, an algorithm would help a clinician appropriately decide at what point a patient with panic symptoms should have a psychopharmacological evaluation, or what factors need to be considered in deciding the appropriate level of intervention for a patient presenting with suicidality. These algorithms will also suggest points at which a case should have clinical review or consultation.

Clinical algorithms also assist in the process of evaluating the relative success of various treatment options and provide feedback loops to systems that are guiding the development of the intake tool, the treatment guidelines, and the case management processes. The goal is to improve quality of care through reduction in unnecessary variability. Thus, a patient in crisis whose clinical profile indicates he or she needs daily contact can be reasonably assured he or she will receive that care and that this care has a reasonable chance of being consistently delivered from site to site. In this way the system is structured to meet the patient with his or her presenting needs. Moreover, staffing patterns and ratios will be less arbitrarily allocated but will fall out of specific indicators of need for program development. Also, work expectations for clinicians are less narrowly defined (e.g., 3–4 new patients per week) but will be tied to treatment planning and guidelines. Thus, clinicians specializing in working with more complex cases can be directly supported in carrying a lower caseload.

Within this new structure, ongoing supervision and education has become centrally important. A work group on training was organized to support the implementation of the redesign project. We have also formalized a staff orientation program in which new staff are introduced to the concepts of managing their practice and to the managed care setting, as well as mastering the concepts of the brief psychotherapies. The program develops skills, teaches systems, and provides a sense of the whole organization. But perhaps most importantly, it communicates a sense of authentic hopefulness from esteemed colleagues that good treatment can be provided to our patients in the managed care setting. For our more experienced clinicians, we have implemented a course curriculum to improve skills in more specialized areas (i.e., forms of brief group therapy, crisis management, psychopharmacology, cognitive behavioral techniques, and advanced techniques of brief psychotherapy). We are also in the process of expanding our postresidency, postdoctoral, and fellowship programs. Our intention is to establish, with the Harvard Medical School, the first psychiatry residency program in the country that offers formal specialization of training in the managed care setting. These programs have been a major source of recruitment and smooth the process of acculturation to the managed care setting.

Summary

Why has the apparently straightforward task of rearticulating the mental health benefit taken almost 5 years, and why is it still not complete? Perhaps the redesign project is, at its core, an effort to clarify our values and establish a collective sense of self. We understand that we cannot promise what we cannot deliver, but we are now more clearly able to say: "This is what we do, and do well, and this is what we do not do." Moreover, the redesign project has naturally led us into a continuous improvement process that will be ongoing. Quality management principles and techniques have recently become an important focus for our mental health managers.

Our newly defined boundaries clarify our purpose, but they necessarily involve certain trade-offs. For example, our reaffirmed commitment to the treatment of those with significant psychiatric problems means that relatively fewer resources are available at this time for supporting the ongoing care of the "worried well." Our commitment to patients who have mental illnesses or who are in acute crisis means that the work lives of some of our clinicians have needed to change. Our commitment to a predictable, consistent assessment instrument in order to decrease variability in treatment planning decisions means that clinicians are burdened with more paperwork. On the other hand, there appears to be considerably more clarity in useful diagnoses and treatment planning and in articulating to patients the rationale for the provision of services that are available to them. The PAT is in need of simplification and further validation, and much work remains to establish working linkages to treatment guidelines.

At this point, our recent data suggest that clinician morale has improved. In addition, a November 1990 formal survey shows members report a significant increase in their overall satisfaction with mental health services at HCHP. Members are particularly pleased with the ability to self-refer and their perception of easier access to care. Employer groups have expressed enthusiasm for our efforts to establish measurable standards for care, and community and state agencies have been appreciative of our efforts to clarify boundaries. On the cost side, we have seen a long-hoped-for leveling in the psychiatric admission rate and a significant decrease in length of stay, particularly for children and adolescents. Substance abuse hospital days per 1,000 members decreased from 31.8 in FY88 to 19.9 in FY91. Savings from inpatient expenditures in 1990 alone amounted to more than $3 million. On the ambulatory side, the ratio of FTE clinicians per 1,000 members has increased from 1:2,900 in FY88 to 1:2,450 in FY92. There has been consensus that the radical decision to lift all benefit restrictions for acute and major mental illness has been an excellent one. On the other hand, there will likely be a need for further benefit modification to reduce disincentives for group therapy.

Much has been accomplished, but significant stresses remain, particularly in the area of offering timely and sufficient services to those with life circumstance and adjustment disorders, as well as those with chronic conditions such as posttraumatic stress disorder, which are currently not typically considered benefit exceptions. Moreover, there is a pressing need to improve management information systems, and ongoing support for effective implementation of programs.

Nonetheless, we are collectively proud of having established a process that has involved all concerned constituencies. A grassroots effort by our clinicians in alliance with a management team has produced a system of service delivery that is more rational and a benefit that is more clearly understood. We have also used this project to move from a greater clarity of values to systematic attention to implementing those values in a structured and managed care setting.

References

American Psychiatric Association: Diagnostic and Statistical Manual of Mental Disorders, 3rd Edition, Revised. Washington, DC, American Psychiatric Association, 1987

Harvard Community Health Plan: HCHP Redesign Project Report, Phase II. Peabody, MA, Harvard Community Health Plan, 1988

✦ Glossary ✦

ADMINISTRATIVELY NECESSARY DAY: Under Medicaid, days of inpatient hospital care that are required to allow time for orderly transfer and discharge of patients who no longer require hospitalization, but who either require care that cannot be provided at home or who have no home to which they can return.

ADVERSE SELECTION: Disproportionate enrollment of insurance risks who are poorer or more prone to suffer more loss or make more claims than the average risk.

ALOS: Average length of stay.

ALTERNATIVE DELIVERY SYSTEMS (ADS):   Health care delivery modes that directly provide or finance delivery of services in innovative ways designed to improve efficiency and/or contain cost.

ASSIGNMENT OF BENEFITS: Written authorization by a subscriber permitting payment of benefits directly to a provider.

AT RISK: The state of being subject to some uncertain event occurring that connotes loss or difficulty. In the financial sense, this refers to an individual, organization, or insurance company assuming the chance of loss through running the risk of having to provide or pay for more services than are paid for through premiums or per capita payments.

BENEFIT: In insurance, a sum of money provided in an insurance policy payable for certain types of loss, or for covered services, under the terms of the policy.

BENEFIT PACKAGE: A contractually defined set of health services, the cost of which is borne in full or in part by a health insurance plan.

Adapted from American Psychiatric Association: An Economic Survival Manual for Private Practice Psychiatrists. Washington, DC, American Psychiatric Association, 1985.

CAFETERIA-STYLE EMPLOYEE BENEFITS: An employer health insurance benefit structure in which employees may choose among an array of health benefits coverages and/or plans, making selections that the individual employees believe best suit their health needs and financial ability.

CAPITATION: A method of health care financing and delivery involving the provision of a specified set of services to an individual for a predetermined periodic payment, without regard to the level and type of actual services provided. Capitation payments are usually figured "per enrolled member."

CARVEOUT: A system in which a health maintenance organization (HMO), usually an individual practice association (IPA), makes all mental health referrals to a specific group practice, rather than to independent practitioners. The group practice is often under a capitation or other contract.

CASE-MIX: The diagnosis-specific makeup of a health program's work load. Case-mix directly influences the length of stay, intensity, cost, and scope of the services provided by a hospital or other health program.

CHAIN ORGANIZATION: A group of two or more health care facilities that are owned, leased, or controlled by one organization. Chain organizations include, but are not limited to, chains operated by proprietary organizations and chains operated by various religions.

CLOSED-PANEL PPO: A preferred provided organization (PPO) variation in which the patient must utilize only member providers in order to receive benefits (also called closed-panel provider or exclusive provider organization).

COINSURANCE: Established percentages indicating the portion of covered expenses, beyond the deductible, to be paid by the insured party.

COMMUNITY RATING: A method of establishing premiums for health insurance in which the premium is based on the average cost of actual or anticipated health care used by all subscribers in a specific geographic area or industry, which does not vary for different groups or subgroups of subscribers, or with such variables as the group's claims experience, age, sex, or health status.

COMORBIDITY: The concurrence of two or more diseases in the same patient (also called complications).

COMPREHENSIVE MEDICAL PLAN (CMP): As defined by Medicare, an organization that provides enrolled members with physician, hospital, and laboratory services on a capitation basis. These services are provided primarily by physicians who are under contract to, employed by, or partners in the CMP. A CMP has fewer restrictions imposed on it than does a federally qualified HMO, but may in fact be a state-licensed HMO.

CONTRACT DISCOUNTS: The reduction in physician or other health service fees that the patient receives as an economic incentive to utilize providers belonging to a specific preferred provider organization (also called Negotiated Discounts).

CONTRACT RATES: The reduction in physician or other health service fee schedule components that results from the contractual agreement between a provider and a PPO (sometimes called alternative rates or negotiated rates).

CONTRIBUTORY INSURANCE: Group insurance in which all or part of the premium is paid by the employee, the remainder, if any, being paid by the employer or union.

COORDINATION OF BENEFITS (COB): Integration of benefits payable under more than one health insurance plan, so that benefits from all sources do not exceed 100% of the total allowable medical expenses.

COPAYMENT: A type of health care cost-sharing whereby the insured or covered person pays a fixed amount per unit of medical service or unit of time (e.g., $2 per physician visit, $10 per inpatient hospital day) and the insurer pays the rest of the cost. The copayment is incurred at the time the service is used, and the amount paid does not vary with the cost of service (unlike coinsurance, which is payment of some percentage of the cost).

COST-BASED REIMBURSEMENT: One method of payment of medical care programs by third parties, typically Blue Cross plans or government agencies, for services delivered to patients. In cost-related systems, the amount of the payment is based on the costs to the provider of delivering the service. The actual payment may be based on any one of several different formulas, such as full cost, full cost plus a percentage, allowable costs, or a fraction of costs (also called retrospective reimbursement).

COST-SHARING: Provisions of a health insurance policy that require the insured or otherwise covered individual to pay some portion of the covered medical expenses. Several forms of cost-sharing are employed, particularly deductibles, coinsurance, and copayments. The amount of the premium is directly related to the benefits provided and hence reflects the amount of cost-sharing required. For a given set of benefits, premiums increase as cost-sharing requirements decrease. In addition to being used to reduce premiums, cost-sharing is used to control utilization of covered services—for example, by requiring a large copayment for a service that is likely to be overused (also called beneficiary cost-sharing).

COVERED DAYS: The number of days that the insurer will accept for services rendered. Covered days may be limited per spell of illness, per year, or per lifetime of the insured or length of the health insurance policy.

COVERED SERVICES: Services and supplies that are covered by a health benefit package or delivery system.

DEDUCTIBLE: A fixed amount that an insured person must expend on medical services before the insurer will pay for the services; may also be the value of specified services (such as 2 days of hospital care or one physician visit). Any amount above the deductible is covered by insurance. Deductibles are usually tied to some reference period over which they must be incurred (e.g., $100 annual deductible means that the consumer pays the first $100 of covered medical services per calendar year, benefit period, or spell of illness).

DISCOUNT: Discounting of fee-for-service charges (ranging from 60%–80%) in return for referrals.

DUAL CHOICE OR DUAL OPTION: Refers to federal legislation requiring that employers give their employees the option to enroll in either an HMO or a conventional employer-sponsored health program.

ENCOUNTER: A face-to-face contact between a patient and a health care provider during which medical, dental, social, or family planning services are provided and documented in the patient's health record. The encounter may be in the health center or at any other location integral to outreach or direct referral service.

ENROLLEE: One who enrolls in a prepaid health program for health services. The terms of enrollment are understood to mean that the health delivery program provides, or contracts for, an agreed-upon list of health services (benefit package) for a given period of time in return for a fixed payment or premium. In most cases, payment may be made directly to the health delivery program by the enrollee; in other cases, payment is made for the enrollee by a third party (e.g., Medicare, an employer, etc.).

EXCLUSIVE PROVIDER ORGANIZATION (EPO): A PPO variation in which the patient must utilize only member providers in order to receive benefits (also called a closed panel PPO).

EXCLUSIVITY CLAUSE: Prohibits physicians from contracting with more than one HMO or PPO.

EXPERIENCE RATING: A method of establishing premiums that is based on the average cost of actual or anticipated health care used by various groups and subgroups of subscribers, and that thus varies with the health experience of groups and subgroups of subscribers, or with such variables as age, sex, or health status. Experience rating is the most common method of establishing premiums for health insurance in private programs. State regulations often do not allow HMOs to use experience rating.

FEE-FOR-SERVICE: A method of reimbursing on the basis of services rendered.

FIRST-DOLLAR COVERAGE: Coverage under an insurance policy that begins with the first dollar of expense incurred by the insured for the covered benefits. Such coverage, therefore, has no deductibles, although it may have copayments or coinsurance.

FOR-PROFIT HOSPITALS: Hospitals owned and/or operated by physicians, other individuals, or a business corporation for the purposes of making a profit (also called investor-owned hospitals).

FREESTANDING FACILITY: This term is usually applied to an ambulatory care facility that has no physical connection with a hospital or other health care unit. Normally, a freestanding facility operates at a distance from any other unit.

GATEKEEPER: A gatekeeper may be a primary care physician or occasionally another specialist or physician extender to whom a defined insured population is assigned and who is required either to provide all health care or to authorize care from other specialists, if necessary, for the assigned individuals. Gatekeepers may or may not be paid on a capitated basis and may or may not be financially at risk for all care provided.

GROUP INSURANCE: Any insurance plan in which a number of employees of an employer (and their dependents) or members of a similar homogeneous group are insured under a single policy, which is issued to their employer or the group with individual certificates of insurance given to each insured individual or family. Individual employees may be insured automatically by virtue of employment, or only on meeting certain conditions (e.g., being employed for longer than a month), or only when they elect to be insured.

GROUP MODEL: An HMO that contracts with physicians in an existing group practice. Physicians are usually paid on a salary-plus-incentive basis.

HEALTH MAINTENANCE ORGANIZATION (HMO): Any organization that, through an organized system of health care, provides or ensures the delivery of an agreed upon set of comprehensive health maintenance and treatment services for an enrolled group of persons under a prepaid fixed sum or capitation arrangement. Services available usually include primary care and rehabilitation. HMOs are also known as prepaid health plans. The HMO must employ or contract with health care providers who undertake a continuing responsibility to provide services to its enrollees. To be considered a federally qualified HMO, the HMO must meet the provisions of Title XIII of the Public Health Service Act.

HOLDBACK: A portion of a clinician's fee held by a HMO in a risk agreement. There is a financial return to the clinician periodically, based on the performance of the organization.

HOLD HARMLESS CLAUSE: A clause meaning that a physician indemnifies or "holds harmless" a PPO or HMO from all costs of defense, settlement, and judgment of patient claims of injury, whether or not these claims result from alleged medical malpractice of the physician. These terms make the physician responsible for alleged injury, even if the injury is caused in whole or in part by the administrative negligence or policies of the PPO or HMO.

INDEMNITY BENEFITS: The provision of benefits on the basis of set dollar allowances for covered services. The indemnity insurance contract usually defines the maximum amounts that will be paid for the covered services.

INDIVIDUAL PRACTICE (OR PRACTITIONER[S]) ASSOCIATION, INDEPENDENT PRACTICE (OR PRACTITIONER[S]) ASSOCIATION, OR INDEPENDENT JOINT VENTURES:
Creation of new entities by hospital and medical staff to operate or negotiate with HMOs. Entities may be 1) for-profit, stock corporations, 2) not-for-profit corporations, 3) general partnerships, or 4) limited partnerships.

IPA MODEL: An HMO that contracts with an association of individual physicians to provide services to the HMO enrollees at a negotiated capitation, flat retainer, or negotiated fee for services.

LAST-DOLLAR COVERAGE: Insurance coverage without upper limits or maximums regardless of the amount of benefits payable.

LENGTH OF STAY (LOS): The length of an inpatient's stay in a hospital, reported as the number of days spent in a facility per admission or discharge. A hospital's overall ALOS is calculated as follows: total number of days in the facility for all discharges occurring during a given period divided by the number of discharges during the same period.

LOCK-IN FEATURE: Individuals who are enrolled in an HMO *must* receive all routine care from the HMO in order to avoid financial liability for the cost of care. These individuals are thus "locked in" to the delivery system, except for urgently needed and emergency care.

MEDICAL NECESSITY: The determination by a health insurer of the need for the medical service(s) in the setting provided, or in accordance with the health insurance policy.

MEMBER: A person who is eligible to receive, or is receiving, benefits from an HMO or insurance policy. Members usually include both those people who have themselves enrolled or subscribed for benefits and their eligible dependents.

MORAL HAZARD: Health insurance risk associated with loss-producing propensities that are subject to the influence of the insured: dishonesty, carelessness, and lack of perspicacity or judgment.

NETWORK MODEL: An HMO that contracts with more than one independent multispecialty group practice.

OPEN ENROLLMENT: A period in which new subscribers may elect to enroll in a health insurance plan or prepaid group practice. Open enrollment periods may be used in the sale of either group or individual insurance and may be the only time of year in which insurance is available to new subscribers. Individuals perceived as high-risk (perhaps because of a preexisting condition) may be subjected to high-risk premiums or exclusions during open enrollment periods.

OPEN PANEL: An HMO that negotiates with individual physicians, small physicians groups, an IPA, or all three on a capitated basis or fee-for-service basis.

OUT-OF-AREA COVERAGE: Payment for medical services out of the geographic area of the provider group. Costs may be the responsibility of the plan or be shared by the provider on a risk-shared basis.

OVERUTILIZATION: Unnecessary or excessive rendering of services by providers or demand for services by patients.

PEER REVIEW: Generally, the evaluation by practicing physicians or other professionals of the effectiveness and efficiency of services ordered or performed by other practicing physicians or other members of the profession whose work is being reviewed (peers). Peer review is usually done by professionals practicing in the same geographic area as the professional whose service is being reviewed.

PENETRATION: In marketing health insurance or HMOs, the percentage of possible subscribers who have in fact contracted for benefits.

PER CAPITA: Payment for health care based on the number of beneficiaries enrolled in the insurer's program, regardless of the number who actually receive services.

PREFERRED PROVIDER ORGANIZATION (PPO): An insurance arrangement whereby insurers contract with providers for certain services based on a fee schedule. Plan members are then encouraged to use these "preferred" providers for necessary services. If the insured chooses to use the services of a provider other than one within the organization, the insured must pay (out of pocket) any difference between actual charges and the approved fee schedule or must pay higher copayments or deductibles.

PREMIUM: The amount of money or consideration that is paid by an insured person or policyholder (or on the policyholder's behalf) to an insurer or third party for health insurance coverage under a health insurance policy. The premium is generally paid in periodic amounts.

PREPAID GROUP PRACTICE: A health plan in which a health organization (or a formal association of three or more physicians) contracts to provide a specified set of services to the health plan enrollees in return for a fixed periodic payment per enrollee, paid in advance of the use of service (also called a group model HMO).

PREPAID HEALTH PLAN (PHP): Generally, a contract between an insurer and a subscriber or group of subscribers whereby the PHP provides a specified set of health benefits in return for a periodic premium.

PRIMARY CARE NETWORK: A method of restricting patient access to specialty care in which a group of primary care providers contracts to serve as gatekeepers for a defined population.

PRIOR AUTHORIZATION: Requirement imposed by a third party, under some systems of utilization review, that a provider must justify before a peer review committee, insurance company representative, or state agent the need for delivering a particular service to a patient, before actually providing the service, in order to be reimbursed (also called preauthorization, precertification, or predetermination).

PRIVATE INSURERS: Refers to nongovernmental insurance firms such as Blue Cross/Blue Shield and commercial insurance companies such as Aetna, Prudential, Nationwide, and Liberty Mutual.

PROSPECTIVE PAYMENT SYSTEM (PPS): The federal medical system that reimburses hospitals for Part A Medicare services based on diagnosis-related groups (DRGs).

PROSPECTIVE REIMBURSEMENT: Any method of paying hospitals or other health programs in which amounts or rates of payment are established in advance for the coming year and the programs paid these amounts regardless of the costs they actually incur.

PROVIDER AGREEMENT: A contractual agreement between a provider or supplier of health services and an insurer of health services, outlining the requirements of the insurance program that the provider or supplier agrees to adhere to when providing services to and billing patients of the insurer.

PROVIDER-BASED PPO: A preferred provider organization (PPO) initiated by providers, physicians, or both. The providers and/or physicians organize a system of other providers and physicians for the purpose of marketing the system to employers or insurers.

QUALITY ASSURANCE: Activities and programs intended to ensure the quality of care in a defined medical setting or program. Such programs must include educational components intended to remedy identified deficiencies in quality, as well as the components necessary to identify such deficiencies (such as peer or utilization review components) and to assess the program's own effectiveness.

RIDER: A legal document that modifies the protection of an insurance policy, either expanding or decreasing its benefits, or adding or excluding certain conditions from the policy's coverage.

RISK: Generally, any chance of loss. In insurance, designates the individual or property insured by an insurance policy against loss from some peril or hazard. Also used to denote the probability that the loss will occur.

RISK SHARING: An arrangement between the program administrator and provider whereby the provider shares any funds remaining at the end of the period that have not been expended for services, and shares in shortages occasioned when spending for program services exceeds the available budget.

SELF-INSURANCE: The practice of an individual, group of individuals, employer, or organization assuming complete responsibility for losses (which could be insured against) such as medical expenses and other losses due to illness.

SERVICE AREA: A geographic area defined and served by a health program or institution, such as a hospital or community mental health center, and delineated on the basis of such factors as population distribution, natural geographic boundaries, and transportation accessibility (also called catchment area).

SKIMMING: The practice in health programs paid on a prepayment or capitation basis, and in health insurance, of seeking to enroll only the healthiest people as a way of controlling program costs. Also, the practice of some providers of offering only those services that are favorably reimbursed by insurers (also called creaming).

SLIDING-FEE SCALE: A schedule of discounts in charges, or a deductible not set at a fixed dollar amount, for services based on the consumer's ability to pay, according to particular income and family size criteria.

STAFF MODEL: An HMO that retains physicians as employees.

SUBSCRIBER: Often used synonymously with the terms member or beneficiary, but in strict sense the term subscriber means only the individual (family head or employee) who has elected to contract for, participate in, or subscribe to an insurance plan or HMO, excluding whatever other persons may also be covered under the plan as a result of the contract.

THIRD-PARTY PAYOR: Any organization, public or private, that pays or insures health or medical expenses on behalf of beneficiaries or recipients (i.e., Blue Cross/Blue Shield, commercial insurance companies, Medicare, and Medicaid). The individual generally pays a premium for such coverage in all private and some public programs. The organization then pays bills on the individual's behalf; such payments are called third-party payments and are distinguished by the separation between the individual receiving the service (the first party), the individual or institution providing it (the second party), and the organization paying for it (the third party).

UTILIZATION: Patterns or rates of use of a single service or type of service (e.g., hospital care, physician visits, prescription drugs). Measurement of utilization of all medical services in combination is usually done in terms of dollar expenditures. Use is expressed in rates per unit of population at risk for a given period (e.g., number of hospital admissions per 1,000 persons over age 65 per year or number of visits to a physician per person per year for family planning services).

UTILIZATION REVIEW (UR):   Evaluation of the necessity, appropriateness, and efficiency of the use of medical services, procedures, and facilities. In a hospital, this includes review of the appropriateness of admissions, services ordered and provided, length of stay, and discharge practices both on a concurrent and retrospective basis. Utilization review may be done by a UR committee, professional standards review organization (PSRO), peer review group, public agency, or private company.

VENDOR: A provider, institution, agency, organization, or individual practitioner who provides health or medical services or equipment.

VERIFICATION OF COVERAGE: Procedures to be followed by hospitals prior to admission of a patient. Usually the hospital must verify that the patient belongs to the HMO by reviewing the membership card or by contacting the plan for a membership number. The admission must be authorized by the primary care physician or his or her designee. Failure to follow procedures will result in loss of payment by the HMO to the hospital.

✦ Index ✦

ϲ